Atrial Natriuretic Factor

FRONTIERS IN PHARMACOLOGY & THERAPEUTICS

FRONTIERS IN PHARMACOLOGY & THERAPEUTICS

Atrial Natriuretic Factor

edited by

Allan D. Struthers

Department of Pharmacology and Clinical Pharmacology,
Ninewells Hospital and Medical School, Dundee DD1 9SY,
Scotland, UK

OXFORD

BLACKWELL SCIENTIFIC PUBLICATIONS

LONDON   EDINBURGH   BOSTON

MELBOURNE   PARIS   BERLIN   VIENNA

© 1990 by
Blackwell Scientific Publications
Editorial Offices:
Osney Mead, Oxford OX2 0EL
25 John Street, London WC1N 2BL
23 Ainslie Place, Edinburgh EH3 6AJ
3 Cambridge Center, Suite 208
  Cambridge, Massachusetts 02142, USA
54 University Street, Carlton
  Victoria 3053, Australia

First published 1990

Set, printed and bound by the
University Press, Cambridge

DISTRIBUTORS

Marston Book Services Ltd
PO Box 87
Oxford OX2 0DT
(*Orders*: Tel: 0865 791155
       Fax: 0865 791927
       Telex: 837515)

USA
Year Book Medical Publishers
200 North LaSalle Street
Chicago, Illinois 60601
(*Orders*: Tel: (312) 726-9733)

Canada
The C.V. Mosby Company
5240 Finch Avenue East
Scarborough, Ontario
(*Orders*: Tel: (416) 298-1588)

Australia
Blackwell Scientific Publications
(Australia) Pty Ltd
54 University Street
Carlton, Victoria 3053
(*Orders*: Tel: (03) 347-0300)

British Library
Cataloguing in Publication Data

Atrial natriuretic factor.
  1. Man. Heart. Atria. Natriuretic
    peptides —
  Bibliographies
  I. Struthers, Allan D.   II. Series
  612.173

ISBN 0-632-02617-0

Contents

    John M. C. Connell and Alan Jardine

10 Biologically active atrial natriuretic factor receptors, 195
    Michael Chinkers

11 Atrial natriuretic factor clearance receptors, 199
    John McMurray and David B. Northridge

12 Urodilatin (hANF 95–126)—characteristics of a new atrial
    natriuretic factor peptide, 209
    *Stephan M. Feller, Hans-Jürgen Mägert, Peter Schulz-Knappe and
    Wolf-Georg Forssmann*

13 Brain natriuretic peptide, 227
    A. D. Struthers

14 Release of atrial natriuretic factor, 235
    A. E. G. Raine

    Concluding remarks, 251

    Index, 253

Contributors

Kenji Ando *Second Department of Internal Medicine, Tokyo Medical and Dental University, Yushima, Tokyo and Kitasato Biochemical Laboratories, Sagamihara, Japan*

Michael Chinkers *Department of Pharmacology and the Howard Hughes Medical Institute, Vanderbilt University School of Medicine, Nashville, Tennessee, TN 37232, USA*

Robert J. Cody *The James II and Ruth J. Wilson Professor of Medicine, Research Director, Division of Cardiology, The Ohio State University Medical School and Hospital, 611 Means Hall, 1654 Upham Drive, Columbus, Ohio, OH 43210, USA*

John M. C. Connell *MRC Blood Pressure Unit, Western Infirmary, Glasgow G11 6NT, UK*

C. F. Deschepper *Department of Physiology, University of California, San Francisco, California, CA 94143, USA*

Stephan M. Feller *Institute for Anatomy and Cell Biology III, University of Heidelberg, INF 307, D-6900 Heidelberg, Federal Republic of Germany*

Wolf-Georg Forssmann *Institute for Anatomy and Cell Biology III, University of Heidelberg, INF 307, D-6900 Heidelberg, Federal Republic of Germany*

D. G. Gardner *Department of Medicine and the Metabolic Research Unit, University of California, San Francisco, California, CA 94143, USA*

R. Green *Department of Physiological Sciences, University of Manchester, Oxford Road, Manchester M13 9PT, UK*

Alan Jardine *MRC Blood Pressure Unit, Western Infirmary, Glasgow G11 6NT, UK*

B. Kovacic-Milivojevic *Department of Medicine and the Metabolic Research Unit, University of California, San Francisco, California, CA 94143, USA*

C. C. Lang *Department of Pharmacology and Clinical Pharmacology, Ninewells Hospital and Medical School, Dundee DD1 9SY, Scotland, UK*

M. C. LaPointe *Department of Medicine and the Metabolic Research Unit, University of California, San Francisco, California, CA 94143, USA*

John McMurray *Department of Cardiology, Western Infirmary, Glasgow G11 6NT, UK*

Hans-Jürgen Mägert *Institute for Anatomy and Cell Biology III, University of Heidelberg, INF 307, D-6900 Heidelberg, Federal Republic of Germany*

Fumiaki Marumo *Second Department of Internal Medicine, Tokyo Medical and Dental University, Yushima, Tokyo 113, Japan*

David B. Northridge *Department of Cardiology, Western Infirmary, Glasgow G11 6NT, UK*

A. E. G. Raine *Department of Nephrology, St Bartholomew's Hospital, West Smithfield, London EC1A 7BE, UK*

A. M. Richards *Departments of Cardiology, Endocrinology and Medicine, The Princess Margaret Hospital, Christchurch 2, New Zealand*

Peter Schulz-Knappe *Institute for Anatomy and Cell Biology III, University of Heidelberg, INF 307, D-6900 Heidelberg, Federal Republic of Germany*

A. D. Struthers *Department of Pharmacology and Clinical Pharmacology, Ninewells Hospital and Medical School, Dundee DD1 9SY, Scotland, UK*

Martin R. Wilkins *Department of Clinical Pharmacology, Royal Postgraduate Medical School, Du Cane Road, London W12 0HS, UK*

Preface

Atrial natriuretic factor (ANF) was first sequenced in 1984. This led to a virtual explosion of interest and activity in ANF research. Over the initial few years, the pace of ANF research was indeed breathtaking. Five years later, ANF research is still continuing at a rapid pace but perhaps not at quite such fever-pitch intensity as in the mid-1980s. We might be said to be in a consolidation phase in ANF research and it therefore appears timely to produce a review monograph.

In this monograph, an international group of experts have written short chapters on their own area of speciality interest and I am extremely grateful to all contributors for producing such high quality chapters. The authors are a mixture of scientists and clinicians and it is therefore hoped that this monograph will appeal to both basic scientists and clinicians.

The chapters in this book fall into two categories. There are long chapters reviewing the extensive literature in specific but major areas for ANF, such as its renal effects or its role in essential hypertension. The second group of chapters are shorter and are devoted to new 'growth' areas for ANF, such as brain natriuretic peptide, urodilatin, clearance receptors and inhibitors of neutral endopeptidase. The second group of chapters give major insight into the future for ANF and how ANF research has already produced novel therapeutic approaches in cardio-vascular medicine.

With ANF there has always been a danger that any monograph would be out of date before it was published. In this case, the publishers have been acutely aware of this possibility, so much so that the time-gap between submission of manuscripts and publication has been reduced to the absolute minimum (i.e. 4 months). We feel therefore that this monograph should be up-to-date, comprehensive and appeal to a wide range of clinicians and scientists.

Allan D. Struthers,
Department of Pharmacology and
  Clinical Pharmacology,
Ninewells Hospital and Medical School,
Dundee

Chronology

1956	Inflation of balloon in RA causes natriuresis
1980/87	Myocardial extracts found to be natriuretic
1984	Human ANF identified and sequenced
1985/86	Biological activity shown for ANF in man
1987	Clearance receptors identified
1988	Urodilatin ANF (95–126) identified
1988	Brain natriuretic peptide (BNP) identified and sequenced
1989	Drugs inhibiting endopeptidase increase biological activity of ANF
1989	Biologically active ANF receptor isolated and sequenced

Conversion factor

Human ANF (99–126)
Molecular weight 3080.5 kDa

1 nmol = 3081 ng
1 pmol = 3.1 ng
1 pmol/l = 3.1 pg/ml

1 μg = 325 pmol
1 ng   = 0.32 pmol
1 pg/ml = 0.325 pmol/l

Chapter 1
Molecular analysis and regulation of the atrial natriuretic factor gene

D. G. Gardner, M. C. LaPointe, B. Kovacic-Milivojevic and C. F. Deschepper

Introduction

Since its discovery (de Bold *et al.*, 1981), atrial natriuretic factor (ANF) has generated an extraordinary level of interest in the scientific and clinical literature. In a sense it represents a true product of the 'new biology' in that its structural gene was cloned and sequenced before the peptide was shown to circulate in plasma (i.e. behave as a true hormone). This review will focus on the subsequent use of this same technology to define the structure and regulation of the ANF gene(s).

Structure of the genes for ANF

Following the initial description of the bioactivity of ANF, several laboratories succeeded in isolating and characterizing biologically active peptides from atrial tissue (Cantin & Genest, 1985; Needleman & Greenwald, 1986). These peptides ranged in size from 21 to 33 amino acids. In general, the mid-region of these peptides shared common amino-acid sequence; heterogeneity appeared to derive from variability in the NH$_2$- or COOH-terminal extensions of this core sequence. This was confirmed with the subsequent cloning of the DNA complement (cDNA) of the ANF mRNA transcript from human (Nakayama *et al.*, 1984; Oikawa *et al.*, 1984; Zivin *et al.*, 1984), rat (Zivin *et al.*, 1984; Maki *et al.*, 1984b; Seidman *et al.*, 1984b; Yamanaka *et al.*, 1984; Flynn *et al.*, 1985), rabbit (Oikawa *et al.*, 1985) and dog (Oikawa *et al.* 1985) atrial tissue. Sequencing of the cDNAs suggested that these peptides arise from a single preproANF molecule translated from the mRNA. PreproANF varies in size from 149–153 amino acids (aa) depending on the species (dog = 149 aa; rat and mouse = 152 aa; cow and human = 151 aa; rabbit = 153 aa). The amino termini of these proteins are rich in hydrophobic amino acids, reflecting the presence of signal sequences responsible for translocating the nascent polypeptide chain across the membrane of rough endoplasmic reticulum (Blobel & Dobberstein, 1975). Removal of the signal peptide results in the generation of a proANF molecule which ranges in size from 126–128 aa depending upon the species. The bioactive peptides are located near the carboxy terminus of the proANF molecule. The extreme carboxy terminus of the proANF molecule from rat, mouse and rabbit, but not human, contains an Arg–Arg dipeptide not present in the biologically active peptides isolated to date, suggesting that it is removed as an early processing event. There is a high degree of conservation of amino-acid sequence among proANF molecules from different species; this homology is most striking across that region harboring the bioactive peptides.

Several heterologous systems have been developed to express the human ANF cDNA in either prokaryotic (Lennick, Haynes & Shen, 1987; Dykes *et al.*, 1988) or eukaryotic cells (Vlasuk *et al.*, 1986a; Iwai *et al.*, 1987). In the bacterial systems the hANF peptide was expressed as a fusion protein linked either to chloramphenicol acetyl transferase (Dykes *et al.*, 1988) or β-galactosidase (Lennick *et al.*, 1987) coding sequence. The β-galactosidase–hANF chimeric protein was shown to yield bona fide hANF (1–28) following enzymatic digestion with endopeptidase Lys-C and carboxypeptidase B (Lennick *et al.*, 1987). hANF has also been expressed in yeast (Vlasuk *et al.*, 1986a) as a fusion protein linking the yeast mating pheromone, α-factor, to a synthetic sequence encoding the biologically active carboxyl-terminal portion of the hANF precursor. In that case only a portion of the processed peptide material appeared to correspond to bona fide hANF (1–28); the major product was a shorter form which lacked the two carboxyl-terminal amino acids of the peptide.

The circulating form of ANF in plasma is predominantly a 28-aa peptide corresponding to positions 123–150 in rat preproANF (Schwartz *et al.*, 1985; positions 90–126 in the prohormone) and 124–151 in the human molecule (Miyata *et al.*, 1987). The major immunoreactive form of ANF in atrial tissue is the proANF molecule and not the shorter peptide (Vuolteenaho, Arjamaa & Ling, 1985). The exact cellular site and mechanism for the processing of the proANF molecule (i.e. cleavage between position Arg_{98} and Ser_{99} of the propeptide) to generate the 28-aa peptide remain unknown. Primary cultures of neonatal rat atrial cardiocytes secrete predominately proANF (Bloch *et al.*, 1985; Glembotski & Gibson, 1985), while *in vitro* perfused heart preparations release exclusively the smaller bioactive peptides (Currie *et al.*, 1984). These data suggest either that processing of proANF in the intact heart is dependent upon non-myocardial cellular elements or enzymatic factors which are absent in the primary cultures, or that myocardial cells lose the native processing function *in vitro*. The latter could result, for example, from the loss of pulsatile tension or an endogenous paracrine factor. The recent demonstration of partial restoration of the processing function to these cells with glucocorticoid treatment (Shields, Dixon & Glembotski, 1988) tends to support the latter model.

The chromosomal genes for cow (Vlasuk *et al.*, 1986b), rat (Argentin *et al.*, 1985), mouse (Seidman *et al.*, 1984a) and human ANF (Greenberg *et al.*, 1984; Nemer *et al.*, 1984; Maki, Parmentier & Inagami, 1984a; Seidman, 1984a) have been isolated and sequenced. The structural features of these genes are quite similar. Each contains three exons separated by two introns. In the rat ANF gene, exon I contains sequence encoding the 5′ untranslated region of the gene, the signal peptide and the amino terminal 16 amino acids of the prohormone. Exon II encodes the majority of the structural sequence of the prohormone and includes most of the bioactive ANF sequence. Exon III harbors the terminal Tyr (aa 151 in the human and dog) or Tyr–Arg–Arg (aa 150–152 in the rat, mouse, rabbit and cow), a translation termination codon and the 3′ untranslated regions. The various ANF genes contain structural features which may impact significantly on their expression. The human gene (Greenberg *et al.*, 1984; Nemer *et al.*, 1984), and to a lesser degree the rat gene (Argentin *et al.*, 1985), contain DNA sequence within the second intron which shows homology with the consensus sequence for the glucocorticoid responsive element (Karin *et al.*, 1984) suggesting the potential for regulation by these steroids. Such regulation has been demonstrated (Gardner *et al.*, 1986b; Day *et al.*, 1987; Gardner *et al.*, 1988a), although the involvement of these specific sequences in mediating the glucocorticoid response remains to be shown. Both the mouse and the human genes contain a short sequence ∼ 250 base pairs (bp) upstream from the transcription start site which share homology with the SV-40 enhancer (Seidman *et al.*, 1984a); however, to date, this sequence has not been shown to possess enhancer-like activity in its native position. The mouse and the rat gene each contain long tracts of alternating (GT) pairs (Seidman *et al.*, 1984a; Argentin *et al.*, 1985). As yet, it is unclear as to what role, if any, these (GT) tracts play in the regulation of ANF gene expression. Alternating purine–pyrimidine tracts like these have been thought to foster the conversion of DNA from its native B conformation to the Z form (Nordeim & Rich, 1983), and may play a role in controlling expression of contiguous genomic sequences. Finally, the human ANF gene is known to contain two Alu-class repeats within its second intron (Greenberg *et al.*, 1984; Nemer *et al.*, 1984; Seidman *et al.*, 1984a). The function of these repeats relative to ANF gene expression remains undefined.

Using *in situ* hybridization and Southern blot analysis of somatic cell hybrid DNAs, the chromosomal locations of two ANF genes have been identified. The mouse gene for ANF is located on chromosome 4 (Yang-Feng *et al.*, 1985; Mullins, Zeng & Gross, 1987) while the human gene is found on the distal short arm of chromosome 1 (Yang-Feng *et al.*, 1985;

Dracopoli *et al.*, 1988). Several allelic polymorphisms have been identified around the hANF gene (Frossard & Coleman, 1986; Nemer, Sirois & Drouin, 1986b, c) but, as yet, these have not been linked to a heritable disorder of fluid and electrolyte metabolism. Analysis of a single restriction fragment length polymorphism in a kindred with Bartter's syndrome failed to establish a linkage (Graham *et al.*, 1986).

Tissue-specific expression of the ANF gene

Expression of the ANF gene, documented by the presence of the ANF mRNA and/or the proANF molecule, has been demonstrated in a number of different tissues. In addition to the cardiac atria (Maki *et al.*, 1984b; Nakayama *et al.*, 1984; Oikawa *et al.*, 1984; Seidman *et al.*, 1984b; Zivin *et al.*, 1984; Yamanaka *et al.*, 1984; Flynn *et al.*, 1985), the cardiac ventricle (Bloch *et al.*, 1986; Gardner *et al.*, 1986a; Nemer *et al.*, 1986a; Hamid *et al.*, 1987), lung (Gardner *et al.*, 1986a), aortic arch (Gardner, Deschepper & Baxter, 1987a), brain (Gardner *et al.*, 1987c; Standaert, Needleman & Saper, 1988), pituitary gland (Gardner *et al.*, 1986a; Morel *et al.*, 1989), autonomic ganglia (Debinski *et al.*, 1986) and the adrenal medulla (Morel *et al.*, 1988) have been shown to be capable of synthesizing the atrial natriuretic peptide(s).

The ANF transcript in the atria of the rat has been reported to be between 950 and 1150 nucleotides long (Maki *et al.*, 1984b; Seidman *et al.*, 1984b; Yamanaka *et al.*, 1984; Flynn *et al.*, 1985; Bloch *et al.*, 1986; Gardner *et al.*, 1986a; Nemer *et al.*, 1986a). Since genomic DNA sequence predicts a coding sequence of $\sim$ 800–900 nucleotides, the remainder presumably reflects polyadenylation of the mRNA at its 3′ terminus. Similar sizes have been reported for ANF transcripts from other species (Nakayama *et al.*, 1984; Oikawa *et al.*, 1984; Zivin *et al.*, 1984). Mapping of the 5′ terminus of the rat atrial ANF transcript using S_1 nuclease protection or primer extension analysis identified a transcript start site 20–25 base pairs (bp) downstream from a genomic TATAAAA sequence (Gardner *et al.*, 1986a). It is this sequence (i.e. the Goldberg–Hogness box) which is believed to position RNA polymerase II for subsequent transcription (Benoist & Chambon, 1981). A second transcription start site, accounting for $\sim$ 5–10 % of total ANF mRNA in the atria, lies approximately 80 bp further upstream. This start, in turn, is located $\sim$ 30 bp downstream from an AT-rich sequence which may subserve a primitive 'TATA box-like' function in fostering transcription. Identical patterns of 5′ start sites have been identified in other tissues expressing the ANF gene (Gardner *et al.*, 1987a,c). A similar approach, employing nuclease S_1 protection, primer extension analysis and RNAse protection, has identified a similar pattern of 5′ termini for the ANF mRNA found in human fetal atria, i.e. a dominant start site $\sim$ 20 bp downstream from a TATAA sequence and a minor start ~ 110 bp further upstream (Gardner et al., 1989).

Mapping of the 3' terminus of the rat ANF mRNA (independent of the poly A+ tail) by S_1 nuclease protection revealed the presence of two independent termini ~ 10 bp apart (Gardner et al., 1987c), each of which was positioned downstream from an AAUAAA sequence. This sequence is thought to provide a major component of the signal dictating cleavage and subsequent polyadenylation of the nascent mRNA transcript (Proudfoot, 1982). These two sites appeared to be employed to a roughly equivalent degree in atrial tissue and were present in all ANF-expressing, extra-atrial tissues which were examined (Gardner et al., 1987c). Topographic localization of ANF gene expression within atrial tissue by immunocytochemistry and in situ hybridization histochemistry demonstrated diffuse expression throughout the entire atrial wall (Gardner et al., 1986a; Nemer et al., 1986a; Hamid et al., 1987; Zeller et al., 1987; Wu, Deschepper & Gardner, 1988).

Despite early reports to the contrary (Nakayama et al., 1984; Yamanaka et al., 1984), several groups (Bloch et al., 1986; Gardner et al., 1986a; Nemer et al., 1986c; Hamid et al., 1987) have succeeded in identifying immunoreactive ANF and ANF mRNA in the cardiac ventricle. Levels of both are extremely low relative to those found in the cardiac atria (i.e. generally < 2% of atrial levels). The ventricular ANF transcripts are similar in overall size, 5'- and 3'-termini to those identified in the cardiac atria. Transcripts are distributed in both ventricular chambers from the apex to the base (Gardner, LaPointe & Wu, 1988c); however, immunocytochemistry (Gardner et al., 1986a; Hamid et al., 1987; Anand-Srivastava et al., 1989), conventional RNA analysis, (Gardner et al., 1988c) and in situ hybridization histochemistry (Hamid et al., 1987; Wu et al., 1988; Anand-Srivastava et al., 1989) indicate that ANF gene expression is particularly active within the ventricular subendocardium. One recent study suggests that this irANF may be localized to the Purkinje cells of the ventricular conduction system (Anand-Srivastava et al., 1989). While most of the studies described above have been performed on rat ventricular tissue, similar findings have been noted in the mouse (Zeller et al., 1987) and human (Gardner et al., 1989) ventricle. Regulation of ventricular ANF gene expression, particularly in pathophysiological states, represents an active area of current investigation and is covered in the following section.

The ontogeny of cardiac ANF gene expression has been investigated in some detail. In the mouse, ANF gene expression appears in the cardiac primordia on roughly day 8 of development (Zeller et al., 1987). Atrial expression continues to increase throughout gestation and into the neonatal period. Ventricular expression appears around day 9, progresses throughout the remainder of pregnancy then recedes in the neonatal period. In the rat, atrial ANF mRNA and irANF levels increase from the late perinatal to the early neonatal period and continue to increase as the animal develops toward adulthood (Wei *et al.*, 1987; Claycomb, 1988; Wu *et al.*, 1988). Ventricular irANF and ANF mRNA levels rise in the late perinatal period, peak on day 1 after birth and then fall during the first 2–3 weeks postpartum (Wei *et al.*, 1987; Claycomb, 1988; Wu *et al.*, 1988). Expression of the ANF gene in the neonatal rat ventricle is localized in a circumferential pattern around the ventricular cavity (Wu *et al.*, 1988). In the adult rat this recedes to subendocardial foci of cells which continue to express the gene (see above). Data on ventricular ANF gene expression in the human foetus is sketchier but basically supports the findings in the mouse and rat models. Ventricular ANF mRNA levels in the mid-gestation foetus are $\sim$ 10–20 % of those found in the foetal atria (Gardner *et al.*, 1989). By a number of different criteria, the ventricular transcripts appear to be identical to those synthesized in the atria. As in the rat, ANF gene expression in the human foetal ventricle exists in a gradient from the subendocardial to the epicardial surface (Gardner *et al.*, 1989) and, again like the rat, ventricular expression decreases as the infant develops through the perinatal period into childhood (Kikuchi *et al.*, 1987; Claycomb, 1988).

Immunoreactive ANF and the ANF mRNA have also been identified in pulmonary tissue (Gardner *et al.*, 1986a), the aortic arch (Gardner *et al.*, 1987a) and the anterior pituitary gland (McKenzie *et al.*, 1985; Gardner *et al.*, 1986a; Morel *et al.*, 1989). In the lung irANF is concentrated in large ovoid cells in the peripheral alveoli, while in the aortic arch it is found concentrated in the vascular adventitia around the bifurcations of the major cephalic vessels, a distribution which mirrors that of the high-pressure aortic baroreceptors. In the pituitary, irANF appears to be localized in cells resembling gonadotropes (McKenzie *et al.*, 1985; Gardner *et al.*, 1986a; Morel *et al.*, 1989) and to a lesser extent in lactotropes and corticotropes (Morel *et al.*, 1989). Recent studies employing *in situ* hybridization histochemistry and *in situ* ANF receptor analysis suggest that gonadotropes are capable of both synthesizing proANF (inferred from the presence of the proANF mRNA) and binding ^{125}I-ANF at the cell surface, presumably through a receptor-dependent mechanism (Morel *et al.*, 1989). At present, the function of ANF in these non-cardiac tissues remains undefined. ANF has been implicated as a modulator of C-fibre activity in vagally dependent reflexes originating in the thorax (Thoren *et al.*, 1986; Imaizumi *et al.*, 1987; Schultz *et al.*, 1988). It is conceivable that ANF present in the aortic arch or lung could be of importance in the endogenous regulation of this reflex activity. The role of ANF in gonadotrope function is similarly undefined. ANF has been shown to regulate gonadotrophin secretion (Standaert, Cicero & Needleman, 1986a; Samson, Aguila & Bianchi, 1988a) as well as the secretion of other pituitary hormones (Iitake *et al.*, 1986; Samson &

Bianchi, 1988; Samson, Bianchi & Mogg, 1988b); however, these effects, in large part, are thought to operate at a hypothalamic level. Of note, the gonadotrope has been shown to harbour a number of components of the renin–angiotensin cascade (Deschepper *et al.*, 1986), a well-known target of ANF bioactivity in other systems (Camargo *et al.*, 1984; Antunes-Rodrigues *et al.*, 1985).

irANF has been shown by conventional radioimmunoassay (Tanaka, Misono & Inagami, 1984) and by immunocytochemistry (Jacobowitz *et al.*, 1985; Saper *et al.*, 1985; Standaert, Needleman & Saper, 1986b) to be present in the preoptic region, hypothalamus and pontine brainstem of the central nervous system (CNS). The former includes the anteroventral third-ventricular region thought to be important in the maintenance of cardiovascular homeostasis (Brody & Johnson, 1980). ANF mRNA has also been identified in tissue samples taken from the hypothalamus and pontine brainstem (Gardner *et al.*, 1987c). These transcripts are identical in overall size, 5′- and 3′-termini and, at least in the case of the hypothalamic transcript, nucleotide sequence to the ANF mRNA synthesized in the cardiac atria. Others have identified proANF (implying endogenous synthesis of the hormone), ANF mRNA and/or ANF receptors in sympathetic and parasympathetic ganglia (Debinski *et al.*, 1986) as well as in the adrenal medulla (Morel *et al.*, 1988).

The potential function of ANF in the CNS is better defined than in other extra-atrial tissues. Central (i.e. intracerebroventricular) administration of ANF results in suppression of vasopressin release from the neurohypophysis (Samson, 1985; Iitake *et al.*, 1986; Januszewicz *et al.*, 1986), inhibition of the thirst mechanism (Antunes-Rodrigues *et al.*, 1985; Nakamura *et al.*, 1985) and salt appetite (Antunes-Rodrigues, McCann & Samson, 1986), and a reduction in sympathetic outflow (Schultz, Steele & Gardner, 1989) and systemic blood pressure (Levin, Weber & Mills, 1988; Schultz *et al.*, 1989). ANF receptors have been identified in the circumventricular organs as well as deeper brain structures (Quirion, Dalpe & Dam, 1986; Saavedra *et al.*, 1986). Some of these receptors appear to be modulated by perturbations in cardiovascular homeostasis (Saavedra *et al.*, 1986). Direct application of ANF in and around the preoptic region of the paraventricular nucleus has been shown to suppress spontaneous neuronal firing rate in these structures (Wong *et al.*, 1986; Standaert *et al.*, 1987). Thus, the accumulated evidence, at this point, argues rather convincingly that ANF plays a key neuromodulatory role in the regulation of CNS activity related to cardiovascular physiology.

Regulation of ANF gene expression

The synthesis and secretion of the atrial peptide(s) are regulated by changes in cardiac haemodynamics and by a number of hormonal factors. Since the control of ANF release is covered elsewhere in this monograph, we will limit our discussion of secretory control to those factors which affect ANF gene expression in parallel.

It is probable that the dominant factor(s) regulating the synthesis and secretion of ANF *in vivo* is wall tension, or stress, which is transmitted in some fashion to the myocardial cell expressing the ANF gene. While the effects of acute volume expansion on ANF gene expression *in vivo* have not been reported, several studies have documented the effects of chronic volume expansion on ANF mRNA levels. In one study chronic administration of a high sodium diet was reported to increase plasma ANF levels as well as the levels of ANF mRNA in the cardiac atria when compared to a low sodium diet (Iwao *et al.*, 1988). However, a second study failed to demonstrate an effect of high sodium intake on ANF mRNA levels (Takayanagi *et al.*, 1985). Reduction of intravascular volume through dehydration (Nakayama *et al.*, 1984; Takayanagi *et al.*, 1985) or salt restriction (Takayanagi *et al.*, 1985) resulted in a decrease in ANF mRNA levels in atrial tissue. Chronic volume expansion through administration of an exogenous mineralocorticoid resulted in significant elevations in plasma ANF levels in the rat (Ballerman *et al.*, 1986), dog (Metzler *et al.*, 1987) and pig (Grekin *et al.*, 1986) and in the relative levels of ANF mRNA in extracts of atrial tissue from the rat (Ballerman *et al.*, 1986) or dog (Metzler *et al.*, 1987). The timing of the increase in plasma ANF levels relative to the re-establishment of Na^+ balance suggests that ANF may play a key role in the phenomenon of mineralocorticoid escape; however, in at least one of these studies, plasma ANF itself accounted for only part of the 'escape' activity (Metzler *et al.*, 1987).

The inability to produce tension reliably on the surface of a culture dish has limited studies of stretch-mediated release in cultured cells. To circumvent this problem, some investigators have attempted to generate myocardial cell tension experimentally by expanding cellular volume in hypo-osmotic media (Greenwald *et al.*, 1989), thereby increasing tension at the cell surface and in the cytoskeleton. This cellular swelling resulted in an increase in the amount of irANF released into the culture medium. A possible problem with these types of studies relates to the potential for osmotically induced cellular damage with release of irANF stores (i.e. proANF), which could erroneously be recorded as 'secretion'. To circumvent this problem, we examined the effects of hypo-osmolar expansion of cellular volume on the expression of the ANF gene, as reflected by ANF mRNA accumulation, in cultured atrial cardiocytes. One would anticipate that cellular damage *per se* would result in a decrease rather than an increase in ANF gene transcription. As shown in Fig. 1.1a, reduction of medium osmolality resulted in a dose-dependent increase in cellular ANF mRNA levels, paralleling the reported effects on secretion.

Several hormones or 'second-messenger equivalents' have been shown to regulate the production and release of ANF *in vivo* and *in vitro*. In

A   **B**

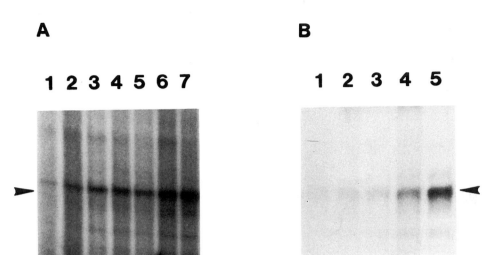

Fig. 1.1 (a) Effect of media osmolarity on ANF gene expression. Neonatal rat atrial cardiocytes were prepared as described previously (Gardner *et al.* 1988a) and cultured for 24 h in Dulbecco's modified Eagles medium containing 5 mM KCl, 44 mM NaHCO$_3$ and 110 mM (lane 1), 107 mM (lane 2), 105 mM (lane 3), 102 mM (lane 4), 99 mM (lane 5), 94 mM (lane 6) or 88 mM(lane 7) NaCl. Cytoplasmic RNA (6 μg) was collected and analysed for ANF mRNA context by nuclease S$_1$ protection. Arrow indicates the position (i.e. $\sim$ 195 nucleotides) of the major fragment protected by the ANF transcript. (b) Effect of ($-$) norepinephrine on ANF gene expression. Cells were cultured in serum-free medium plus 0.1 mM ascorbate (lane 1) and 10^{-9} M (lane 2), 10^{-8} M (lane 3), 10^{-7} M (lane 4) or 10^{-6} M (lane 5) ($-$) norepinephrine. Cytoplasmic RNA (4 μg) was collected 24 h later and analysed as described above.

addition to the mineralocorticoid hormones mentioned above, thyroid hormone (Gardner, Gertz & Hane, 1987b; Ladenson, Bloch & Seidman, 1988), glucocorticoids (Gardner *et al.*, 1986b; Day *et al.*, 1987; Gardner *et al.*, 1988a), α- and β-adrenergic agonists (Sonnenberg & Veress, 1984; Currie & Newman, 1986; Schiebinger, Baker & Linden, 1987), cholinergic agonists (Sonnenberg & Veress, 1984; Schiebinger *et al.*, 1987) and an as yet undefined pituitary factor (Zamir *et al.*, 1987) have been shown to regulate the secretion of ANF and/or the accrual of ANF mRNA in relevant expressing tissues.

Triiodothyronine (T$_3$), the bioactive form of thyroid hormone *in vivo*, increased plasma levels of circulating ANF *in vivo* (Gardner *et al.*, 1987b; Ladenson *et al.*, 1988) and the secretion of irANF from cultured atrial and ventricular myocytes *in vitro* (Gardner *et al.*, 1987b). This was accompanied by an increase in atrial ANF mRNA levels at a relative (Gardner *et al.*, 1987b) as well as an absolute (Ladenson *et al.*, 1988) level. Increments in tissue irANF and ANF mRNA levels were directly proportional to the level of thyroid hormone bioactivity. Interestingly, T$_3$ also activated ANF gene expression in normally quiescent ventricular tissue (Gardner *et al.*, 1987b; Ladenson *et al.*, 1988). The relative

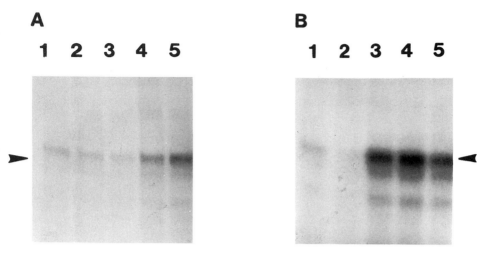

Fig. 1.2   (a) Effect of dexamethasone on ANF gene expression in neonatal rat cardiocytes. Atrial cardiocytes were cultured for 24 h in glucocorticoid-free media (lane 1) or 10^{-10} M (lane 2), 10^{-9} M (lane 3), 10^{-8} M (lane 4) or 10^{-7} M (lane 5) dexamethasone. Cytoplasmic RNA (5 μg) was isolated and analysed by S_1 nuclease protection. The arrow indicates the position of the DNA fragment protected by the ANF mRNA. (b) Ventricular cardiocytes were treated with increasing concentrations of dexamethasone as described for (a). Cytoplasmic RNA (10 μg) was analysed by S_1 nuclease protection.

induction of ANF mRNA levels in ventricular tissue was even higher than that seen with atrial tissue, perhaps reflecting the higher level of 'basal' gene activity in the latter. Taken together, the experimental data support a role for thyroid hormone in controlling ANF production. Based on the in vitro data it seems clear that at least a portion of this effect derives from direct interaction of thyroid hormone with the myocardial cell exclusive of changes in central haemodynamics.

Glucocorticoids regulate the synthesis and release of ANF from cardiac cells *in vivo* (Gardner *et al.*, 1986b; Day *et al.*, 1987) and *in vitro* (Gardner *et al.*, 1988a). In the intact rat, dexamethasone (Dex, 1 mg/day) increased plasma ANF levels and atrial and ventricular ANF mRNA levels ~ twofold relative to the sham-injected controls (Gardner *et al.*, 1986b). The glucocorticoid effect was synergistic with that of increased afterload in promoting ventricular ANF gene expression (Day *et al.*, 1987). Dex also increased release of irANF from primary cultures of neonatal cardiocytes *in vitro* (Matsubara *et al.*, 1987; Gardner *et al.*, 1988a) and the accumulation of ANF mRNA within these cells (Gardner *et al.*, 1988a). One study (Matsubara *et al.*, 1987) suggested that secretion of ANF from ventricular cells may be more sensitive to the effects of glucocorticoids than that from atrial cardiocytes. As shown in Fig. 1.2 this finding appears to be borne out at the level of ANF gene expression. The dexamethasone dose-response for ANF mRNA accumulation is clearly shifted to the left in ventricular vs. atrial cardiocytes indicating increased

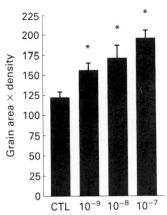

Fig. 1.3 *In situ* hybridization histochemistry for ANF mRNA. Atrial cells were cultured on Lab-Tek culture slides (Nunc, Naperville, Illinois), fixed with 4% paraformaldehyde and hybridized to a ^{3}H-labelled ANF cRNA probe. After autoradiography, the slides were analysed in a Zeiss photomicroscope coupled to a computerized image analyser (SMI, Atlanta, Georgia). This system allowed us to visualize labelled cells on a monitor, define the cytoplasmic boundaries of each cell with a cursor and calculate two values: (i) the percentage of cytoplasmic area covered by silver grains and (ii) the relative density of the grain-covered area. The product of the two values was taken as a quantitative estimate of the amount of ANF mRNA in each cell. Quantitative analysis was performed on 15 cells from four different groups, i.e. control cells (CTL) and cells treated with dexamethasone at three different concentrations (i.e. 10^{-9} M, 10^{-8} M and 10^{-7} M). The bar graph depicts the mean value in each group$\pm$SEM; $P < 0.01$ vs. control. We have determined previously that the percentage of labelled cells was similar in each group (Gardner *et al.*, 1988a).

glucocorticoid activity at lower concentrations of the steroid in the ventricular cells. The increase in ANF mRNA levels was specific for glucocorticoids and resulted largely from increased transcription of the ANF gene from the dominant promoter locus (Gardner *et al.*, 1988a). While the steroid appeared to have a modest effect on the half-life of the ANF mRNA (i.e. an increase from 18 to 30 h), this difference did not reach statistical significance. *In situ* hybridization analysis indicated that the increase in ANF gene expression resulted from enhanced mRNA production in previously expressing cells rather than from recruitment of otherwise quiescent cells into the ANF gene-expressing pool. As with the increment in relative ANF mRNA levels, the increase in ANF gene expression per cell was a direct function of steroid concentration (Fig. 1.3). Glucocorticoids also appear to have a second, and largely independent effect, on the production of bioactive ANF. These steroids stimulate the processing of proANF to ANF in primary cultures of neonatal rat myocardial cells (Shields *et al.*, 1988). Thus, glucocorticoids may act at several levels to promote ANF activity at the periphery.

Extracellular calcium has been reported to increase (LaPointe &

Gardner, 1988) or decrease (Greenwald *et al.*, 1989) ANF secretion. Calcium is clearly required for optimal ANF gene expression, and calcium channel antagonists are potent suppressants of ANF secretion and ANF mRNA levels in cultured cardiocytes *in vitro* (Gardner *et al.*, 1988a). Further study will be required to resolve the discrepant findings regarding ANF secretion.

Vasopressin has been shown to foster secretion of ANF *in vitro* (Sonnenberg & Veress, 1984) and *in vivo* (Manning *et al.*, 1985). In the latter case this appears to be related, in large part, to the vasoactive properties of the peptide with attendant changes in central haemodynamics. Of interest, two recent studies (Lavigne *et al.*, 1988; Ruskoaho *et al.*, 1989) of ANF gene expression in the vasopressin-deficient Brattleboro rat suggest that ANF immunoreactivity and ANF mRNA accumulate to higher levels in the atrial and ventricular cardiocytes of these animals when compared to the vasopressin-replete Long–Evans controls. These increases were observed in the absence of overt ventricular hypertrophy and despite the fact that circulating plasma ANF levels were similar between the two strains. The authors suggested a possible disruption of the linkage between synthesis and secretion in the Brattleboro strain.

Several neurotransmitters, including α- and β-adrenergic and cholinergic agonists, have been shown to regulate ANF secretion. α-agonists promote release of irANF from the isolated perfused heart (Currie & Newman, 1986), from atrial fragments (Sonnenberg & Veress, 1984) from perfused atria under tension (Schiebinger *et al.*, 1987) and from cultured atrial cells (Shields & Glembotski, 1989). β-adrenergic and cholinergic agonists have been reported to increase ANF release in some systems (Sonnenberg & Veress, 1984; Schiebinger *et al.*, 1987) yet suppress it in others (Schiebinger *et al.*, 1987; Shields & Glembotski, 1989). Norepinephrine, the predominant endogenous catecholamine in the heart, promotes the release of ANF, at least in part through activation of the α_1-adrenergic receptor (Currie & Newman, 1986; Shields & Glembotski, 1989). This agonist also effects an increase in the ANF mRNA levels (Fig. 1.1b) suggesting that long-term stimulation with catecholamines is capable of driving the synthesis as well as the secretion of the ANF peptide. Among the second messenger systems which mediate hormone and neurotransmitter activity, the phorbol ester, TPA, a potent activator of protein kinase C, has been reported to increase ANF release *in vitro* (Ruskoaho, Toth & Lang, 1985; Matsubara *et al.*, 1988; Shields & Glembotski, 1989) and to activate ANF gene expression either alone or in combination with the calcium ionophore A23187 (LaPointe & Gardner, 1988). These studies suggest that agonists which foster phosphoinositide turnover within myocardial cells should be effective stimulators of ANF synthesis and secretion, a hypothesis which is supported by the observation made with the α_1-adrenergic agonists above.

Kohtz *et al.* (1989) recently reported the isolation of several presumptive human cardiac myoblast cell lines which continue to replicate in continuous culture. When these cells were placed in mitogen-free medium for several days, they acquired a more differentiated myogenic phenotype which included the expression of the ANF gene. Increased levels of the ANF mRNA in the 'differentiated' cells reflected predominantly enhanced transcription of the ANF gene. Of interest, while cells derived from the right atria or the right ventricle accrued substantial levels of hANF mRNA, cells derived form the left ventricle showed little accrual of the transcript despite a high level of ANF gene transcription. This latter finding suggests that some of the differences in the relative levels of ANF gene expression among individual cardiac cell populations may derive from variable post transcriptional processing of the ANF mRNA. This same group identified a soluble factor produced by a neuroblastoma cell line which accentuated ANP gene expression in co-cultured myocardial cells. The responsible factor was capable of penetrating a 3.0 μm filter but appeared to be larger than a conventional neurotransmitter molecule. Exact identification of this factor awaits definition.

As discussed above, expression of the ANF gene in the cardiac ventricle is, in general, only a fraction of that present in the cardiac atria under physiological conditions. However, activation of ventricular expression occurs in a number of different pathophysiological states. These include states of thyroid (Gardner *et al.*, 1987b; Ladenson *et al.*, 1988) and glucocorticoid hormone (Gardner *et al.*, 1986b; Day *et al.*, 1987; Gardner *et al.*, 1988a) excess, as described in the preceding section, as well as a number of situations characterized by haemodynamic overload of the ventricular chamber(s).

Experimental manipulations resulting in volume or pressure overload of the ventricular chamber lead to dramatic increases in ANF gene expression, inferred from the accumulation of the proANF precursor protein and/or the ANF mRNA within ventricular cardiocytes. Volume overload, resulting from placement of an A–V fistula, effected a significant increment in ventricular ANF gene expression, as assessed by conventional RNA analysis and *in situ* hybridization histochemistry (Lattion *et al.*, 1986). Pressure overload of the left ventricle, created by banding the aorta of otherwise normal rats, led to a dramatic increase in left ventricular ANF mRNA levels (Day *et al.*, 1987; Izumo, Nadal-Ginard & Mahdavi, 1988) and promoted the accumulation of irANF within the ventricular myocardium (Day *et al.*, 1987). These latter effects were additive with those resulting from glucocorticoid treatment (Day *et al.*, 1987).

Pressure overload due to genetic hypertension results in a similar increase in ANF gene expression. The spontaneously hypertensive rat (SHR) at 26 weeks of age has a mean arterial blood pressure, plasma ANF level and ventricular ANF mRNA level which are significantly elevated when compared with the normotensive Wistar–Kyoto (WKY) control (Arai *et al.*, 1988). These differences are exaggerated to an even greater degree in the more severely hypertensive SHR-stroke-prone strain yet largely absent in 7-week-old animals, an age at which the blood pressure differences between the SHR and WKY strains are minimal. Left atrial ANF mRNA levels were also shown to be elevated selectively (vs. the right atrium) in the older SHR rat when compared to the WKY (Arai *et al.*, 1987). These findings suggest that hypertension, with the accompanying increase in afterload, results in a diffuse activation of ANF gene expression in the left side of the SHR heart.

There is a similar blood-pressure-dependent increase in plasma ANF and ventricular ANF mRNA levels in the Dahl salt-sensitive rat when compared to the Dahl salt-resistant (R) strain. Again, these differences were only apparent following the onset of hypertension in the Dahl S strain (Dene & Rapp, 1987). In this study atrial ANF mRNA levels in the S strain were not different from those in the R strain despite the presence of hypertension.

Ventricular ANF immunoreactivity as well as ANF mRNA levels are increased in states of cardiac hypertrophy and congestive heart failure both in animal models (Ding *et al.*, 1987; Cantin *et al.*, 1988; Lee *et al.*, 1988) and in humans (Nemer, Lavigne & Drouin, 1987; Saito *et al.*, 1987; Edwards *et al.*, 1988; Gutkowska *et al.*, 1989), again presumably reflecting the effects of increased wall tension in the hypertrophied and/or dilated cardiomyopathic ventricle. The coexistence of elevated ventricular ANF production and plasma ANF levels suggests that the ventricle contributes a larger percentage of ANF to the circulating pool in these states. In the case of the cardiomyopathic hamster (Gutkowska *et al.*, 1989) the lung appears to represent another major contributor to plasma ANF levels.

Ventricular ANF gene expression has also been shown to increase following myocardial infarction both in humans (Galipeau, Nemer & Drouin, 1988) and in animal models (Mendez *et al.*, 1987). In the latter case ANF levels correlated directly with the severity of the infarct. Ischemia, *per se*, has been shown to increase release of irANF from isolated perfused hearts (Baertschi *et al.*, 1986; Lew & Baertschi, 1989) and in human hearts subjected to diminished coronary perfusion (Gasser *et al.*, 1989); however, it remains unclear what fraction of the increased ANF gene expression seen in the postinfarct ventricle results from ischemia *per se* vs. abnormal contractile tension placed upon the secretory cells as the infarcted heart attempts to compensate for the loss of functional myocardium. Chronic hypoxia, induced by exposing rats to a 10% oxygen environment for 3 weeks, resulted in right ventricular hypertrophy and significant increases in irANP and ANP mRNA concentration in that chamber (Stockmann *et al.*, 1988). The effects on ANP synthesis were reversible following alleviation of the hypoxia despite the persistence of right ventricular hypertrophy.

Molecular determinants of ANF gene expression

A key unanswered question regarding ANF gene expression relates to the molecular mechanisms whereby atrial, and in some instances ventricular, cells are afforded the capacity to express the gene at such a high level relative to non-cardiac tissue.

Using a conventional gene transfection approach, we (LaPointe *et al.*, 1988; Wu *et al.*, 1989), as well as others (Seidman *et al.*, 1988), have attempted to identify *cis*-acting elements in the 5'FS of the ANF gene capable of promoting tissue-specific expression. LaPointe *et al.*, (1988) linked ~ 2500 bp of 5'FS from the human ANF gene to a bacterial chloramphenicol acetyl transferase reporter gene which is not expressed in eukaryotic cells. This construction, as well as the intact hANF gene, was expressed following introduction into primary cultures of neonatal rat atrial cells. Sensitive protection assays revealed that transcripts derived from these transfected plasmids arose from the predicted ANF-promoter-dependent transcription start site. Little or no expression of these plasmids was observed following transfection into ventricular cells. When the -2500 hANF CAT construction was truncated to 409 bp of 5'FS, the high level of expression persisted. However, when the construction was deleted to -337, expression fell dramatically suggesting the presence of an atrial-specific, *cis*-acting element in this region of the gene. No further reduction in expression could be documented as the truncation was pushed closer to the CAP site (i.e. position -182). When the DNA fragment lying between -400 and -337 was excised from the hANF gene and placed upstream of a heterologous neutral promoter (i.e. the promoter for viral thymidine kinase, TK) linked to CAT coding sequences, it proved capable of augmenting reporter gene expression in both atrial and ventricular cardiocytes but not in cardiac mesenchymal cells derived from the same primary cultures (Wu *et al.*, 1989). This fragment was active only when placed in the transcriptionally correct orientation upstream from the TK promoter. Placing the fragment in an inverted orientation upstream of the TK promoter or downstream of the CAT coding sequences failed to activate CAT expression (Wu *et al.*, 1989).

Current models of gene expression suggest that *cis*-acting DNA elements accrue their activity by virtue of their ability to interact with soluble proteins found in the cell nucleus (i.e. *trans*-acting factors). The bioactive 64-bp fragment lying between -400 and -337 in the hANF gene was shown to associate with protein(s) in cardiocyte (i.e. atrial or ventricular) nuclear extracts in a sequence- and tissue-specific fashion. More definitive analysis using DNAse I footprinting and methylation interference analysis indicated that the key region of DNA–protein interaction was located between -373 and -355 in the hANF gene 5'FS (Wu *et al.*, 1989). Taken together these data imply the presence of a cardiac-specific element within the proximal 5'FS of the hANF gene which may acquire this activity by virtue of its ability to associate with nuclear proteins found largely in myocardial cells.

Seidman *et al.* (1988) have localized a similar atrial-specific element in the rat ANF gene. Using a deletion mutation approach similar to that described above, they identified a *cis*-acting element between -2427 and -638 relative to the CAP site which was capable of driving reporter gene expression in atrial but not ventricular cells. A somewhat longer chimeric construction (i.e. 3412 bp of rANF 5′FS linked to CAT coding sequence) also demonstrated sensitivity to glucocorticoid regulation implying the presence of a hormone-response element in this region (i.e. between positions -3412 to $+61$) of the rat gene.

In summary, the gene encoding the ANF mRNA is highly conserved among different species. While the cardiac atria represent the predominant site of ANF gene expression in the intact animal, ANF mRNA transcripts can be identified in a number of extra-atrial locations. Several of these lie in or around key cardiovascular regulatory structures raising the possibility that ANF may play a role in modulating cardiovascular function independent of atrial ANF secretion. Ventricular ANF gene expression, which is usually very low in the basal state, can be activated by hormonal stimuli (e.g. glucocorticoid or thyroid hormone) or by factors which act to promote functional overload of the ventricular chambers. In the latter case, it is conceivable that the ventricle could contribute a significant portion of total cardiac ANF secretion to the circulating plasma pool. Finally, at least two *cis*-acting genomic elements have been identified on separate ANF genes. One of these appears to be capable of associating with myocardial cell nuclear proteins in a highly specific fashion. These elements may account for a significant portion of this gene's atrial specific expression.

Acknowledgements

The authors are grateful to Mrs Ann Bull for preparation of the manuscript. This work was supported by NIH grants HL35753 (DGG) and HL 38774 (CFD) and by a Grant-in-Aid from the American Heart Association with partial support form the Redwood Empire Chapter. DGG is an Established Investigator of the American Heart Association.

References

Antunes-Rodrigues, J., McCann, S. M., Rogers, L. C. & Samson, W. K. (1985). Atrial natriuretic factor inhibits dehydration- and angiotensin II-induced water intake in the conscious, unrestrained rat. *Proc. Nat. Acad. Sci. USA* **82**: 8720–3.

Antunes-Rodrigues, J., McCann, S. M. & Samson, W. K. (1986). Central administration of atrial natriuretic factor inhibits saline preference in the rat. *Endocrinology* **118**: 1726–8.

Anand-Srivastava, M. B., Thibault, G., Sola, C., Fon, E., Ballah, M., Charbonneau, C. *et al.* (1989). Atrial natriuretic factor in Purkinje fibers of rabbit heart. *Hypertension* **13**: 789–98.

Arai, H., Nakao, K., Saito, Y., Morii, N., Sugawara, A., Yamada, T., Itoh, H. *et al.* (1987). Simultaneous measurement of atrial natriuretic polypeptide (ANP) messenger RNA and ANP in rat heart—evidence for a preferentially increased synthesis and secretion of ANP in left atrium of spontaneously hypertensive rats (SHR). *Biochem. Biophys. Res. Commun.* **148**: 239–45.

Arai, H., Nakao, K., Saito, Y., Morii, N., Sugawara, A., Yamada, T., Itoh, H. *et al.* (1988). Augmented expression of atrial natriuretic polypeptide gene in ventricles of spontaneously hypertensive rats (SHR) and SHR-stroke prone. *Circulation Res.* **62**: 926–30.

Argentin, S., Nemer, M., Drouin, J., Scott, G., Kennedy, B. & Davies, P. (1985). The gene for rat atrial natriuretic factor. *J. Biol. Chem.* **260**: 4568–71.

Baertschi, A. J., Hausmaninger, C., Walsh, R. S., Mentzer, R. M. Jr., Wyatt, D. A. & Pence, R. A. (1986). Hypoxia-induced release of atrial natriuretic factor (ANF) from the isolated rat and rabbit heart. *Biochem. Biophys. Res. Commun.* **140**: 427–33.

Ballerman, B. J., Bloch, K. D., Seidman, J. G. & Brenner, B. M. (1986). Atrial natriuretic peptide transcription, secretion, and glomerular activity during mineralocorticoid escape in the rat. *J. Clin. Invest.* **78**: 840–3.

Benoist, C. & Chambon, P. (1981). *In vivo* sequence requirements of the SV40 early promoter region. *Nature* **290**: 304–10.

Blobel, G. & Dobberstein, B. (1975). Transfer of proteins across membranes. Reconstitution of functional rough microsomes from heterologous components. *J. Cell Biol.* **67**: 852–62.

Bloch, K. D., Scott, J. A., Zisfein, J. B., Fallon, J. T., Margolies, M. N., Seidman, C. E., Matsueda, G. R. *et al.* (1985). Biosynthesis and secretion of proatrial natriuretic factor by cultured rat cardiocytes. *Science* **230**, 1168–71.

Bloch, K. D., Seidman, J. G., Naftilan, J. D., Fallon, J. T. & Seidman, C. E. (1986). Neonatal atria and ventricles secrete atrial natriuretic factor via tissue-specific secretory pathways. *Cell* **47**: 695–702.

Brody, M. J. & Johnson, A. K. (1980). Role of the AV3V region in fluid and electrolyte balance, arterial pressure regulation and hypertension. In: *Frontiers in Neuroendocrinology*, Vol. 6 (Martini, L. & Ganong, W. F., eds). London: Oxford University Press, pp. 249–93.

Camargo, M. J. F., Kleinert, H. D., Atlas, S. A., Sealey, J. E., Laragh, J. H. & Maack, T. (1984). Ca-dependent hemodynamic and natriuretic effects of atrial extract in isolated rat kidney. *Am. J. Physiol.* **246**: F447–56.

Cantin, M. & Genest, J. (1985). The heart and the atrial natriuretic factor. *Endocrine Rev.* **6**: 107–27.

Cantin, M., Thibault, G., Ding, J., Gutkowska, J., Garcia, R., Jasmin, G., Hamet, P., Genest, J. (1988) ANF in experimental congestive heart failure. *Am. J. Pathol.* **13**: 552–68.

Claycomb, W. C. (1988). Atrial natriuretic factor mRNA is developmentally regulated in heart ventricles and actively expressed in cultured ventricular cardiac muscle cells of rat and human. *Biochem. J.* **255**: 617–20.

Currie, M. G. & Newman, W. H. (1986). Evidence for α-adrenergic receptor regulation of atriopeptin release from the isolated rat heart. *Biochem. Biophys. Res. Commun.* **137**: 94–100.

Currie, M. G., Sukin, D., Geller, D. M., Cole, B. R. & Needleman, P. (1984). Atriopeptin release from the isolated perfused rabbit heart. *Biochem. Biophys. Res. Commun.* **124**: 711–17.

Day, M. L., Schwartz, D., Wiegand, R. C., Stockman, P. T., Brunnert, S. R., Tolunay, H. E., Currie, M. G. *et al.* (1987). Ventricular atriopeptin: Unmasking of messenger RNA and peptide synthesis by hypertropy or dexamethasone. *Hypertension* **9**: 485–91.

Debinski, W., Gutkowska, J., Kuchel, O., Racz, K., Buu, N. T., Cantin, M. & Genest, J. (1986). ANF-like peptides in the peripheral autonomic nervous system. *Biochem. Biophys. Res. Commun.* **134**: 279–84.

deBold, A. J., Borenstein, H. B., Veress, A. T. & Sonnenberg, H. (1981). A rapid and potent natriuretic response to intravenous injection of atrial myocardial extract in rats. *Life Sci.* **28**: 89–94.

Dene, H. & Rapp, J. P. (1987). Quantification of messenger ribonucleic acid for atrial natriuretic factor in atria and ventricles of Dahl salt-sensitive and salt-resistant rats. *Molec. Endocrinol.* **1**: 614–20.

Deschepper, C. F., Mellon, S. H., Cumin, F., Baxter, J. D. & Ganong, W. F. (1986). Analysis by immunocytochemistry and *in situ* hybridization of renin and its mRNA in kidney, testis, adrenal, and pituitary of the rat. *Proc. Nat. Acad. Sci. USA* **83**: 7552–6.

Ding, J., Thibault, G., Gutkowska, J., Garcia, R., Karabatsos, T., Jasmin, G., Genest, J. *et al.* (1987). Cardiac and plasma atrial natriuretic factor in experimental congestive heart failure. *Endocrinology* **121**: 248–57.

Dracopoli, N. C., Stanger, B. Z., Ito, C. Y., Call, K. M., Lincoln, S. E., Lander, E. S. *et al.* (1988). A genetic linkage map of 27 loci from PNP to FY on the short arm of human chromosome I. *Am. J. Human Genet.* **43**: 462–70.

Dykes, C. W., Bookless, A. B., Coomber, B. A., Noble, S. A., Humber, D. C. & Holden, A. N. (1988). Expression of atrial natriuretic factor as a cleavable fusion protein with chloramphenicol acetyltransferase in *Escherichia coli*. *Eur. J. Biochem.* **174**: 411–16.

Edward, B. S., Ackermann, D. M., Lee, M. E., Reeder, G. S., Wold, L. E. & Burnett, J. C., Jr. (1988). Identification of atrial natriuretic factor within ventricular tissue in hamsters and humans with congestive heart failure. *J. Clin. Invest.* **81**: 82–6.

Flynn, T. G., Davies, P. L., Kennedy, B. P., deBold, M. L. & deBold, A. J. (1985). Alignment of rat cardionatrin sequences with the preprocardionatrin sequence from complementary cDNA. *Science* **228**: 323–5.

Frossard, P. M. & Coleman, R. T. (1986). Human atrial natriuretic peptide (ANP) gene locus: Bgl I RFLP. *Nucleic Acids Res.* **14**: 9223.

Galipeau, J., Nemer, M. & Drouin, J. (1988). Ventricular activation of the atrial natriuretic factor gene in acute myocardial infarction. *New Engl. J. Med.* **319**: 654–5.

Gardner, D. G., Deschepper, C. F. & Baxter, J. D. (1987a). The gene for the atrial natriuretic factor is expressed in the aortic arch. *Hypertension* **9**: 103–6.

Gardner, D. G., Deschepper, C. F., Ganong, W. F., Hane, S., Fiddes, J., Baxter, J. D. & Lewicki, J. (1986a). Extra-atrial expression of the gene for atrial natriuretic factor. *Proc. Nat. Acad. Sci. USA* **83**: 6697–701.

Gardner, D. G., Gertz, B. J., Deschepper, C. F. & Kim, D. Y. (1988a). Gene for the rat atrial natriuretic peptide is regulated by glucocorticoids *in vitro*. *J. Clin. Invest.* **82**: 1275–81.

Gardner, D. G., Gertz, B. J. & Hane, S. (1987b). Thyroid hormone increases rat atrial natriuretic peptide messenger ribonucleic acid accumulation *in vivo* and *in vitro*. *Molec. Endocrinol.* **1**: 260–5.

Gardner, D. G., Hane, S., Trachewsky, D., Schenk, D. & Baxter, J. D. (1986b). Atrial natriuretic peptide mRNA is regulated by glucocorticoids *in vivo*. *Biochem. Biophys. Res. Commun.* **139**: 1047–54.

Gardner, D. G., Hedges, B. K., Wu, J., LaPointe, M. C. & Deschepper, C. F. (1989). Expression of the atrial natriuretic peptide gene in human fetal heart. *J. Clin. Endocrinol. Metab.* **69**: 729–37.

Gardner, D. G., LaPointe, M. C., Wu, J., Baxter, J. D. & Gertz, B. J. (1988b). Hormonal regulation of the atrial natriuretic peptide gene. In: *Biologically Active Atrial Peptides*, Vol. II (Brenner, B. & Laragh, J., eds). New York: Raven Press, pp. 9–13.

Gardner, D. G., LaPointe, M. C. & Wu, J. (1988c). Expression and regulation of the gene for atrial natriuretic factor. In: *Frontiers of Neuroendocrinology*, Vol. 10 (Martini, L. & Ganong, W. F., eds). New York: Raven Press, pp. 45–61.

Gardner, D. G., Vlasuk, G. P., Baxter, J. D., Fiddes, J. C. & Lewicki, J. A. (1987c). Identification of atrial natriuretic factor transcripts in the central nervous system of the rat. *Proc. Nat. Acad. Sci. USA*, **84**: 2175–9.

Gasser, R., Dusleag, J., Eber, B., Rotman, B., Weinrauch, V., Brussee, E., Schaffer, E. *et al.* (1989). Plasma levels of atrial natriuretic peptide in transient left ventricular ischemia. *New Engl. J. Med.* **320**: 1752.

Glembotski, C. & Gibson, T. R. (1985). Molecular forms of immunoactive atrial natriuretic peptide released from cultured rat atrial myocytes. *Biochem. Biophys. Res. Commun.* **132**: 1008–17.

Graham, R. M., Bloch, K. D., Dehaney, V. B., Bourke, E. & Seidman, J. G. (1986). Bartter's syndrome and the atrial natriuretic factor gene. *Hypertension* **8**: 549–51.

Greenberg, B., Bencen, G., Seilhamer, J., Lewicki, J. & Fiddes, J. (1984). Nucleotide sequence of the gene encoding human ANF precursor. *Nature*, **312**: 656–8.

Greenwald, J. E., Apkon, M., Hruska, K. A. & Needleman, P. (1989). Stretch-induced atriopeptin secretion in the isolated rat myocyte and its negative modulation by calcium. *J. Clin. Invest.* **83**: 1061–5.

Grekin, R. J., Ling, W. D., Shenker, Y. & Bohr, D. F. (1986). Immunoreactive atrial natriuretic hormone levels increase in deoxycorticosterone acetate treated pigs. *Hypertension* **8** (Suppl. II): II16–20.

Gutkowska, J., Nemer, M., Sole, M. J., Drouin, J. & Sirois, P. (1989). Lung is an important source of atrial natriuretic factor in experimental cardiomyopathy. *J. Clin. Invest.* **83**: 1500–4.

Hamid, Q., Wharton, J., Terenghi, G., Hassall, C. J. S., Aimi, J., Taylor, K. M., Nakazato, H. *et al.* (1987). Localization of atrial natriuretic peptide mRNA and immunoreactivity in the rat heart and human atrial appendage. *Proc. Nat. Acad. Sci. USA* **84**: 6760–4.

Iitake, K., Share, L., Crofton, J. T., Brooks, D. P., Ouchi, Y. & Blaine, E. H. (1986). Central atrial natriuretic factor reduces vasopressin secretion in the rat. *Endocrinology* **119**: 438–40.

Imaizumi, T., Takeshita, A., Higashi, H. & Nakamura, M. (1987). α-ANP alters reflex control of lumbar and renal sympathetic nerve activity and heart rate. *Am. J. Physiol.* **253**: H1136–40.

Iwai, N., Matsunaga, M., Ogawa, K., Matsumori, A., Yoshida, H., Ohta, E. & Kawai, C. (1987). Expression of human atrial natriuretic polypeptide gene in Cos 7 cells. *Biochem. Biophys. Res. Commun.* **143**: 288–93.

Iwao, H., Fukui, K., Kim, S., Nakayama, K., Ohkubo, H., Nakanishi, S. & Abe, Y. (1988). Sodium balance effects on renin, angiotensinogen, and atrial natriuretic polypeptide mRNA levels. *Am. J. Physiol.* **255**(2): E129–36.

Izumo, S., Nadal-Ginard, B. & Mahdavi, V. (1988). Protooncogene induction and re-programming of cardiac gene expression produced by pressure overload. *Proc. Nat. Acad. Sci. USA* **85**: 339–43.

Jacobowitz, D. M., Skofitsch, G., Keiser, H. R., Eskay, R. L. & Zamir, N. (1985). Evidence for the existence of atrial natriuretic factor-containing neurons in the rat brain. *Neuroendocrinology* **40**: 92–4.

Januszewicz, P., Thibault, G., Garcia, R., Gutkowska, J., Genest, J. & Cantin, M. (1986). Effect of synthetic atrial natriuretic factor on arginine vasopressin release by the rat hypothalamo-neuropophyseal complex in organ culture. *Biochem. Biophys. Res. Commun.* **134**: 652–8.

Karin, M., Haslinger, A., Holtgreve, H., Richards, R. I., Krauter, P., Westphal, H. M. & Beato, M. (1984). Characterization of DNA sequences through which cadmium and glucocorticoid hormones induce human metallothionein II$_A$ gene. *Nature* **308**: 513–19.

Kikuchi, K., Nakao, K., Hayashi, K., Morii, N., Sugawara, A., Sakamoto, M., Imura, H. *et al.* (1987). Ontogeny of atrial natriuretic polypeptide in the human heart. *Acta Endocrinol.* (Copenhagen) **115**: 211–17.

Kohtz, D. S., Dische, N. R., Inagami, T. & Goldman, B. (1989). Growth and partial differentiation of presumptive human cardiac myoblasts in culture. *J. Cell Biol.* **108**: 1067–78.

Ladenson, P. W., Bloch, K. D. & Seidman, J. G. (1988). Modulation of atrial natriuretic factor by thyroid hormone: Messenger ribonucleic acid and peptide levels in hypothyroid, euthyroid, and hyperthyroid rat atria and ventricles. *Endocrinology* **123**: 652–7.

LaPointe, M. C., Deschepper, C. F., Wu, J., Gardner, D. G. (1990). Extracellular calcium regulates expression of the gene for atrial natriuretic factor. *Hypertension* **15**: 20–8.

LaPointe, M. C., Wu, J., Greenberg, B. & Gardner, D. G. (1988). Upstream sequences confer atrial-specific expression on the human atrial natriuretic factor gene. *J. Biol. Chem.* **263**: 9075–8.

Lattion, A.-L., Michel, J.-B., Arnauld, E., Corvol, P. & Soubriers, F. (1986). Myocardial recruitment during ANF mRNA increase with volume overload in the rat. *Am. J. Physiol.* **251**: H890–6.

Lavigne, J. P., Drouin, J., Ding, J., Thibault, G., Nemer, M. & Cantin, M. (1988). Atrial natriuretic factor (ANF) gene expression in the Brattleboro rat. *Peptides* **9**: 817–24.

Lee, R. T., Bloch, K. D., Pfeffer, J. M., Pfeffer, M. A., Neer, E. J. & Seidman, C. E. (1988). Atrial natriuretic factor gene expression in ventricles of rats with spontaneous biventricular hypertrophy. *J. Clin. Invest.* **81**: 431–4.

Lennick, M., Haynes, J. R. & Shen, S.-H. (1987). High-level expression of α-human atrial natriuretic peptide from multiple joined genes in *Escherichia coli. Gene* **61**: 103–12.

Levin, E. R., Weber, M. A. & Mills, S. (1988). Atrial natriuretic factor-induced vasodepression occurs through central nervous system. *Am. J. Physiol.* **255**: H616–22.

Lew, R. A. & Baertschi, A. J. (1989). Mechanisms of hypoxia-induced atrial natriuretic factor release from rat hearts. *Am. J. Physiol.* **257**: H147–56.

Maki, M., Parmentier, M. & Inagami, T. (1984a). Cloning of the genomic DNA for human ANF. *Biochem. Biophys. Res. Commun.* **125**: 797–802.

Maki, M., Takayanagi, R., Misono, K. S., Pandey, K. N., Tibbetts, C. & Inagami, T. (1984b). Structure of rat ANF precursor deduced from cDNA sequence. *Nature* **309**: 722–4.

Manning, P. T., Schwartz, D., Katsube, N. C., Holmberg, S. W. & Needleman, P. (1985). Vasopressin-stimulated release of atriopeptin: Endocrine antagonists in fluid homeostasis. *Science* **229**: 395–7.

Matsubara, H., Hirata, Y., Yoshimi, H., Takata, S., Takagi, Y., Umeda, Y., Yamane, Y. *et al.* (1988). Role of calcium and protein kinase C in ANP secretion by cultured rat cardiocytes. *Am. J. Physiol.* **255**: H405–9.

Matsubara, H., Hirata, Y., Yoshimi, H., Takata, S., Takagi, Y., Yamane, Y., Umeda, Y. *et al.* (1987). Ventricular myocytes from neonatal rats are more responsive to dexamethasone than atrial myocytes in synthesis of atrial natriuretic peptide. *Biochem. Biophys. Res. Commun.* **148**: 1030–8.

McKenzie, J. C., Tanaka, I., Misono, K. S. & Inagami, T. (1985). Immunocytochemical localization of atrial natriuretic factor in the kidney, adrenal medulla, pituitary and atrium of the rat. *J. Histochem. Cytochem.* **33**: 828–32.

Mendez, R. E., Pfeffer, J. M., Ortola, F. V., Bloch, K. D., Anderson, S., Seidman, J. G. & Brenner, B. M. (1987). Atrial natriuretic peptide transcription, storage, and release in rats with myocardial infarction. *Am. J. Physiol.* **253**: H1449–55.

Metzler, C. H., Gardner, D. G., Keil, L. C., Baxter, J. D. & Ramsay, D. G. (1987). Increased synthesis and release of atrial peptide during mineralocorticoid escape in conscious dogs. *Am. J. Physiol.* **252**: R188–92.

Miyata, A., Toshimori, T., Hashiguchi, T., Kangawa, K. & Matsuo, H. (1987). Molecular form of atrial natriuretic polypeptides circulating in human plasma. *Biochem. Biophys. Res. Commun.* **142**: 461–7.

Morel, G., Chabot, J.-G., Garcia-Caballero, T., Gossard, F., Dihl, F., Belles-Isles, M. & Heisler, S. (1988). Synthesis, internalization and localization of atrial natriuretic peptide in rat adrenal medulla. *Endocrinology* **123**: 149–58.

Morel, G., Chabot, J.-G., Gossard, F. & Heisler, S. (1989). Is atrial natriuretic peptide synthesized and internalized by gonadotrophs? *Endocrinology* **124**: 1703–10.

Mullins, J. J., Zeng, Q. & Gross, K. W. (1987). Mapping of the mouse atrial natriuretic factor gene. Evidence for tight linkage to the *Fr-1* locus. *Hypertension* **9**: 518–21.

Nakayama, K., Ohkubo, H., Hirose, T., Inayama, S. & Nakanishi, S. (1984). mRNA sequence for human cardiodilatin-atrial natriuretic factor precursor and regulation of precursor mRNA in rat atria. *Nature* **310**: 699–701.

Nakamura, M., Katsuura, G., Nakao, K., Imura, H. (1985). Antidipsogenic action of a human atrial natriuretic polypeptide administered intracerebroventricularly in rats: *Neuroscience Letts* **58**: 1–6.

Needleman, P. & Greenwald, J. E. (1986). Atriopeptin: A cardiac hormone intimately involved in fluid, electrolyte and blood-pressure homeostasis. *New Engl. J. Med.* **314**: 828–34.

Nemer, M., Chamberland, M., Sirois, D., Argentin, S., Drouin, J., Dixon, R. A. F., Zivin, R. A. *et al.*, (1984). Gene structure of human cardiac hormone precursor, pronatriodilatin. *Nature* **312**: 654–6.

Nemer, M., Lavigne, J.-P. & Drouin, J. (1987). Ventricles are a major site of ANF gene expression in congestive heart failure. *J. Molec. Cell Cardiol.* **19** (Suppl. IV): 45.

Nemer, M., Lavigne, J.-P., Drouin, J., Thibault, G., Gannon, M. & Antakly, T. (1986a). Expression of atrial natriuretic factor gene in heart ventricular tissue. *Peptides* **7**: 1147–52.

Nemer, M., Sirois, D. & Drouin, J. (1986b). Taq polymorphism at the 3′ end of the human pronatriodilatin gene (hPND). *Nucleic Acids Res.* **14**: 8697.

Nemer, M., Sirois, D. & Drouin, J. (1986c). Xho I polymorphism at the human pronatriodilatin (hPND) gene locus. *Nucleic Acids Res.* **14**: 8696.

Nordeim, A. & Rich, A. (1983). Negatively supercoiled simian virus 40 DNA contains DNA segments within transcriptional enhancer sequences. *Nature* **303**: 674–9.

Oikawa, S., Imai, M., Inuzuka, C., Tawaragi, Y., Nakazato, H. & Matsuo, H. (1985). Structure of dog and rabbit precursors of atrial natriuretic polypeptides deduced from nucleotide sequence of cloned cDNA. *Biochem. Biophys. Res. Commun.* **132**: 892–9.

Oikawa, S., Imai, M., Ueno, A., Tanaka, S., Noguchi, T., Nakazato, N., Kangawa, K. *et al.* (1984). Cloning and sequence analysis of cDNA encoding a precursor for human ANP. *Nature* **309**: 724–6.

Proudfoot, N. (1982). The end of the message. *Nature* **298**: 516–17.

Quirion, R., Dalpe, M. & Dam, T.-V. (1986). Characterization and distribution of receptors for the atrial natriuretic peptides in mammalian brain. *Proc. Nat. Acad. Sci. USA* **83**: 174–8.

Ruskoaho, H., Taskinen, T., Pesonen, A., Vuolteenaho, O., Leppaluoto, J. & Tuomisto, J. (1989). Atrial natriuretic peptide in plasma, atria, ventricles, and hypothalamus of Long-Evans and vasopressin-deficient Brattleboro rats. *Endocrinology* **124**: 2595–603.

Ruskoaho, H., Toth, M. & Lang, R. E. (1985). Atrial natriuretic peptide secretion: Synergistic effect of phorbol ester and A23187. *Biochem. Biophys. Res. Commun.* **133**: 581–8.

Saavedra, J. M., Correa, F. M. A., Plunkett, L. M., Israel, A., Kurihara, M. & Shigematsu, K. (1986). Binding of angiotensin and atrial natriuretic peptide in brain of hypertensive rats. *Nature* **320**: 758–60.

Saito, Y., Nakao, K., Arai, H., Sugawara, A., Morii, N., Yamada, T., Itoh, H. *et al.* (1987). Atrial natriuretic polypeptide (ANP) in human ventricle—increased gene expression of ANP in dilated cardiomyopathy. *Biochem. Biophys. Res. Commun.* **148**: 211–17.

Samson, W. K. (1985). Atrial natriuretic factor inhibits dehydration and hemorrhage-induced vasopressin release. *Neuroendocrinology* **40**: 277–9.

Samson, W. K., Aguila, M. C. & Bianchi, R. (1988a). Atrial natriuretic factor inhibits luteinizing hormone secretion in the rat: Evidence for a hypothalamic site of action. *Endocrinology* **122**: 1573–82.

Samson, W. K. & Bianchi, R. (1988). Further evidence for a hypothalamic site of action of atrial natriuretic factor: Inhibition of prolactin secretion in the conscious rat. *Can. J. Physiol. Pharmacol.* **66**: 301–5.

Samson, W. K., Bianchi, R. & Mogg, R. (1988b). Evidence for a dopaminergic mehcanism for the prolactin inhibitory effect of atrial natriuretic factor. *Neuroendocrinology* **47**: 268–71.

Saper, C. B., Standaert, D. G., Currie, M. G., Schwartz, D., Geller, D. M. & Needleman, P. (1985). Atriopeptin-immunoreactive neurons in the brain: presence in cardiovascular regulatory areas. *Science* **227**: 1047–9.

Schiebinger, R. J., Baker, M. Z. & Linden, J. (1987). Effect of adrenergic and muscarinic cholinergic agonists on atrial natriuretic peptide secretion by isolated rat atria. *J. Clin. Invest.* **80**: 1687–91.

Schultz, H. D., Gardner, D. G., Deschepper, C. F., Coleridge, H. M. & Coleridge, J. C. G. (1988). Vagal C-fiber blockade abolishes sympathetic inhibition by atrial natriuretic factor. *Am. J. Physiol.* **255**: R6–R13.

Schultz, H. D., Steele, M. K. & Gardner, D. G. (1989). Renal, sympathetic and cardiovascular responses to central administration of angiotensin II (AII) and atrial natriuretic peptide. *FASEB J.* **3**: A1008.

Schwartz, D., Geller, D. M., Manning, P. T., Siegel, N. R., Fok, F., Smith, C. E. & Needleman, P. (1985). Ser-Leu-Arg-Arg-Atriopeptin III: The major circulating form of atrial peptide. *Science* **229**: 397–400.

Seidman, C., Bloch, K., Klein, K., Smith, J. & Seidman, J. (1984a). Nucleotide sequences of the human and mouse atrial natriuretic factor genes. *Science* **226**: 1206–9.

Seidman, C. E., Duby, A. D., Choi, E., Graham, R. M., Haber, E., Homcy, C., Smith, J. A. & Seidman, J. G. (1984b). Structure of rat pre-proatrial natriuretic factor as defined by a complementary DNA clone. *Science* **225**: 324–6.

Seidman, C. E., Wong, D. W., Jarcho, J. A., Bloch, K. D. & Seidman, J. G. (1988). Cis-acting sequences that modulate atrial natriurctic factor gene expression. *Proc. Nat. Acad. Sci. USA* **85**: 4104–8.

Shields, P. P., Dixon, J. E. & Glembotski, C. C. (1988). The secretion of atrial natriuretic factor-(99–126) by cultured cardiac myocytes is regulated by glucocorticoids. *J. Biol. Chem.* **263**, 12619–28.

Shields, P. P. & Glembotski, C. C. (1989). Regulation of atrial natriuretic factor-(99–126) secretion from neonatal rat primary atrial cultures by activators of protein kinases A and C. *J. Biol. Chem.* **264**: 9322–8.

Sonnenberg, H. & Veress, A. T. (1984). Cellular mechanism of release of atrial natriuretic factor. *Biochem. Biophys. Res. Commun.* **124**(2): 443–9.

Standaert, D. G., Cechetto, D. F., Needleman, P. & Saper, C. B. (1987). Inhibition of the firing of vasopressin neurons by atriopeptin. *Nature* **329**: 151–3.

Standaert, D. G., Cicero, T. & Needleman, P. (1986a). Atriopeptin inhibits the release of luteinizing hormone. *Fed. Proc.* **45**: 174 (abstract).

Standaert, D. G., Needleman, P. & Saper, C. B. (1986b). Organization of atriopeptin-like immunoreactive neurons in the central nervous system of the rat. *J. Comp. Neurol.* **253**: 315–41.

Standaert, D. G., Needleman, P. & Saper, C. B. (1988). Atriopeptin: Neuromediator in the central regulation of cardiovascular function. In: *Frontiers in Neuroendocrinology*, Vol. 10 (Martini, L. & Ganong, W. F., eds). New York: Raven Press, pp. 45–61.

Stockmann, P. T., Will, D. H., Sides, S. D., Brunnert, S. R., Wilner, G. D., Leaky, K. M., Wiegand, R. C. *et al.* (1988). Reversible induction of right ventricular atriopeptin synthesis in hypertrophy due to hypoxia. *Circulation Res.* **63**: 207–13.

Takayanagi, R., Tanaka, I., Maki, M. & Inagami, T. (1985). Effects of changes in water-sodium balance on levels of atrial natriuretic factor messenger RNA and peptide in rats. *Life Sci.* **36**: 1843–8.

Tanaka, I., Misono, K. S. & Inagami, T. (1984). Atrial natriuretic factor in rat hypothalamus, atria and plasma: Determination by specific radioimmunoassay. *Biochem. Biophys. Res. Commun.* **124**: 663–8.

Thoren, P., Mark, A. L., Morgan, D. A., O'Neill, T. P., Needleman, P. & Brody, M. J. (1986). Activation of vagal depressor reflexes by atriopeptins inhibits renal sympathetic nerve activity. *Am. J. Physiol.* **251**: H1252–9.

Vlasuk, G. P., Bencen, G. H., Scarborough, R. M., Tsai, P.-K., Whang, J. L., Maack, T.,

Camargo, M. J. F. *et al.* (1986a). Expression and secretion of biologically active human atrial natriuretic peptide in *Saccharomyces cerevisiae*. *J. Biol. Chem.* **261**: 4789–96.

Vlasuk, G., Miller, J., Bencen, G. & Lewicki, J. (1986b). Structure and analysis of the bovine atrial natriuretic peptide precursor gene. *Biochem. Biophys. Res. Commun.* **136**: 396–403.

Vuolteenaho, O., Arjamaa, O. & Ling, N. (1985). Atrial natriuretic polypeptides (ANP): Rat atria store high molecular weight precursor but secrete processed peptide of 25–35 amino acids. *Biochem. Biophys. Res. Commun.* **129**: 82–8.

Wei, Y., Rodi, C. P., Day, M. L., Wiegand, R. C., Needleman, L. D., Cole, B. R. & Needleman, P. (1987). Developmental changes in the rat atriopeptin hormonal system. *J. Clin. Invest.* **79**: 1325–9.

Wong, M., Samson, W. K., Dudley, C. A. & Moss, R. L. (1986). Direct neuronal action of atrial natriuretic factor in the rat brain. *Neuroendocrinology* **44**: 49–53.

Wu, J., Deschepper, C. F. & Gardner, D. G. (1988). Perinatal expression of the atrial natriuretic factor gene in rat cardiac tissue. *Am. J. Physiol.* **255**: E388–96.

Wu, J., LaPointe, M. C., West, B. L. & Gardner, D. G. (1989). Tissue-specific determinants of human atrial natriuretic factor gene expression in cardiac tissue. *J. Biol. Chem.* **264**: 6472–9.

Yamanaka, M., Greenberg, B., Johnson, L., Seilhamer, J., Brewer, M., Friedmann, T., Miller, J. *et al.* (1984). Cloning and sequence analysis of the cDNA for the rat ANF precursor. *Nature* **309**: 719–22.

Yang-Feng, T. L., Floyd-Smith, G., Nemer, M., Drouin, J. & Francke, U. (1985). The pronatriodilatin gene is located on the distal short arm of human chromosome 1 and on mouse chromosome 4. *Am. J. Human Genet.* **37**: 1117–28.

Zamir, N., Haass, M., Dave, J. R. & Zukowska-Grojec, Zofia. (1987). Anterior pituitary gland modulates the release of atrial natriuretic peptides from cardiac atria. *Proc. Nat. Acad. Sci. USA* **84**: 541–5.

Zeller, R., Bloch, K. D., Williams, B. S., Arceci, R. J. & Seidman, C. E. (1987). Localized expression of the atrial natriuretic factor gene during cardiac embryogenesis. *Genes Develop.* **1**: 693–8.

Zivin, R., Condra, J., Dixon, R., Seidah, N. G., Chretien, M., Nemer, M., Chamberland, M. *et al.* (1984). Molecular cloning and characterization of DNA sequences encoding rat and human ANF. *Proc. Nat. Acad. Sci. USA* **81**: 6325–9.

Chapter 2
Molecular forms of atrial natriuretic factor
Fumiaki Marumo and Kenji Ando

Introduction

In 1984, Kangawa and Matsuo (1984) identified three distinct types of human atrial natriuretic factor (ANF): α- (28 residues, 99–126 ANF), β- (56 residues, antiparallel dimer of α-ANF), and γ-ANF (126 residues, ANF 1–126), from a human atrium obtained at autopsy. Soon after their report, synthesized α- and β-ANF became commercially available. Thus, a number of antibodies were made by independent researchers using commercially synthesized α-ANF. Radioimmunoassay (RIA) has been widely used to measure the concentrations of ANF. Major analytical methods estimating molecular forms of ANF include gel permeation chromatography (GPC) and reverse-phase high-performance liquid chromatography (RP-HPLC) coupled with RIA. Sensitivities and specificities of the antisera of RIA have caused different results, and the pretreatment of samples, such as heat inactivation of tissue, has affected the estimation of molecular forms of ANF.

Since ANF content in the atrium is sufficient to be measured, the molecular forms of ANF can be estimated by either assay method. Estimation of molecular forms of ANF from the ventricle and brain tissue, which contains much less ANF than the atrium, is not difficult, since enough tissue mass can be obtained for measurement. ANF contents in the plasma, urine, or cerebrospinal fluid are much lower than in the atrium, and also the size of these samples is restricted. Thus, the data from body fluid depend on the assay method or specificities of ANF antibody.

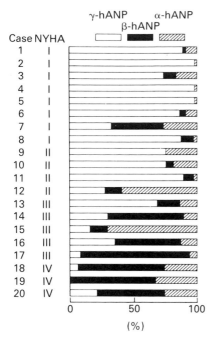

Fig. 2.1 Percentages of α-, β-, and γ-ANF from atrial tissue as related to the severity of CHF, classified by the functional classification of NYHA. (Sugawara *et al.* 1988, with permission of the authors.)

Molecular forms of ANF in tissues

It has been well known that tissue ANF content is highest in the atrium. In healthy persons, ANF content in the ventricle is almost three times lower than that in the atrium. In the atrium, the presence of three components of ANF (α-, β- and γ-ANF) was first reported by Kangawa & Matsuo (1984). In congestive heart failure (CHF), the distribution of the three components of ANF in the atrium changes remarkably from the condition without CHF. As shown in Fig. 2.1, Sugawara *et al.* (1988) reported that the absolute content and percentage of three components of ANF dramatically changed in accordance with the advance of chronic heart failure stage, classified by the functional classification of the New York Heart Association (NYHA). This finding is consistent with our observation that an elevated plasma ANF concentration decreased as the severity of CHF reduced and that β-ANF was absent or decreased when CHF was successfully treated (Marumo *et al.*, 1988). ANF content in the ventricle increases quantitatively in CHF patients (Edwards *et al.*, 1988; Saito *et al.*, 1989). Saito *et al.* (1989) reported that in six patients with left ventricular aneurysm, tissue ANF concentrations (mean ± SEM) were 17.5 ± 6.9 ng/g in normal ventricle, 660 ± 122 ng/g in left ventricular aneurysm tissues, and 3100 ± 1600 ng/g in biopsy specimens of the dilated cardiomyopathy (DCM) ventricle. The levels in ventricular aneurysm tissue and DCM ventricles were 40 and 200 times those of the normal ventricle. The ANF-mRNA level in the left ventricular aneurysm showed a tenfold increase compared with that in the normal heart, reaching 23 % of that in the atrium of the same heart. A similar increase in the ANF-mRNA level was observed in the entire ventricle of DCM. These data clearly showed that the expression of the ANF gene in the ventricle is augmented in the failing heart in accordance with the severity of heart failure. In the atrium of the failing heart, ANF and ANF-mRNA levels were only 2 times higher than those in the normal atrium. Thus, the augmented expression of the ANF gene was more prominent in the ventricle than the atrium.

Akimoto *et al.* (1988) presented interesting results that show that molecular forms of ANF in the atrium of CHF patients change with age. They obtained parts of operated right atrium from 35 patients suffering from various forms of heart failure, with the patients' ages ranging from 1 month to 65 years. They were divided into three age groups: group 1, 1 month to 3 years; group 2, 3 to 20 years; and group 3, more than 20 years. In group 1, four out of nine patients showed α-, β- and γ-ANF type while five showed only γ-ANF. In group 2, β- and γ-ANF type and α-, β- and γ-ANF type were found in only one case each of a group total of 14, and 12 showed only γ-ANF. In group 3, five out of 12 patients showed α-, β- and γ-ANF type, and four showed only γ-ANF type. Thus, they concluded that the major component was γ-ANF in patients younger than 20 years old, while α- and β-ANF appeared more frequently and their contents increased in older patients, and that the differences in the content and forms of ANF in atrial tissue reflect the pathological state in patients with cardiovascular disease.

Molecular forms of ANF in brain tissue are different from those in the atrium and ventricle. Compared with the heart, in which γ-ANF constitutes most ANF components, the brain has mainly low-molecular-mass ANF in such animals as the rat (Glembotski, Wildey & Bibson, 1985; Morii *et al.*, 1985; Shiono *et al.*, 1986), dog (Fujuio *et al.*, 1987; Marumo *et al.*, 1988b), and monkey (Itoh *et al.*, 1988). However, the molecular form of ANF in the human brain has not been established (Itoh *et al.*, 1988). Varying ANF components observed in the plasma, cerebrospinal fluid, atrium, and hypothalamus of dogs are shown in Fig. 2.2.

Molecular forms of ANF in plasma

The circulatory ANF in normal persons was first reported to be only α-ANF (Miyata *et al.*, 1986). In 1986 we reported that healthy persons have either α-ANF or α- and γ-ANF in their plasma (Marumo *et al.*, 1986), as

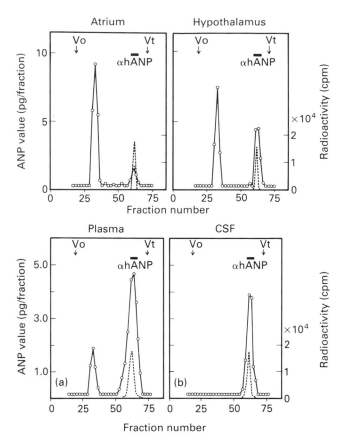

Fig. 2.2 Gel permeation profile of ANF. Upper panel: atrium and hypothalamus; lower panel: plasma and CSF. The solid lines represent ANF activity, the broken lines radioactivity of ^{125}I-α-ANF added to the samples. α-hANP represents authentic human α-ANF (Marumo *et al.*, 1988b).

summarized in Table 2.1. Twelve out of 25 persons had both α- and γ-ANF in their plasma. Miyata *et al.* (1987) found not only α-ANF but also β-ANF in the plasma of two out of eight healthy persons. Gutkowska *et al.* (1987) mentioned in their review that the major circulating form of ANF is the 28-amino-acid peptide Ser 99–Tyr 126, with a minor form probably due to degradation in plasma. Recently, it was reported that two peptides of 1–30 and 31–67 residues in the N-terminal end segment of the proANF, in addition to ANF (99–126), were found to circulate in 54 normal human volunteers (Winters *et al.*, 1988). Mukoyama recently recognized the presence of γ-ANF in normal human plasma (Mukoyama *et al.*, 1989). Differences in specificities of antibodies have probably produced this confusion in the molecular forms of ANF in plasma. However, at present many researchers agree with the presence of only an α-ANF or α- and γ-ANF in the plasma of healthy persons.

Table 2.1 Plasma ANF molecular forms in healthy persons (Marumo *et al.*, 1988a)

Case	ANP (pg/ml)	Molecular form
1	32.8	$\alpha\gamma$
2	43.8	$\alpha\gamma$
3	55.6	$\alpha\gamma$
4	58.1	α
5	79.1	α
6	43.9	α
7	22.8	$\alpha\gamma$
8	102.3	$\alpha\gamma$
9	45.9	α
10	71.4	$\alpha\gamma$
11	28.6	$\alpha\gamma$
12	54.3	$\alpha\gamma$
13	185	$\alpha\gamma$
14	123	$\alpha\gamma$
15	100.7	α
16	30.1	α
17	17.5	α
18	33.6	α
19	48.9	α
20	79.5	$\alpha\gamma$
21	45.5	α
22	42.0	α
23	66.1	α
24	33.8	$\alpha\gamma$
25	34.4	α

Bovine and canine ANF were identical with human ANF, but rat, mouse, and rabbit ANF substituted Ile for Met at the 110 position (Gutkowska *et al.*, 1987). There has been no report that β-ANF, an antiparallel dimer, is present in the rat, mouse or rabbit. These different molecular forms of ANF may reflect some pathophysiological condition(s). In the following sections, we discuss human, bovine, and canine ANF, with particular emphasis on human ANF components and their pathophysiological significance.

Patients with various diseases

Plasma ANF concentrations in CHF patients are known to be higher than those in normal subjects (Burnett *et al.*, 1986; Katoh *et al.*, 1986). Changes in circulatory ANF in CHF patients were first noted independently, by German and Japanese groups. Arendt *et al.* (1986) reported that γ-ANF in addition to α-ANF was detected in plasma of hypertensive patients, and in trace amounts in cirrhotic patients as well, and that in some CHF patients, elevated plasma ANF levels predominantly comprised γ-ANF, in

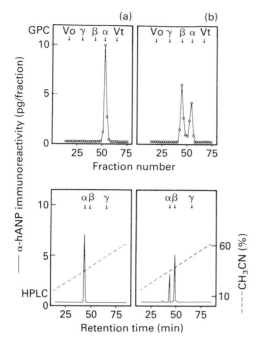

Fig. 2.3 Changes of ANF molecular forms in CHF before and after successful treatment. The patient, with ischaemic heart disease after acute myocardial infraction, was class IV on admission (*B*) and class I (NYHA) after treatment (*A*). The β-ANF peak disappeared with treatment.

addition to considerable amounts of ANF immunoreactivity, presumably bound to larger proteins that eluted in the void volume. They concluded that a disregulation of posttranslational processing of ANF may contribute to the pathophysiology of cardiovascular disease.

   Yoshinaga *et al.* (1986) found two major components with 99–126 and 94–126 ANF in GPC from CHF patients with high plasma ANF levels. Yandle *et al.* (1986) also detected smaller molecule materials (about 1600 Da) in addition to 99–126 ANF in pooled plasma obtained from CHF patients. They mentioned that the amount of α-ANF was larger than that of smaller components in plasma extracts obtained from the coronary sinus. They found 106–126 and 99–105 ANF in addition to 99–126 ANF in the plasma of CHF patients (Yandle *et al.*, 1987). Due to the moderate sensitivity of RIA, they had to use pooled plasma, not an individual sample, to obtain chromatographs by GPC and RP-HPLC.

   Using highly sensitive RIA (Marumo *et al.*, 1986), we could estimate circulatory forms of ANF obtained from individual peripheral blood samples. The plasma ANF concentration was extremely elevated in CHF patients of classes III or IV, NYHA criteria, but it decreased to a moderately elevated or normal level when the patient's condition was restored to classes I or II with successful treatment (Katoh *et al.*, 1986). In our earlier observation, large β-ANF components were usually noted in advanced CHF patients with class IV NYHA criteria, but they either disappeared or became much smaller when patients were successfully treated to class I (Fig. 2.3; Marumo *et al.*, 1988).

Recently we calculated the percentages of each circulatory form per total α-ANF-like immunoreactivity (LI) on 50 chromatograms of plasma and 30 of urine from CHF patients. As shown in the upper panel of Fig. 2.4, only α-ANF was noticed in 10 out of 14 chromatograms of patients classified as class I NYHA, in five out of 16 of class II, and in no chromatograms of classes III and IV. β-ANF was observed in all chromatograms of classes III and IV, and the mean average β-ANF percentage was extremely high in these NYHA criteria classes. In the urine, β-ANF was observed in class III and class IV patients, but not in classes I and II, as shown in the lower panel of Fig. 2.4. These results suggest that β-ANF may be an indicator of the severity of CHF.

While β-ANF has been recognized as a specific human component of ANF, Takemura *et al.* (1990) recently reported that immunoreactive materials coeluting with authentic human β-ANF and/or γ-ANF were detected in addition to α-ANF obtained from the plasma of cattle with dilated cardiomyopathy (DCM).

Conversion of 1–126 ANF to more active forms is probably taking place upon its secretion from the atrium. An enzyme which specifically cleaves the Arg^{98}–Ser^{99} bond has been found in an atrial homogenate (Imada, Takayanagi & Inagami, 1987). Multistep affinity purification yields a polymeric enzyme with *Mr.* 560 kDa consisting of several 28 kDa protomers. This enzyme is presumably located on plasma membrane and converts 1–126 ANF to 99–126 ANF during the exocytic secretion of 1–126 ANF from its storage vesicles (Imada, Takayanagi & Inagami, 1988). Inagami (1989) supposed that the presence of β-ANF in the atria of CHF patients may be explained by the involvement of degenerating heart tissue. The mechanism of its formation and release into the circulation are not yet clear.

β-ANF was slowly converted into a smaller peptide corresponding to α-ANF *in vitro* (Itoh *et al.*, 1987). The administration of authentic β-ANF into healthy volunteers resulted in a longer retention of the ANF-LI level in the plasma, compared with that of α-ANF administration (Itoh *et al.*, 1988). This finding suggests that β-ANF may be converted into α-ANF *in vivo*. However, the elution profiles of β-ANF components and the elution profiles from the coronary sinus and superior vena cava of CHF patients were essentially the same (Marumo *et al.*, 1988). This suggests that conversion of β- to α-ANF *in vivo* is slow and that one blood circulation cycle does not affect molecular forms.

While the presence of β-ANF in the atrium is accepted in CHF patients

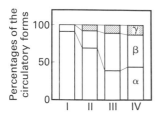 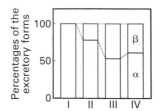

Fig. 2.4 Percentages of α-, β-, and γ-ANF in the total ANF-LI in the plasma and urine of CHF patients as related to disease severity. Left-hand panel: percentages of molecular forms in the total ANF-LI in the plasma; right-hand panel: percentages of molecular forms in the total ANF-LI in urine.

(Akimoto *et al.*, 1988; Sugawara *et al.*, 1988; Saito *et al.*, 1989), Akimoto *et al.* (1988) observed only α-ANF in the plasma of CHF patients. Arendt *et al.* (1986) found γ-ANF in the plasma of CHF patients. Thus, the frequency and significance of β-ANF in plasma should be studied further.

Renal diseases

Circulatory ANF in patients with renal diseases has not been reported in detail, as in heart failure. There are two conflicting results regarding the plasma ANF concentration in non-dialysed chronic renal failure (CRF) patients. Several researchers (Anderson *et al.*, 1986; Hasegawa *et al.*, 1986; Predel *et al.*, 1988) reported that plasma ANF concentrations increase in CRF patients. Sudsfjord *et al.* (1988) reported that the plasma concentration of 1–98 ANF increased in both CHF and CRF patients, and that 1–98 ANF was cosecreted with 99–126 ANF. In their CRF patients, the ANF 1–98 concentration in plasma was higher than that of ANF 99–126, suggesting a different elimination process for ANF 1–98 than for ANF 99–126 mediated, at least in part, by the kidney. However, the half-life of ANF 1–98 in rats was found to be 8 times longer than that of its C-terminal counterpart (2.5 min vs. 20 s). Similarly, the elimination time of human ANF 1–98 may be much longer (Sundsfjord *et al.*, 1988). In discussing the plasma ANF concentration in CRF patients, the half-life of ANF, including its degraded fragments, should be taken into consideration.

Other researchers (Marumo *et al.*, 1988c; Ong, De Lean & Gagnon, 1988) found no increase in plasma ANF concentration due to decreased renal function itself and it may be the volume overload which normally accompanies CRF which causes plasma ANF to be elevated.

The major circulatory ANF in CRF patients has been reported to be α-ANF (Anderson *et al.*, 1986; Hasegawa *et al.*, 1986). Predel *et al.* (1988) observed γ-ANF in addition to α-ANF. A typical elution profile of plasma from a CRF patient in our study is shown in Fig. 2.5. The creatinine

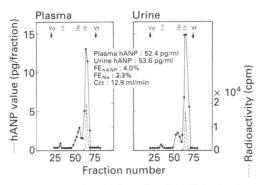

Fig. 2.5 A typical GPC profile of ANF in the plasma and urine of a non-dialysed patient.

clearance of this patient was 12.0 ml/min, and the fractional excretion of ANF (FE_{ANF}) was 4.0%. FE_{ANF} in healthy persons is $0.70 \pm 0.05\%$ (Marumo *et al.*, 1988c). In our observation, β-ANF as well as α- and γ-ANF were noted in the chromatograms of six out of 10 CRF patients (Marumo *et al.*, 1990).

In patients with nephrotic syndrome, no report regarding the molecular forms of ANF has appeared except ours (Marumo *et al.*, 1990). In our study, the plasma ANF concentrations in 11 patients with nephrotic syndrome were variable (mean $\pm$ SD, 57.9 ± 70.9, ranging from 10.5 to 265.0 pg/ml). This may be due to an altered extracellular fluid volume and circulating blood volume, depending on the stage of disease. In the plasma of seven out of 11 patients, α- and γ-ANF were observed in the chromatograms, while in the rat only α-ANF, was found (Marumo *et al.*, 1990).

It is well known in haemodialysis (HD) that plasma ANF concentrations before dialysis are due to the expanded extracellular fluid volume (Hasegawa *et al.*, 1986; Kurokawa *et al.*, 1987; Saxenhofer *et al.*, 1987). While some (Anderson *et al.*, 1986; Hasegawa *et al.*, 1986) reported α-ANF as the predominant circulating form in the plasma of HD patients, we found β- and/or γ-ANF in addition to α-ANF (Akiba, Ando & Marumo, 1990; Marumo *et al.*, 1990). In addition, molecular forms of plasma ANF often change after HD. As shown in Table 2.2, some components disappeared after HD, and others changed in their percentages in ANF-LI (Akiba *et al.*, 1990). A typical elution profile change is shown in Fig. 2.6. In this case, a predialysis sample showed α-, β-, and γ-ANF, while, α-ANF disappeared in the postdialysis plasma. This patient was maintained on regular HD for 5 years and was diagnosed as class I heart failure by NYHA criteria. The HD was carried out for 4 h each day, 3 times a week, using a hollow fibre-type dialyser and dialysate containing bicarbonate. These results indicate that long-term metabolic

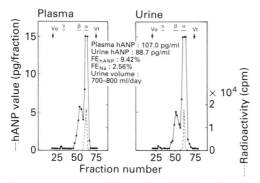

Fig. 2.6 A typical GPC profile of ANF in the plasma and urine of a haemodialysed patient.

Table 2.2 Influences on molecular forms of ANF by a single dialysis (Akiba *et al.*, 1990).

	Age	Sex	Predialysis					Postdialysis				
			Plasma ANP (pg/ml)	Molecular forms				Plasma ANP (pg/ml)	Molecular forms			
1	38	F	145.9	α				33.6	α			
2	31	F	380	α			γ	80.0	α			γ
3	34	M	243	α			γ	60.2	α			γ
4	51	M	211	α				32.5	α			
5	26	M	137.2	α	β		γ	58.6	α			
6	37	M	236	α			γ	47.4	α			γ
7	21	F	107.6	α	β		γ	47.0			β	γ
8	37	M	80.1	α			γ	32.4	α			γ
9	30	M	199	α	β		γ	91.4			β	γ
10	71	F	369	α	β		γ	233	α		β	γ

disorders may change the secreting form of ANF by affecting the heart muscle and/or the processing enzyme of proANF. Case 10 in the table had both class III CHF and CRF. Her plasma ANF concentration was extremely elevated, and her molecular forms of ANF, including α-, β-, and γ-ANF, did not change by a single dialysis.

Molecular forms of ANF in urine and cerebrospinal fluid

The presence of ANF in urine has been reported by a few researchers (Hartter *et al.*, 1986; Marumo *et al.*, 1986). Only α-ANF was present in normal urine.

Suzuki *et al.* (1988) measured plasma and urine concentrations of ANF in patients with diabetes mellitus. They found that ANF concentrations in the plasma and urine increased as diabetic nephropathy advanced, and that the major component was α-ANF in both plasma and urine.

Ando *et al.* (1988) reported that urinary ANF excretion in normal persons was 2.5 ± 1.34 ng/day ($n = 65$), and that the increased urinary ANF concentration in CHF patients decreased from 119.2 to 53.3 ng/day ($n = 14$) after successful treatment. Urinary ANF was stable even at room temperature, and FE_{ANF} was almost constant in CHF patients. Thus the amount of ANF in 24-h urine may also reflect plasma ANF in these patients, as shown in Fig. 2.4.

As mentioned above, only α-ANF was noted in the urine of healthy persons. In nephrotic patients, α-ANF and/or α- and γ-ANF was observed in the urine. Six of 11 urine samples had both α- and γ-ANF. β-ANF was not observed in the urine or the plasma. All six patients whose urine samples had γ-ANF showed α- and γ-ANF in the plasma (Marumo *et al.*, 1990). CRF patients had β and/or γ-ANF in the urine as well as in the plasma, as shown in Fig. 2.5. In CRF, α- and β-ANF were noticed in the plasma and urine.

In dialysed patients, if patients can excrete urine, β- and/or γ-ANF in addition to α-ANF is found in both plasma and urine. A typical case is shown in Fig. 2.6. In this case, α-, and β-, and γ-ANF were noticed in the chromatograms of plasma and urine. In renal failure patients, the molecular forms of plasma and urine usually present the same patterns in both. They always have high FE_{ANF}. γ-ANF may appear in the urine of these cases. Part of plasma ANF may pass through renal tubules without being degraded.

Schulz-Knappe *et al.* (1988) recently reported the presence of a new polypeptide (urodilatin) of 32 amino-acid residues (95–126) in urine. The molecule has an N-terminally extended structure compared to circulatory ANF 99–126. They suggest that the analysed urinary peptide is not the residual plasma form, filtrated and renally cleaved from blood, but is probably a polypeptide produced and processed in the kidney tubules and cleaved by a different posttranslational process. Dörner *et al.* (1989) recently reported that elution positions of ANF, urodilatin and brain natriuretic peptide (BNP) are different.

The presence of ANF in cerebrospinal fluid (CSF) in humans (Marumo, Masuda & Audo, 1987; Levin, 1988) and canines (Masuda, Audo & Marumo, 1988) has been reported. The ANF content in CSF of humans or canines was one level of magnitude lower than that in plasma. The molecular form is only α-ANF (Marumo *et al.*, 1987; Levin, 1988; Masuda *et al.*, 1988), as shown in Fig. 2.2.

Other vasoactive substances newly found (endothelin)

Recently Masaki and associates (Yanagisawa *et al.*, 1988) identified a
novel vasoactive peptide, endothelin, from porcine aortic endothelial cells.
Porcine endothelin (pET) consists of 21 amino-acid residues containing
two intramolecular disulphide linkages, and it is derived from preproET
with 203 amino-acid residues through an unusual proteolytic processing.
Ando *et al.* (1989) recently established a highly sensitive and specific RIA
for human ET (hET), and the plasma concentration in normal subjects
was 1.5 ± 0.5 pg/ml. An elution profile of pooled human plasma extracts
on RP-HPLC shows that two major components of hET-LI were
observed: one component eluted in the position of standard ET-1 while
the other component, representing about two-thirds of the total hET-LI,
eluted earlier than the hET standard. Suzuki *et al.* (1989) reported that the
human plasma concentration of hET was 1.6 ± 0.3 pg/ml, measured by a
sensitive sandwich enzyme immunoassay method.

ET and ANF have quite opposite biological actions. While ANF
shows natriuretic and vasodilatory action, ET shows vasoconstrictive
action and reduces the glomerular filtration rate. A stimulative effect of
pET on the release of rat ANF in cultured neonatal rat atrial cardiocytes
has been reported (Fukuda *et al.*, 1988). Hirata *et al.* (1989) also reported
that long-term pretreatment of cultured rat vascular smooth muscle cells
with angiotensin and vasopressin induced a marked reduction of the
maximal binding capacity of ANF receptors, and that down-regulation of
the receptors induced by vasoconstrictors was concomitantly associated
with an attenuation of ANF-stimulated cGMP accumulation. Their
results suggest that vasoconstrictor-induced activation of protein kinase C
is involved in the mechanism of heterologous down-regulation of vascular
ANF receptors.

Problems regarding analytical methods

To estimate molecular forms of ANF, GPC and/or RP-HPLC coupled
with RIA is usually performed. The concentrations of proteins, salts,
and/or ions in samples affect the immunoreactivity in RIA and other
immunoassays. It should at least be confirmed that the dilution curves of
eluates obtained from GPC and RP-HPLC are parallel to that of standard
ANF on RIA, and that non-specific binding in eluates is negligible. In
addition, the condition of the reacting mixture in RIA using the same
antibody depends on the immunological cross-reactivity (Amit *et al.*,
1985). The specificity of antiserum should be examined independently.
Kangawa, Fukuda & Matsuo (1985) successfully identified ANF by
boiling samples into inactive proteolytic enzyme. Different pretreatments
of samples have produced varying results in analyses of molecular profiles

of ANF. Depending on procedures employed through extraction, chromatography analysis and RIA, we and others (Kangawa, 1988) have experienced lower recoveries of γ-ANF due to its significant adsorption on to glass equipment, and of β-ANF, which may possibly cleave to fragments. Sufficient recoveries of α-, β-, and γ-ANF throughout all analytical procedures are essential in estimating molecular forms of ANF.

Summary

Molecular forms of ANF components in the plasma, urine, and CSF of healthy persons and patients are discussed. In addition to ANF, endothelin was also mentioned. In healthy persons, α- and γ-ANF are present in the plasma, while only the α-ANF form is in the urine or CSF. In patients with CHF, β-ANF is the predominant molecular form in heart muscle, plasma, and urine. When CHF improved, β-ANF peaks in chromatograms disappeared or decreased significantly. Thus, presence of β-ANF may be a good indicator reflecting the severity of CHF.

In renal diseases, α- or α- and γ-ANF were found in the plasma and urine of nephrotic patients. α-, β-, and γ-ANF were sometimes found in the plasma and urine of CRF patients. Molecular forms change according to the condition of CRF. Molecular forms of haemodialysed patients were affected by a single dialysis.

β-ANF may appear in heart tissue, plasma, and urine in heart failure with volume overload, or in metabolic heart disorders. γ-ANF may appear in the plasma and urine in metabolic disorders, with high FE_{ANF}. However, the mechanisms of these changes in ANF molecular forms observed in tissue, plasma, and urine have not been established. Further studies should establish the overall significance of these different molecular forms.

References

Akiba, T., Ando, K. & Marumo, F. (1990). Changes in molecular pattern of atrial natriuretic peptide in hemodialysis patients. *Klin. Wochenschr.* (in press).

Akimoto, K., Miyata, A., Kangawa, K., Koga, Y., Hayakawa, K. & Matsuo, H. (1988). Molecular forms of atrial natriuretic peptide in the atrium of patients with cardiovascular disease. *J. Clin. Endocrinol. Metab.* **64**: 93–7.

Amit, A. G., Mariuzza, R. A., Phillips, S. E. V. & Poljak, R. J. (1985). Three-dimensional structure of an antigen–antibody complex at 6 Å resolution. *Nature* **313**: 156–8.

Anderson, J. V., Raine, A. E. G., Proudler, A. & Bloom, S. R. (1986). Effect of hemodialysis on plama concentrations of atrial natriuretic peptide in adult patients with chronic renal failure. *J. Endocrinol.* **110**: 193–6.

Ando, K., Hirata, Y., Shichiri, M., Emori, T. & Marumo, F. (1989). Presence of immunoreactive endothelin in human plasma. *FEBS Lett.* **245**: 164–6.

Ando, K., Umetani, N., Kurosawa, T., Takeda, S., Katoh, Y. & Marumo, F. (1988). Atrial natriuretic peptide in human urine. *Klin. Wochenschr.* **66**: 768–72.

Arendt, R. M., Gerbes, A. L., Ritter, D. & Stangl, E. (1986). Molecular weight heterogeneity of plasma-ANF in cardiovascular disease. *Klin. Wochenschr.* **64** (Suppl. VI): 97–102.

Burnett, J. C. Jr., Kao, P. C., Hu, D. C., Heser, D. W., Heublein, D., Granger, J. P., Opgenorth,

T. J. & Reeder, G. S. (1986). Atrial natriuretic peptide elevation in congestive heart failure in the human. *Science* **231**: 1145–7.

Dörner, T., Gagelmann, M., Hock, D., Herbst, F. & Forssmann, W. G. (1989). Separation of synthetic cardiodilatin/atrial natriuretic factor and related peptides by reverse-phase high-performance liquid chromatography. *J. Chromatogr.* **490**: 411–17.

Edwards, B. S., Ackeramm, D. M., Lee, M. E., Reeder, G. S., Wold, L. E. & Burnett, J. C. Jr. (1988). Identification of atrial natriuretic factor within ventricular tissue in hamsters and humans with congestive heart failure. *J. Clin. Invest.* **81**: 82–6.

Fukuda, Y., Hirata, Y., Yoshimi, H., Kojima, T., Kobayashi, Y., Yanagisawa, M. & Masaki, M. (1988). Endothelin is a potent secretagogue for atrial natriuretic peptide in cultured rat atrial natriuretic peptide in cultured rat atrial myocytes. *Biochem. Biophys. Res. Commun.* **155**: 167–72.

Fujino, N., Ohashi, M., Nawata, H., Kato, K., Tateishi, J., Matsuo, H. & Ibayashi, H. (1987). Unique distributions of natriuretic hormones in dog brain. *Reg. Peptides* **18**: 131–7.

Glembotski, C. C., Wildey, G. M. & Bibson, T. R. (1985). Molecular forms of immunoreactive atrial natriuretic peptide in the rat hypothalamus and atrium. *Biochem. Biophys. Res. Commun.* **129**: 671–8.

Gutkowska, J., Genest, J., Thibault, G., Garcia, R., Larochelle, P., Cusson, J. R., Kuchel, O., Hamet, P., Deän, A. & Cantin, M. (1987). Circulating forms and radioimmunoassay of atrial natriuretic factor. *Endocrinol. Metab. Clin. N. Am.* **16**: 183–98.

Hartter, E., Pacher, R., Frass, M., Woloszczuk, W. & Leithner, C. (1986). Plasma levels of atrial natriuretic peptide (ANP) in volume expanded patients: response to fluid removal by continuous pump driven hemofiltration. *Klin. Wochenschr.* **64** (Suppl. VI): 112–14.

Hasegawa, K., Matsushita, Y., Inoue, T., Morii, H., Ishibashi, M. & Yamaji, T. (1986). Plasma levels of atrial natriuretic peptide in patients with chronic renal failure. *J. Clin. Endocrinol. Metab.* **63**: 813–22.

Hirata, Y., Emori, T., Ohta, K., Shichiri, M. & Marumo, F. (1989). Vasoconstrictor-induced heterologous down-regulation of vascular atrial natriuretic peptide receptor. *Eur. J. Pharmacol.* **164**: 603–6.

Imada, T., Takayanagi, R. & Inagami, T. (1987). Identification of a peptidase which processes atrial natriuretic factor precursor to its active form with 28 amino acid residues in particulate fractions of rat atrial homogenate. *Biochem. Biophys. Res. Commun.* **143**: 587–92.

Imada, T., Takayanagi, R. & Inagami, T. (1988). Atrioactivase, a specific peptidase in bovine atria for the processing of pro-atrial natriuretic factor. *Biochem. Biophys. Res. Commun.* **143**: 587–92.

Imada, T., Takayanagi, R. & Inagami, T. (1988). Atrioactivase, a specific peptidase in bovine atria for the processing of pro-atrial natriuretic factor. *J. Biol. Chem.* **263**: 9515–19.

Inagami, T. (1989). Atrial natriuretic factor. *J. Biol. Chem.* **264**: 3043–6.

Itoh, H., Nakao, K., Mukoyama, M., Hosoda, K., Shiono, S., Morii, N., Yamada, T. *et al.* (1988). Peptides derived from atrial natriuretic polypeptide precursor in human and monkey brains. *J. Hypertension* **6** (Suppl. 4): S309–13.

Itoh, H., Nakao, K., Mukoyama, M., Shiono, S., Morii, N., Sugawara, A., Yamada, T. *et al.* (1988). Effects of intravenously administered beta-human atrial natriuretic polypeptide in humans. *Hypertension* **11**: 697–702.

Itoh, H., Nakao, K., Shiono, S., Mukoyama, M., Morii, N., Sugawara, A., Yamada, T. *et al.* (1987). Conversion of beta-human atrial natriuretic polypeptide in human plasma *in vitro*. *Biochem. Biophys. Res. Commun.* **143**: 560–9.

Kangawa, K. (1988). Identification of ANP. In: *Atrial Natriuretic Peptide* (Saito, J. & Imai, T., eds). Japan: Chugai-Igakusha, pp. 23–4 (in Japanese).

Kangawa, K., Fukuda, A. & Matsuo, H. (1985). Structural identification of beta- and gamma-human atrial natriuretic polypeptides. *Nature* **313**: 397–400.

Kangawa, K. & Matsuo, H. (1984). Purification and complete amino acid sequence of alpha-human atrial natriuretic polypeptide (alpha-hANP). *Biochem. Biophys. Res. Commun.* **118**: 131–9.

Kurokawa, S., Katoh, Y., Sugiyama, T., Kurosawa, T., Takeda, S., Sakamoto, H., Marumo, F. & Kikawada, R. (1987). Correlation of decreased plasma atrial natriuretic peptide level with left atrial diameter in chronic hemodialysis. *Am. J. Cardiol.* **60**: 1135.

Katoh, Y., Kurosawa, T., Takeda, S., Kurokawa, S., Sakamoto, H., Marumo, F. & Kikawada, R. (1986). Atrial natriuretic peptide levels in treated congestive heart failure. *Lancet* **i**: 851.

Levin, E. R. (1988). Atrial natriuretic factor is detectable in human cerebrospinal fluid. *J. Clin. Endocrinol. Metab.* **66**: 1080–3.

Marumo, F., Kurosawa, T., Takeda, S., Katoh, Y., Hasegawa, N. & Ando, K. (1988a). Changes of molecular forms of atrial natriuretic peptide after treatment for congestive heart failure. *Klin. Wochenschr.* **66**: 675–81.

Marumo, F., Masuda, T. & Ando, K. (1987). Presence of the atrial natriuretic peptide in human cerebrospinal fluid. *Biochem. Biophys. Res. Commun.* **143**: 813–18.

Marumo, F., Masuda, T., Masaki, Y. & Ando, K. (1988b). The presence of atrial natriuretic peptide in canine cerebrospinal fluid and its possible origin in the brain. *J. Endocrinol.* **119**: 127–31.

Marumo, F., Sakamoto, H., Ando, K., Ishigami, T. & Kawakami, M. (1986). A highly sensitive radioimmunoassay of atrial natriuretic peptide (ANP) in human plasma and urine. *Biochem. Biophys. Res. Commun.* **137**: 231–6.

Marumo, F., Sakamoto, H., Umetani, N. & Okubo, M. (1988c). Atrial natriuretic peptide in kidney of renal disease patients and healthy persons. *Endocrinol. Japon.* **35**: 523–9.

Marumo, F., Shichiri, M., Emori, T., Umetani, N., Kurosawa, T. & Ando, K. (1990). Molecular forms of atrial natriuretic peptide in health and renal diseases. *Peptide* (in press).

Masuda, T., Ando, K. & Marumo, F. (1988). The existence of low concentrations of atrial natriuretic peptide (ANP) in canine cerebrospinal fluid which does not correlate with plasma ANP levels. *Neurosci. Lett.* **88**: 93–9.

Miyata, A., Kangawa, K., Yoshimori, T., Hatoh, T. & Matsuo, H. (1986). Molecular forms of atrial natriuretic polypeptides in mammalian tissues and plasma. *Biochem. Biophys. Res. Commun.* **129**: 248–55.

Miyata, A., Toshimori, T., Hashiguchi, T., Kangawa, K. & Matsuo, H. (1987). Molecular forms of atrial natriuretic polypeptides circulating in human plasma. *Biochem. Biophys. Res. Commun.* **142**: 461–7.

Morii, N., Nakao, K., Sugawara, A., Sakamoto, M., Suda, M., Shimokura, M., Kiso, Y. *et al.* (1985). Occurrence of atrial natriuretic polypeptide in brain. *Biochem. Biophys. Res. Commun.* **127**: 413–19.

Mukoyama, M., Nakao, K., Yamada, T., Itoh, H., Saito, Y., Arai, H., Hosoda, K. *et al.* (1989). Application of monoclonal antibodies against atrial natriuretic polypeptide: Direct sandwich enzyme immunizes for plasma alpha, beta, and gamma-ANP. *Fourth Scientific Meeting of the American Society of Hypertension*, New York, Abstract No. 1364.

Ong, H., DeLean, A. & Gagnon, C. (1988). A highly specific radioreceptor assay for the active circulating form of atrial natriuretic factor in human plasma. *Clin. Chem.* **34**: 2275–9.

Predel, H. G., Kipnowski, J., Becker, A., Stelkens, H., Jürgens, U., Düsing, R. & Kramer, H. J. (1988). Erhöhte plasmaspiegel und heterogenität von humanem atrialen natriuretischen Peptid bei patienten mit progressivem chronischen nierenversagen. *Z. Kardiol.* **77** (Suppl. 2): 65–71.

Saito, Y., Nakao, K., Arai, H., Nishimura, K., Okumura, K., Obata, K. *et al.* (1989). Augmented expression of atrial natriuretic polypeptide gene in ventricle of human failing heart. *J. Clin. Invest.* **83**: 298–305.

Saxenhofer, H., Gnadinger, M. P., Weidmann, P., Shaw, S., Schohn, D., Hess, C., Uehlinger, D. E. *et al.* (1987). Plasma levels and dialysance of atrial natriuretic peptide in terminal renal failure. *Kidney Int.* **32**: 554–61.

Schulz-knappe, P., Forssmann, K., Herbst, F., Hock, D., Pipkorn, R. & Forssmann, W. G. (1988). Isolation and structural analysis of "Urodilatin", a new peptide of Cardiodilatin-(ANP)-family, excreted from human urine. *Klin. Wochenschr.* **66**: 752–9.

Shiono, S., Nakao, K., Morii, N., Yamada, T., Itoh, H., Sakamoto, M., Sugawara, A. *et al.* (1986). Nature of atrial natriuretic polypeptide in rat brain. *Biochem. Biophys. Res. Commun.* **135**: 728–34.

Sugawara, A., Nakao, K., Morii, N., Yamada, T., Itoh, H., Shiono, S., Saito, Y. *et al.* (1988). Synthesis of atrial natriuretic polypeptide in human failing hearts. *J. Clin. Invest.* **81**: 1962–70.

Sundsfjord, J. A., Thibault, G., Larochelle, P. & Cantin, M. (1988). Identification and plasma concentrations of the N-terminal fragment of proatrial natriuretic factor in man. *J. Clin. Endocrinol. Metab.* **66**: 605–10.

Suzuki, N., Matsumoto, H., Kitada, C., Masaki, T. & Fujino, M. (1989). A sensitive sandwich-enzyme immunoassay for human endothelin. *J. Immunol. Methods* **118**: 245–50.

Suzuki, Y., Suzuki, H., Ohtake, R., Tsuchiya, T., Muramatsu, H., Hashigami, Y., Kobori, H. *et al.* (1988). Plasma and urine concentrations of atrial natriuretic peptide in patients with diabetes mellitus. *Pancreas* **3**: 404–8.

Takemura, N., Koyama, H., Sako, T., Ando, K., Motoyoshi, S. & Marumo, F. (1990). Bovine atrial natriuretic peptide (ANP) in heart failure. *J. Endocrinol.* **124**: 463–7

Winters, C. J., Sallman, A. L., Meadows, J., Rico, D. M. & Vesely, D. L. (1988). Two hormones: Prohormone atrial natriuretic peptides 1–30 and 31–67 circulate in man. *Biochem. Biophys. Res. Commun.* **150**: 231–6.

Yanagisawa, M., Kurihara, H., Kimura, S., Tomobe, Y., Kobayashi, M., Mitsui, Y., Yazaki *et al.* (1988). A novel potent vasoconstrictor peptide produced by vascular endothelial cells. *Nature* **332**: 411–15.

Yandle, T., Crozier, I., Nicholls, M. G., Espiner, E., Carne, A. & Brennan, S. (1987). Amino acid sequence of atrial natriuretic peptides in human coronary sinus plasma. *Biochem. Biophys. Res. Commun.* **146**: 832–9.

Yandle, T. G., Espiner, E. A., Nicholls, M. G. & Duff, H. (1986). Radioimmunoassay and characterization of atrial natriuretic peptide in human plasma. *J. Clin. Endocrinol. Metab.* **63**: 72–9.

Yoshinaga, E., Yamaguchi, K., Abe, K., Miyata, Y., Otsubo, K., Hori, S., Oono, H. *et al.* (1986). Determination of atrial natriuretic polypeptide (ANP) in human plasma. *Biomed. Res.* **7**: 173–9.

Chapter 3
Physiological role of atrial natriuretic factor in volume regulation
Martin R. Wilkins

Introduction

Sodium is a major determinant of extracellular fluid (ECF) volume and ECF volume homeostasis is dependent upon the ability of the kidney to regulate urinary sodium excretion. Conversely, as proposed by Starling (1909) and later Peters (1935), renal sodium and water secretion is 'conditioned by the volume of body fluids'.

While the extravascular compartment may contribute, the intravascular compartment appears to be the critical site for assessing the adequacy of ECF volume. For example, immersion to the neck in water, which increases 'effective blood volume' but not total ECF volume, is associated with a rise in sodium excretion (Epstein, 1978). Although the kidney perceives changes in 'effective blood volume' directly through changes in perfusion pressure, studies such as those first performed by Henry and colleagues (1956) established that the cardiac atria also have a prominent role in sensing perturbations of intravascular volume and initiating a renal response to restore balance. Thus, inflation of a balloon within the right atrium, even in the absence of ECF volume expansion, results in a natriuresis and diuresis (Henry et al., 1956); on the other hand, expansion of ECF volume fails to elicit a diuresis if atrial stretch is prevented (Goetz et al., 1970). Data such as these have led to the concept that the atria act as non-renal volume receptors which communicate with the kidney via neural and humoral pathways (Fig. 3.1).

The cardiac nerves are an important component of the volume regulatory pathway linking heart and kidney. Stimulation of atrial stretch receptors increases vagal nerve activity which inhibits vasopressin

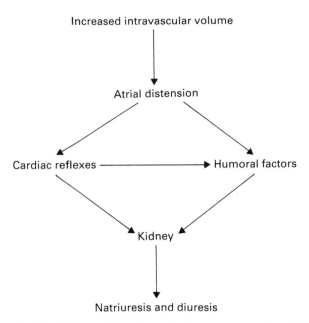

Increased intravascular volume

Atrial distension

Cardiac reflexes   Humoral factors

Kidney

Natriuresis and diuresis

Fig. 3.1 Outline of the interrelationship between heart and kidney in intravascular volume regulation.

secretion from the pituitary and reduces renal sympathetic nerve activity (Gauer, Henry & Behn, 1970; Linden & Kappagoda, 1982). The renal nerves in turn regulate renin secretion from the juxtaglomerular apparatus and may have a direct effect on sodium reabsorption from the proximal tubule (DiBona, 1982). For many years, however, several investigators have argued the existence of a natriuretic hormone stimulated by intravascular volume expansion (deWardener & Clarkson, 1985). The concept of such a hormone evolved into one of an endogenous inhibitor of sodium–potassium adenosine triphosphatase (Na^+/K^+-ATPase) but its precise identity proved elusive. The discovery that the cardiac atria are the site of synthesis, storage and release of a peptide—atrial natriuretic factor or ANF—with natriuretic and diuretic properties fuelled speculation that this peptide might be 'natriuretic hormone'. Early studies clearly demonstrated that ANF does not inhibit Na^+/K^+-ATPase but the idea that it is involved in the regulation of intravascular volume appeared logical and has prevailed. This review focuses on the contribution of circulating ANF to sodium excretion and leaves detailed discussion of the mechanism of its renal effects (haemodynamic v. tubular, interactions with renin and aldosterone, etc.) to other reviewers.

Plasma ANF levels and intravascular volume status

ANF secretion

The cardiac atria are very active in transcribing the ANF gene, as 1–3 % of mRNA contained in atrial myocytes represents ANF prohormone mRNA (Seidman *et al.*, 1984; Lewicki *et al.*, 1986) and the heart is thought to be the principle source of peptide circulating in plasma. Although a number of pharmacological stimuli of ANF release have been identified, the major physiological stimulus of ANF secretion is atrial distension. Soon after the discovery of ANF, Dietz (1984) demonstrated release of a natriuretic factor in response to an increase in venous return and atrial stretch in an isolated rat heart–lung preparation. In the following year, Lang *et al.* (1985) reported that increases in left atrial volume stimulated release of immunoreactive ANF from the isolated rat heart perfused according to a modified Langendorff protocol. *In vivo* left atrial distension in anaesthetized dogs (Ledsome *et al.*, 1986) and either left or right atrial distension in conscious dogs (Goetz *et al.*, 1986; Metzler *et al.*, 1986) increases circulating ANF levels. Goetz (1988) has calculated that for each 1 mmHg rise in atrial pressure (left or right) plasma ANF levels increase acutely $\sim$ 10 to 15 pmol/l. As suggested by *in vitro* studies, this response is independent of the cardiac nerves as it is not affected by chronic cardiac denervation (Goetz *et al.*, 1986).

Acute volume expansion

Compatible with a role as a circulating hormone regulating sodium excretion, most studies show that plasma ANF levels rise with volume expansion and fall with fluid volume depletion. The range of plasma values for healthy human subjects sitting or standing at rest varies amongst different laboratories but a reasonable working range is 3–25 pmol/l. Intravenous administration of a saline load of 2 l over 60 min produces a two- to threefold increase in plasma ANF levels (Sagnella *et al.*, 1985; Singer *et al.*, 1987; Lewis *et al.*, 1988). Similarly 3-h immersion to the neck in water, which is equivalent to a 10 % expansion of ECF volume with saline (2 l/120 min) produces a prompt threefold rise in plasma ANF levels which is maintained for the duration of immersion (Epstein *et al.*, 1987). Conversely bolus administration of frusemide reduces circulating levels in healthy volunteers that have previously been volume-expanded with saline (Kimura *et al.*, 1986). In the absence of cardiac tamponade, the plasma ANF response to acute volume expansion correlates well with changes in atrial pressure (Anderson *et al.*, 1986b; Salazar *et al.*, 1986) but can be dissociated from changes in plasma osmolality, sodium concentration and vasopressin activity (Salazar *et al.*,

1986; Dietz, 1987). Indeed, if atrial pressure is prevented from increasing during volume expansion, plasma ANF levels do not rise (Barbee & Trippodo, 1987). When atrial distension is inhibited, acute volume loading does not increase ANF levels despite a rise in atrial pressure (Mancini et al., 1987). Thus the effects of acute volume expansion on circulating ANF levels appears to be mediated via changes in atrial distension.

Chronic volume expansion

Healthy individuals on a high salt diet (Sagnella et al., 1987) or receiving mineralocorticoids (Miyamori et al., 1987) develop a sustained two- to threefold elevation of plasma ANF levels. Pathological disturbances of sodium and water balance provide a particularly useful insight into the relationship between plasma ANF and chronic volume expansion. Abnormally high circulating levels are found in congestive cardiac failure (Burnett et al., 1986; Raine et al., 1986), chronic renal failure (Wilkins et al., 1986) primary aldosteronism (Tunny, Higgins & Gordon, 1986), and the syndrome of inappropriate secretion of antidiuretic hormone (Cogan et al., 1986). Reduced metabolism of the peptide might contribute to the elevated levels in some of these conditons but there remains a close relationship with the degree of fluid overload. In heart failure, plasma levels are proportional to the elevation of atrial pressure (Raine et al., 1986) and decline as patients respond to treatment (Katoh et al., 1986). Similarly levels fall in chronic renal failure as fluid is removed by ultrafiltration or haemodialysis (Wilkins et al., 1986).

   In health, levels of ventricular ANF mRNA are $\sim 1\%$ of those in atria (Lewicki et al., 1986). In animal models and disease states associated with chronic fluid retention, ventricular ANF mRNA and immunoreactivity increase substantially. Rats with aortocaval fistula show striking ventricular hypertrophy and an 11-fold increase in mRNA has been observed (Stockman & Needleman, 1988, unpublished observations). In the cardiomyopathic hamster ventricular ANF mRNA and immunoreactivity increase with increasing severity of congestive heart failure (Edwards et al., 1988; Franch et al., 1988; Thibault et al., 1989). Data is now emerging from patients with congestive cardiac failure. Saito et al. (1989) have reported a 10-fold increase in ANF mRNA and a 200-fold increase in ANF levels in patients with dilated cardiomyopathy and a positive correlation between pulmonary capillary wedge pressure and ventricular ANF levels in patients with left ventricular aneurysms. This study also showed that augmentation of gene expression was more prominent in ventricle than atrium. Taking account of tissue weight, ANF mRNA content of ventricle of the failing heart approached that of the atrium. The ventricle may therefore be a substantial contributor to total circulating ANF levels in heart failure (Thibault et al., 1989; Yasue et al., 1989). The recruitment of the ventricle for ANF synthesis in chronic volume overload is a strong argument that ANF may have a physiological role in the regulation of sodium and water balance.

Plasma ANF levels and natriuretic response

Short duration studies

Early studies reporting a brisk and sizeable natriuretic response to ANF administration employed high doses of the peptide which elevated plasma levels into the pathological or pharmacological range (Richards *et al.*, 1985; Anderson *et al.*, 1986b). More recent studies have used lower doses and raised plasma ANF to levels produced by physiological stimuli. Biollaz *et al.* (1986) gave salt-loaded healthy volunteers an ANF analogue at a low infusion rate for 4 h and found a significant rise in sodium excretion after 60 min. Other authors report that a continuous infusion of human ANF (99–126), 1.2–2 pmol/kg/min in salt-replete, hydrated subjects increases plasma ANF levels two- to fourfold during the first hour and leads to a progressive rise in sodium excretion which becomes significantly elevated above control values during the second hour (Anderson *et al.*, 1987; Richards *et al.*, 1988a; Solomon *et al.*, 1988). Thus, rises in plasma ANF concentration within the stimulated physiological range are natriuretic but under the conditions of these experiments, small sustained changes in concentration lead to a gradual rather than rapid end-organ response.

Direct comparison of the renal response to ANF and the response to acute volume expansion reveals some important differences. The delayed natriuresis during low-dose ANF infusion contrasts with the rapid rise in sodium excretion that follows acute volume loading. Richards *et al.* (1988b) have given an infusion of ANF to healthy volunteers to match the natriuresis produced by an infusion of saline (15 ml/kg/h) and found that the two infusions were associated with markedly different plasma ANF concentrations and profiles of urinary electrolyte excretion. Reddy *et al.* (1988) have compared maximal doses of ANF with sustained volume expansion with saline (~ 1.3 ml/kg/min for 1 h) in anaesthetized rats. They found that the saline load was more natriuretic than ANF and less affected by a reduction in renal perfusion pressure. These differences indicate that the natriuresis of volume expansion is not solely ANF-induced and therefore the peptide can account for only part of the renal response to this stimulus.

The same conclusion may be drawn from examining the temporal relationship between the change in plasma ANF and the natriuresis following an acute volume load. Homer Smith (1957) recognized that 'the half-life of a litre of saline in man is generally a good many hours, even after intravenous infusion'; in comparison, the rise in plasma ANF is transient (Singer *et al.*, 1987; Lewis *et al.*, 1988). In attempts to quantitate the contribution from ANF, the peptide has been infused in doses calculated to reproduce the plasma levels stimulated by acute volume expansion. Kaneko *et al.* (1987) gave ANF 4 pmol/min for 60 min to anaesthetized euvolaemic rats and produced a rise in plasma ANF levels ($\sim$ threefold) which was similar to that seen after semi-acute volume expansion with saline (2.5% body weight over 60 min), but whereas the saline increased sodium excretion twofold, the ANF infusion was not natriuretic. The authors concluded that ANF cannot be critical for the induction of natriuresis in volume expansion. However, a more significant role for ANF is suggested by studies which have employed more substantial volume expansion protocols. Khraibi *et al.* (1987) found that ANF in a dose of 0.7 nmol/kg/h in anaesthetized rats produced plasma levels comparable to a large saline load (5% body weight in 30 min) and estimated that ANF might account for 40% of the early (30 min from the start of volume loading) natriuretic response to volume expansion. Barbee & Trippodo (1987) arrived at a similar figure. These authors gave a graded dose infusion of ANF to anaesthetized rats during volume expansion with blood (6% body weight in 15 min) while controlling right atrial pressure with a caval snare (to inhibit homeostatic mechanisms triggered by a rise in atrial pressure). They reproduced the plasma levels seen in another group of rats similarly volume-expanded but whose atrial pressure was allowed to rise and found that the ANF infusion produced approximately 34% of the natriuresis seen in the control group. Furthermore, when the natriuretic response was arbitrarily divided into early (0–45 min) and intermediate (45–90 min) stages from the start of the volume load, the increase in circulating ANF accounted for $\sim$ 20% and 56% of the two periods respectively. Recently, Pichet *et al.* (1989) have given infusions of ANF (3.7 pmol/kg/min for 30 min) to conscious dogs and elevated plasma ANF concentration two- to threefold, equivalent to the effect of rapid volume expansion with 3% dextran in saline (18 ml/kg over 2 to 3 min). The authors estimated that 23% of sodium excretion within 30 min of volume expansion could be accounted for by the plasma ANF response to this stimulus.

It is possible that studies comparing an infusion of ANF with volume expansion underestimate the physiological role of ANF. First, several factors influence the natriuretic activity of ANF, in particular renal perfusion pressure, the renin–aldosterone system and renal sympathetic nerve activity, that in volume expansion are adjusted in a direction which facilitates the action of this peptide. Indeed the threshold dose of ANF required to stimulate a natriuresis is lower in volume-expanded than euvolaemic animals (Metzler & Ramsay, 1989; Soejima *et al.*, 1988) and Reddy *et al.* (1988) have reported that volume expansion has a synergistic effect on the natriuretic response to ANF. Secondly, investigators often used saline rather than donor blood as the agent for inducing volume expansion and this introduces a confounding factor, namely haemodilution. The latter may itself promote sodium excretion and thus reduce the apparent contribution of ANF to the overall response. This is the argument used by Paul, Ferguson & Navar (1988) to explain their finding that the addition of volume expansion with equilibrated blood (1.5% body weight over 15 min) to an infusion of ANF 133 pmol/kg/min in anaesthetized rats produced no further rise in sodium excretion and vice versa, suggesting that the two stimuli act on the kidney through a similar saturable mechanism.

On the other hand, it cannot be overlooked that some studies, notably conducted in conscious animals, in which plasma ANF levels have been related to renal response have suggested a very limited role for the peptide in mediating the natriuresis of acute volume expansion. Sakata, Greenwald & Needleman (1988) gave 4% albumin in saline (1.5 ml/kg/min over 15 min) to conscious rats and observed a sharp rise in sodium excretion but no significant change in plasma ANF levels. This contrasts with a fivefold rise in plasma ANF recorded when the stimulus was repeated in the same rats anaesthetized with chloral hydrate. Certain anaesthetics, chloral hydrate included, have been shown to increase plasma ANF levels (Horky et al., 1985) and this may explain in part why volume expansion of anaesthetized rats was associated with higher plasma ANF levels. None the less, it does not explain the lack of response of this peptide to volume loading in conscious rats. Cowley, Anderas & Skelton (1988) have reported a similar observation, that is natriuresis following a saline load (400 ml in 10 min) without a change in plasma ANF concentration, in conscious dogs. However, while these studies may emphasize the role of factors other than ANF in the natriuresis of volume expansion with saline in conscious animals, the findings must be viewed in the context of a two- to threefold rise in plasma ANF reported by other investigators in conscious dogs (Miki et al., 1986; Verburg et al., 1986; Pichet et al., 1988) and healthy human subjects volume-expanded to a similar degree (Sagnella et al., 1985; Singer et al., 1987; Lewis et al., 1988).

The converse observation has been made by Goetz et al. (1986). These authors found that cardiac denervation of conscious dogs inhibited the natriuresis but not the rise in plasma ANF produced by inflating a balloon in the left atrium, thus dissociating a rise in circulating levels from a natriuresis. This study affirms the importance of cardiac innervation in mediating the natriuresis of atrial distension and, by implication, volume expansion, but does not rule out a contribution from ANF. It is possible that ANF acts in synergy with other factors under the influence of the cardiac nerves to promote sodium excretion during volume expansion, as suggested by Reddy et al., (1988).

Supportive evidence that ANF is a mediator of the natriuresis of volume expansion in both conscious and anaesthetized states comes from measurements of urinary guanosine $3':5'$-cyclic monophosphate (cyclic GMP) excretion. Cyclic GMP has emerged as the most likely candidate for second messenger of ANF (Leitman et al., 1987). Consistent with this role, ANF increases cyclic GMP levels in renal and other target tissues (Leitman & Murad 1987) and the nucleotide reproduces the effect of the peptide on glomerular filtration rate (Huang, Ives & Cogan, 1986) and cation transport in inner medullary collecting ducts (Light et al., 1989). Administration of ANF in vivo is accompanied by marked rises in urinary cyclic GMP excretion (Gerzer et al., 1985) which is thought to reflect renal levels and the natriuretic effect of the peptide (Wong et al., 1988). An important observation therefore is that urinary cyclic GMP levels rise in man following an acute volume load (Lewis et al., 1988) and immersion to the neck in water (Gerbes et al., 1988) and excretion of the nucleotide follows the plasma ANF response to these stimuli (Lewis et al., 1988). Moreover immunological blockade of ANF activity during volume expansion of rats completely inhibits the rise in urinary cyclic GMP excretion (Stasch et al., 1986), suggesting that ANF is the major determinant of this effect.

Long-term studies

Garcia and colleagues (1985a, b; 1986) and others (Yasujima et al., 1985) have administered low doses of ANF (100 ng to 2 μg/h) for periods up to 1 week by osmotic minipump to normotensive and hypertensive rats. Only one of the hypertensive groups (Garcia et al., 1985b) and none of the normotensive groups increased their 24-h urinary sodium output during the infusion period. Unfortunately, sodium intake was not monitored or controlled in any of these experiments which makes the presence or absence of any specific effect of ANF difficult to discern.

    In studies in which sodium intake has been controlled, an increase in sodium excretion in the first few hours of ANF infusion has been detected but then output returns to match intake. Granger et al. (1986) placed dogs on a sodium-deficient diet and provided sodium via a constant infusion of saline. ANF 16 pmol/kg/min for 4 days increased plasma levels 10-fold and appeared to increase sodium excretion on the first day, but this was not maintained. Janssen et al. (1989) gave ANF 67 pmol/min for 4 days to six patients with essential hypertension on a constant sodium diet (150 mmol/day). Plasma ANF levels increased twofold for the duration of the study. Sodium excretion increased within 4 h and continued to exceed baseline values for the first 24 h amounting to a net negative sodium balance of 72 mmol. Thereafter, sodium output equalled sodium intake. Both studies suggested that the accompanying fall in blood pressure was an element in attentuating the natriuretic effect of chronic ANF administration but the multifactorial nature of sodium homeostasis means that more than one factor may be responsible.

Effect of reducing ANF secretion or inhibiting its activity

An alternative approach to infusing ANF to assess its contribution to sodium and water homeostasis is to reduce secretion of the peptide or inhibit its activity. In the absence of a specific pharmacological agent, investigators have had to rely on surgical techniques and immunological blockade, and this has restricted studies to animals.

Atrial appendectomy

Removal of one or both atrial appendages significantly reduces atrial tissue mass but leaves the majority of atrial stretch receptors intact and has little effect on basal circulating ANF levels. Only one study has reported a fall in basal urinary sodium excretion in the period following this procedure (Villarreal et al., 1986). On the other hand, a consistent finding in rats is that atrial appendectomy reduces the natriuresis of acute volume expansion. Right atrial appendectomy reduces the natriuretic response to an iso-oncotic albumin—saline infusion (6% body weight over 15 min) in anaesthetized rats by $\sim 50\%$ (Veress & Sonnenberg, 1984; Schwab et al., 1986). Bilateral atrial appendectomy has been reported to have a greater effect ($\sim 80\%$ reduction) on the response to a smaller volume load (1% body weight over 30 min) of saline (Villarreal et al., 1986). These observations extend to conscious rats studied 2–4 weeks after surgery (Korbin et al., 1985; Sakata et al., 1988). The right atrial appendage may be more important than the left but both appear to contribute to the rise in sodium excretion (Sakata et al., 1988). In anaesthetized rats, the attenuated natriuretic response is not affected by vagotomy (Veress & Sonnenberg, 1984) but is associated with a smaller rise in plasma ANF (Schwab et al., 1986; Villarreal et al., 1986). Thus, the smaller natriuresis may be attributable to a reduction in ANF secretion. The underlying mechanism in conscious rats is less clear. Sakata et al. (1988) found no rise in plasma ANF in either sham-operated or appendisectomized rats following volume expansion. In their control experiments they demonstrated preservation of neurally mediated cardiac responses and postulated that atrial appendectomy might have reduced secretion of another natriuretic factor (independent of ANF) residing in atrial tissue.

While the atrial appendages may be important to the natriuresis of volume expansion in rats, they appear to have a less significant role in dogs. Kinter et al. (1986) found that chronic (15 to 29 days) bilateral atrial appendectomy did not affect the natriuresis following iso-oncotic volume expansion in conscious dogs. Benjamin, Metzler & Peterson (1987) confirmed these findings but also demonstrated that the procedure had no effect on the rise in plasma ANF associated with volume loading. This may reflect a difference in the distribution of ANF in the atrium of dogs compared to rats (Cernacek *et al.*, 1988), such that atrial appendectomy leads to a greater depletion of ANF stores in the rat.

Immunological blockade

Passive immunization of anaesthetized rats with polyclonal antisera directed against ANF has been reported to reduce basal urinary sodium excretion by 50 to 60% (Naruse *et al.*, 1985; Sasaki *et al.*, 1987). The effect was transient, lasting 20 to 30 min. Naruse *et al.* (1985) recorded an associated rise in plasma renin activity and found that the effect on sodium excretion was more pronounced in rats treated with deoxy-corticosterone acetate.

More striking is the effect of immunological blockade of ANF activity during acute volume expansion. Hirth *et al.* (1986) found that anaes-thetized rats immunized with a monoclonal antibody raised against ANF were unable to increase sodium and water excretion during the first 20–40 min after acute volume expansion with homologous blood (20 ml/kg bolus injection). This finding is rather surprising as it implies that ANF is totally responsible for the early natriuresis and diuresis following an acute volume load. However, the authors have subsequently repeated their observations in conscious rats; administration of mono-clonal antibody with saline volume load (20 ml/kg bolus injection) completely inhibited the rise in sodium excretion and urinary cyclic GMP excretion seen during the ensuing 60 min in a control group.

Sakata *et al.* (1988) addressed the same question using a group of rats made autoimmune to ANF but found a difference between the conscious and the anaesthetized state. Anaesthetized ANF-autoimmune rats showed marked blunting of natriuresis and diuresis following a 15-min 4% albumin–saline infusion (1.5 ml/kg/min) but the same rats showed no impairment of response to the same stimulus when conscious. While this result is compatible with the rest of their report suggesting a very limited physiological role for ANF in regulating sodium and water excretion in conscious rats, it is not clear why anaesthesia should unmask a prominent role for the peptide.

The author has repeated the study of Hirth and colleagues (1986) in conscious rats using a different monoclonal antibody directed against ANF. The dose of antibody chosen for these experiments was sufficient to inhibit the natriuretic effect of a 15-min infusion of ANF 200 pmol/kg/min. Given 90 min prior to volume expansion with 4% albumin–saline (1.0 ml/kg/min over 15 min) it completely inhibited the rise in urinary cyclic GMP excretion during the ensuing 60 min, suggesting effective antagonism of circulating ANF, and reduced sodium excretion

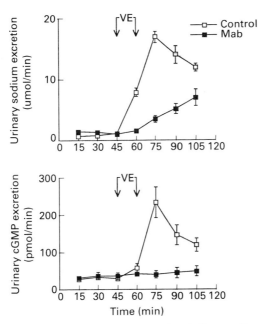

Fig. 3.2 Effect of volume expansion (VE) on sodium excretion (top) and urinary cyclic GMP excretion (bottom) in conscious rats that have received vehicle (control, □) or monoclonal antibody directed against ANF (Mab, ■) 1 h prior to volume loading. $n = 6$ in each group.

by $\sim 66\%$ compared with the control group (Fig. 3.2). Thus, the consensus from these experiments with immunological blockade must be that ANF plays a significant role in the early natriuresis of acute volume expansion in both conscious and anaesthetized rats.

With one exception, chronic immunological inhibition of ANF activity has been shown to have little effect on long-term sodium and water homeostasis. Greenwald *et al.* (1988) found no difference in daily urinary sodium excretion between ANF autoimmune and non-immune rats, and when stressed with a high (8%) salt diet or mineralocorticoid administration, no impairment of adaptation was demonstrated. Itoh *et al.* (1989) passively immunized spontaneously hypertensive, DOCA-salt and normotensive rats with high-affinity blocking or low-affinity non-blocking anti-ANF monoclonal antibody for 4 weeks. Only the DOCA-salt rats treated with blocking antibody showed reduced 24-h urinary sodium excretion at the end of this period when compared with appropriate controls, and even these animals showed no excess gain in body weight. Doubt has been cast on the efficacy of immunization as a technique for chronically antagonizing ANF; the criticism is that once the anti-ANF antibodies are saturated by the peptide the circulating free ANF level is re-established. However, evidence that this approach does work is provided by Itoh *et al.* (1989) who used the technique to accelerate the development of hypertension in spontaneously hypertensive and DOCA-salt rats. The apparent lack of effect of chronic antagonism of the peptide on sodium excretion may indicate that prolonged ANF deficiency is not harmful but does not exclude a role for ANF in day-to-day regulation of sodium and water balance. As pointed out by Smith (1957) 'where multiple controls are superimposed on a function, such as sodium excretion, it is conceived that normal regulatory mechanisms may be obscured by compensatory mechanisms'.

Effect of enhancing endogenous ANF levels and bioactivity

Multidisciplinary interest in ANF has allowed rapid progress in our understanding of the mechanisms underlying ANF clearance and activity. This in turn has afforded pharmacological opportunities for the manipulation of endogenous ANF levels and activity.

One important pathway of ANF clearance appears to involve degradation by neutral endopeptidase. In support of this, ANF has been shown to be a substrate for this enzyme *in vitro* (Olins *et al.*, 1987) and inhibitors of the enzyme (for example, thiorphan, SQ 29072) enhance the natriuretic and cyclic GMP response to low-dose ANF infusion in conscious and anaesthetized rats (Trapani *et al.*, 1989; Seymour, Fennell & Swerdel, 1989). The author has recently examined the effect of neutral endopeptidase inhibition during volume expansion of conscious rats. Thiorphan 30 mg/kg or saline vehicle was administered 15 min prior to volume expansion with 4% albumin in saline (1% body weight over 15 min). Thiorphan-treated rats showed a 64% increase in peak urinary sodium excretion over vehicle-treated rats (Fig. 3.3). This was associated with a urinary cyclic GMP response which was greater than the sum of the effect of volume expansion and thiorphan administration alone, suggesting that the facilitated natriuresis was mediated by augmentation of the ANF response to the volume load.

Another approach to enhancing the natriuretic activity of ANF is to manipulate renal cyclic GMP levels. Co-administration of low doses of the peptide and a cyclic GMP-specific phosphodiesterase inhibitor (M + B 22948) to conscious rats greatly potentiates the rise in urinary sodium and cyclic GMP excretion seen with either compound alone (Wilkins, Settle & Needleman, 1989). To investigate the effect of this manipulation on volume expansion, the phosphodiesterase inhibitor was given to rats prior to and during acute volume loading with 4% albumin in saline (1% body weight over 15 min). The rise in sodium excretion in the animals that received the enzyme inhibitor was nearly threefold greater than in the control group and was accompanied by a twofold greater rise in urinary cyclic GMP excretion (Wilkins *et al.*, 1989). The protocol was then repeated in rats that had been predosed with monoclonal antibody directed against ANF; the antibody markedly attenuated the natriuretic

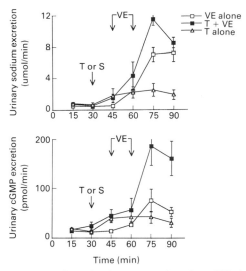

Fig. 3.3 Effect of volume expansion alone (VE alone), thiorphan plus volume expansion (T + VE) and thiorphan alone (T alone) on sodium excretion (top) and urinary cyclic GMP excretion (bottom) in conscious rats. Thiorphan (T) or saline (S) was administered as a bolus injection at 30 min. $n = 6$ in each group.

response in both the phosphodiesterase inhibitor treated group and the control group and completely blocked the rise in urinary cyclic GMP excretion. These data suggest that the phosphodiesterase inhibitor was dependent on the ANF-driven surge in cyclic GMP levels associated with volume loading for its striking effect on sodium excretion and provides another argument that ANF (and cyclic GMP) plays an active role in mediating the natriuretic of acute volume expansion.

Final analysis

The preservation of the structure of ANF across species lines, the abundance of ANF mRNA in atrial tissue and the recruitment of the ventricle for ANF synthesis in conditions inducing ventricular hypertrophy all suggest that ANF is a physiologically important substance. Consistent with a role in blood volume regulation, plasma ANF levels rise with intravascular volume expansion and fall with volume depletion. The profile of biological activity of ANF provides further support for such a role; thus ANF is natriuretic at 'physiological' as well as pharmacological plasma levels and the peptide has been shown to interact with other hormones that regulate blood volume, such as renin, aldosterone and arginine vasopressin. Unfortunately, the lack of a specific pharmacological antagonist and the multifactorial regulation of sodium balance has meant that the precise contribution of ANF to sodium and water homeostasis is difficult to define.

It is tempting to accept that the major role of ANF is to off-load the heart in conditions associated with acute volume expansion. Differences between the renal response to an acute volume load and low-dose ('physiological') ANF infusions and the time-course of changes in plasma ANF and urinary cyclic GMP levels during acute volume expansion indicate that the peptide can account for only part of the effect of this stimulus. Infusions of ANF that achieve plasma levels comparable to an acute volume load suggest that ANF may be responsible for 20–40 % of the early natriuresis (30 to 60 min). Atrial appendectomy and passive immunization experiments argue for a more critical role for ANF, particularly in rats.

It is likely that ANF also contributes to day-to-day sodium and water excretion. The rise in plasma ANF during such chronic stimuli as high salt diet and mineralocorticoid administration and the natriuretic (and urinary cyclic GMP) effect of neutral endopeptidase inhibitors provide evidence of this. However, the lack of effect of chronic immunological blockade of ANF on long-term sodium and water balance indicate that other factors involved in regulating sodium and water excretion are capable of compensating for prolonged ANF deficiency.

The discovery of ANF held the potential of a new therapeutic agent, but its short half-life in circulation and the problems of chronic administration of peptides mean that the peptide itself (or analogues) is unlikely to find its way into our therapeutic armoury. On the other hand, the presence of ANF as an endogenous circulating substance with its own mechanism for regulating release, metabolism and activity provides alternative measures for enhancing ANF activity. The demonstration that inhibitors of neutral endopeptidase are natriuretic and that phosphodiesterase inhibition potentiates the renal effects of ANF may yet give rise to novel strategies for the management of disorders of sodium and water balance.

Acknowledgements

This article was written while the author was a British–American Research Fellow of the American Heart Association (AHA) and the British Heart Foundation (BHF) in the Department of Pharmacology at Washington University Medical School, St Louis, Missouri. During this period he was supported by the excellent technical skills of Steven L. Settle and received encouragement and expert guidance from Philip Needleman, and he is indebted to both.

References

Anderson, J., Struthers, A., Christofides, N. & Bloom, S. (1986a). Atrial natriuretic peptide: an endogenous factor enhancing sodium excretion in man. *Clin. Sci.* **60**: 327–31.

Anderson, J. V., Donckier, J., McKenna, W. J. & Bloom, S. R. (1986b). The plasma release of atrial natriuretic peptide in man. *Clin. Sci.* **71**: 151–5.

Anderson, J. V., Donckier, J., Payne, N. N., Beacham, J., Slater, J. D. H. & Bloom, S. R. (1987). Atrial natriuretic peptide: evidence of action as a natriuretic hormone at physiological plasma concentrations in man. *Clin. Sci.* **72**: 305–12.

Barbee, R. W. & Trippodo, N. C. (1987). The contribution of atrial natriuretic factor to acute volume natriuresis in rats. *Am. J. Physiol.* **253**: F1129–35.

Benjamin, B. A., Metzler, C. H. & Peterson, T. V. (1987). Renal response to volume expansion in atrial-appendectomized dogs. *Am. J. Physiol.* **253**: R786–93.

Biollaz, J., Nussberger, J., Poschet, M., Burnner-Ferber, F., Otterbein, E., Gomez, H., Waeber, B. *et al.* (1986). Four-hour infusions of synthetic atrial natriuretic peptide in normal volunteers. *Hypertension* **8**: (Suppl. II): II-96–105.

Burnett, J. C., Kao, P. C., Hu, D. C. *et al.* (1986). Atrial natriuretic peptide elevation in congestive heart failure in the human. *Science* **231**: 1145–7.

Cernacek, P., Maher, E., Crawhall, J. C. & Levy, M. (1988). Molecular forms of atrial natriuretic peptides in dog atrium and plasma. *Life Sci.* **42**: 2533–9.

Chinkers, M., Garbers, D. L., Chang, M.-S., *et al.* (1989). A membrane form of guanylate cyclase is an atrial natriuretic peptide receptor. *Nature* **338**: 78–83.

Cogan, E., Debiève, M., Philipast, I., Pepersack, T. & Abramow, M. (1986). High plasma levels of atrial natriuretic factor in SIADH. *New Engl. J. Med.* **314**: 1258.

Cowley, A. W., Anderas, P. R. & Skelton, M. M. (1988). Acute saline loading in normal and bilaterally atrial-resected conscious dogs. *Am. J. Physiol.* **255**: H144–52.

DeWardener, H. E. & Clarkson, E. M. (1985). Concept of natriuretic hormone. *Physiol. Rev.* **65**: 658–759.

DiBona, G. F. (1982). The functions of the renal nerves. *Rev. Physiol. Biochem. Pharmacol.* **94**: 75–181.

Dietz, J. R. (1984). Release of natriuretic factor from rat heart–lung preparation by atrial distension. *Am. J. Physiol.* **247**: R1093–6.

Dietz, J. R. (1987). Control of atrial natriuretic factor release from a rat heart–lung preparation. *Am. J. Physiol.* **235**: R498–502.

Edwards, B. S., Ackermann, D. M., Lee, M. E., Reeder, G. S., Wold, L. E. & Burnett, J. C. (1988). Identification of atrial natriuretic factor within ventricular tissue in hamsters and humans with congestive heart failure. *J. Clin. Invest.* **81**: 82–6.

Epstein, M. (1978). Renal effects of head-out of water immersion in man: implications for an understanding of volume homeostasis. *Physiol. Rev.* **58**: 529–81.

Epstein, M., Loutzenhiser, R., Friedland, E., Aceto, R. M., Camargo, M. J. F. & Atlas, S. A. (1987). Relationship of increased plasma atrial natriuretic factor and renal sodium handling during immersion-induced central hypervolaemia in normal humans. *J. Clin. Invest.* **79**: 738–45.

Franch, H. A., Dixon, R. A. F., Blaine, E. H. & Siegel, P. K. S. (1988). Ventricular atrial natriuretic factor in the cardiomyopathic hamster model of congestive heart failure. *Circulation Res.* **62**: 31–6.

Garcia, R., Gutkowska, J., Genest, J., Cantin, M. & Thibault, G. (1985a). Reduction of blood pressure and increased diuresis and natriuresis during chronic infusion of atrial natriuretic factor (ANF Arg[101]–Tyr[126]) in conscious one-kidney, one-clip hypertensive rats. *Proc. Soc. Exp. Biol. Med.* **179**: 539–45.

Garcia, R., Thibault, G., Gutkowska, J. & Cantin, M. (1986). Effect of chronic infusion of atrial natriuretic factor on plasma and urinary aldosterone, plasma renin activity, blood pressure and sodium excretion in 2-K, 1-C hypertensive rats. *Clin. Exp. Hypertension: Part A. Theory Prac.* **8**: 1127–47.

Garcia, R., Thibault, G., Gutkowska, J. *et al.* (1985b). Chronic infusion of low doses of atrial natriuretic factor (ANF Arg[101]–Tyr[126]) reduces blood pressure in conscious SHR without apparent changes in sodium excretion. *Proc. Soc. Exp. Biol. Med.* **179**: 396–401.

Gauer, O. H., Henry, J. P. & Behn, C. (1970). The regulation of extracellular fluid volume. *Ann. Rev. Physiol.* **32**: 547–95.

Gerbes, A. L., Arendt, R. M., Gerzer, R. *et al.* (1988). Role of atrial natriuretic factor, cyclic GMP, and the renin–aldosterone system in acute volume regulation of healthy human subjects. *Eur. J. Clin. Invest.* **18**: 425–29.

Gerzer, R., Witzgall, H., Tremblay, J., Gutkowska, J. & Hamet, P. (1985). Rapid increase in plasma and urinary cyclic GMP after bolus injection of atrial natriuretic factor in man. *J. Clin. Endocrinol. Metab.* **61**: 1217–19.

Goetz, K. L. (1988). Physiology and pathophysiology of atrial peptides. *Am. J. Physiol.* **254**: E1–15.

Goetz, K. L., Hermreck, A. S., Slick, G. L. & Starke, H. S. (1970). Atrial receptors and renal function in conscious dogs. *Am. J. Physiol.* **219**: 1417–23.

Goetz, K. L., Wang, B. C., Geer, P. G., Leadley, R. J. & Reinhardt, H. W. (1986). Atrial stretch increases sodium excretion independently of release of atrial peptides. *Am. J. Physiol.* **250**: R946–50.

Granger, J. P., Opgenoth, T. J., Salazar, J., Romero, J. C. & Burnett, J. C. (1986). Long-term hypotensive and renal effects of atrial natriuretic factor. *Hypertension* **8** (Suppl. II): II-112–16.

Greenwald, J. E., Sakata, M., Michener, M. L., Sides, S. D. & Needleman, P. (1988). Is atriopeptin a physiological or pathophysiological substance? Studies in the autoimmune rat. *J. Clin. Invest.* **81**: 1036–41.

Henry, J. P., Gauer, O. H. & Reeves, J. L. (1956). Evidence of the atrial location of receptors influencing urine flow. *Circulation Res.* **4**: 85–90.

Hirth, C., Stasch, J.-P., John, A., Kazda, S., Morich, F., Neuser, D. & Wohlfeil, S. (1986). The renal response to acute hypervolemia is caused by atrial natriuretic peptides. *J. Cardiovasc. Pharmacol.* **8**: 268–75.

Horky, K., Gutkowska, J., Garcia, R., Thibault, G., Genest, J. & Cartin, M. (1985). Effect of different anesthetics on immunoreactive atrial natriuretic factor concentrations in rat plasma. *Biochem. Biophys. Res. Commun.* **129**: 651–7.

Huang, C.-L., Ives, H. E. & Cogan, M. G. (1986). *In vivo* evidence that cGMP is the second messenger for atrial natriuretic factor. *Proc. Nat. Acad. Sci. USA* **83**: 8015–18.

Itoh, H., Nakao, K., Mukoyama, M., Yamada, T., Hosoda, K., Shirakami, G. *et al.* (1989). Chronic blockade of endogenous atrial natriuretic polypeptide (ANP) by monoclonal antibody against ANP accelerates the development of hypertension in spontaneously hypertensive and deoxycorticosterone acetate-salt-hypertensive rats. *J. Clin. Invest.* **84**: 145–54.

Janssen, W. M. T., deZeeuw, D., Van der Hen, G. K. & de Jong, P. E. (1989). Antihypertensive effect of a 5-day infusion of atrial natriuretic factor in humans. *Hypertension* **13**: 640–6.

Kaneko, K., Okada, K., Ishikawa, S., Kuzuya, T. & Saito, T. (1987). Role of atrial natriuretic peptide in natriuresis in volume-expanded rats. *Am. J. Physiol.* **253**: R877–922.

Katoh, Y., Kurosawa, T., Takeda, S., Kurokawa, S., Sakamotom, H., Marumo, F. & Kikawada, R. (1986). Atrial natriuretic peptide levels in treated congestive heart failure. *Lancet* **i**: 851.

Khraibi, A. A., Granger, J. P., Burnett, J. C., Walker, K. R. & Knox, F. G. (1987). Role of atrial natriuretic factor in the natriuresis of acute volume expansion. *Am. J. Physiol.* **252**: R921–4.

Kimura, T., Abe, K., Ota, K., Omata, K., Shosi, M., Kudo, K., Matsui, K. *et al.* (1986). Effects of acute water load, hypertonic saline infusion and furosemide administration on atrial natriuretic peptide and vasopressin release in humans. *J. Clin. Endocrinol. Metab.* **62**: 1003–10.

Kinter, L. B., Kopia, G., DePalma, D., Brennan, F., Landi, M. & Inagami, T. (1986) Chronic bilateral atrial appendectomy does not affect salt excretion in dogs *J. Hypertens.* **4** (Suppl. 5): S80–82.

Kobrin, I., Kardon, M. B., Trippodo, N. C., Pegram, B. L. & Frohlich, E. D. (1985). Renal responses to acute volume overload in conscious rats with atrial appendectomy. *J. Hypertens.* **3**: 145–8.

Lang, R. E., Tholker, H., Ganten, D., Luft, F. C., Ruskoaho, H. & Unger, T. (1985). Atrial natriuretic factor—a circulating hormone stimulated by volume loading. *Nature* **324**: 264–6.

Ledsome, J. R., Wilson, N., Courneya, C. A. & Rankin, A. J. (1985). Release of atrial natriuretic peptide by atrial distension. *Canad. J. Physiol. Pharmacol.* **63**: 739–42.

Leitman, D. C. & Murad, F. (1987) Atrial natriuretic factor receptor heterogeneity and stimulation of particulate guanylate cyclase and cyclic GMP accumulation. *Endocrinol. Metab. Clin. N. Am.* Atrial Natriuretic Factor. M. Rosenblatt & J. W. Jacobs (eds). **16**(1), 79–105 W. B. Saunders Co., Philadelphia.

Lewicki, J. A., Greenberg, B., Yamanaka, M. *et al.* (1986). Cloning, sequence analysis and processing of the rat and human atrial natriuretic peptide precursors. *Fed Proc* **45**: 2086–90.

Lewis, H. M., Wilkins, M. R., Selwyn, B. M., Yelland, V. J., Griffith, M. E. & Bhoola, K. D. (1988). Urinary guanosine 3′:5′-cyclic monophosphate but not tissue kallikrein follows the plasma atrial natriuretic factor response to acute volume expansion with saline. *Clin. Sci.* **75**: 489–94.

Light, D. B., Schweibert, E. M., Karlson, K. H. & Stanton, B. A. (1989). Atrial natriuretic peptide inhibits a cation channel in renal inner medullary collecting duct cells. *Science* **243**: 383–5.

Linden, R. J. & Kappagoda, C. T. (1982). *Atrial Receptors*. Cambridge University Press.

Mancini, G. B. J., McGillen, M. J., Bates, E. R., Weder, A. B., DeBoe, S. F. & Grekin, R. J. (1987). Hormonal responses to cardiac tamponade: inhibition of release of atrial natriuretic factor despite elevation of atrial pressures. *Circulation* **76**: 884–90.

Metzler, C. H., Lee, M., Thrashner, T. N. & Ramsey, D. J. (1986). Increased right or left atrial pressure stimulated release of atrial natriuretic peptides in conscious dogs. *Endocrinology* **119**: 2396–8.

Metzler, C. H. & Ramsay, D. J. (1989). Atrial peptide potentiates renal responses to volume expansion in conscious dogs. *Am. J. Physiol.* **256**: R284–9.

Miki, K., Hajduczok, G., Klocke, M. R., Krasney, J. A., Hong, S. K. & deBold, A. J. (1986). Atrial natriuretic factor and renal function during head-out of water immersion in conscious dogs. *Am. J. Physiol.* **251**: R1000–8.

Miyamori, I., Ikeda, M., Matsubara, T. *et al.* (1987). Human atrial natriuretic polypeptide during escape from mineralocorticoid excess in man. *Clin. Sci.* **73**: 431–6.

Morice, A., Pepke-Zaba, J., Loyser, E. *et al.* (1988). Low dose infusion of atrial natriuretic peptide causes salt and water excretion in normal man. *Clin. Sci.* **74**: 359–63.

Naruse, M., Obara, K., Naruse, K. *et al.* (1985). Antisera to atrial natriuretic factor reduces urinary sodium excretion and increases plasma renin activity in rats. *Biochem. Biophys. Res. Commun.* **132**: 954–60.

Olins, G. M., Spear, K. L., Siegel, N. R. & Zurcher-Neely, H. A. (1987). Inactivation of atrial natriuretic factor by the renal brush border. *Biochem. Biophys. Acta* **901**: 97–100.

Paul, R. V., Ferguson, T. & Navar, L. G. (1988). ANF secretion and renal responses to volume expansion with equilibrated blood. *Am. J. Physiol.* **255**: F936–43.

Peters, J. P. (1935). *Body water*. Springfield, Illinois: Charles C. Thomas, p. 288.

Pichet, R., Cantin, M., Thibault, G. & Lavallée, M. (1989). Hemodynamic and renal responses to physiological levels of atrial natriuretic factor in conscious dogs. *Hypertension* **14**: 104–10.

Pichet, R., Gutkowska, J., Cantin, M. & Lavallée, M. (1988). Hemodynamic and renal responses to volume expansion in dogs with cardiac denervation. *Am. J. Physiol.* **254**: F780–6.

Raine, A. E. G., Erne, P., Burgisser, E. *et al.* (1986). Atrial natriuretic peptide and atrial pressure in patients with congestive heart failure. *New Engl. J. Med.* **315**: 533–7.

Reddy, S., Kelly, D., Cochineas, C. & Gyory, A. Z. (1988). Additive and synergistic interaction of atrial natriuretic peptide and volume expansion. *Am. J. Physiol.* **255**: F66–73.

Richards, A. M., Nicholls, M. G., Ikram, H., Webster, M. W., Yandle, T. G., Espiner, E. A. (1985). Renal, haemodynamic and hormonal effects of human alpha atrial natriuretic peptide in healthy volunteers. *Lancet* **i**: 545–9.

Richards, A. M., Tonolo, G., Montorsi, P., Finlayson, J., Fraser, R., Inglis, G., Tourie, A. *et al.* (1988a). Low dose infusions of 26- and 28-amino acid human atrial natriuretic peptides in normal man. *J. Clin. Endocrinol. Metab.* **66**: 465–72.

Richards, A. M., Tonolo, G., Polonia, J. & Montorsi, P. (1988b). Contrasting plasma atrial natriuretic factor concentrations during comparable natriuresis with infusions of atrial natriuretic factor and saline in normal man. *Clin. Sci.* **75**: 455–62.

Sagnella, G. A., Markardu, N. D., Shore, A. C. & MacGregor, G. A. (1985). Effects of changes in dietary sodium intake and saline infusion on immunoreactive atrial natriuretic peptide in human plasma. *Lancet* **ii**: 1206–11.

Sagnella, G. A., Markardu, N. D., Shore, A. C. & MacGregor, G. A. (1987). Plasma immuno-reactive atrial natriuretic peptide and changes in dietary sodium intake in man. *Life Sci.* **40**: 139.

Saito, Y., Nakao, K., Atai, H., Nishimura, K., Okumura, K., Obata, K., Takemura, G. *et al.* (1989). Augmented expression of atrial natriuretic polypeptide gene in ventricle of human failing heart. *J. Clin. Invest.* **83**: 298–305.

Sakata, M., Greenwald, J. E. & Needleman, P. (1988). Paradoxical relationship between atriopeptin plasma levels and diuresis–natriuresis induced by acute volume expansion. *Proc. Nat. Acad. Sci. USA* **85**: 3155–9.

Salazar, F. J., Granger, J. P., Joyce, M. L. M., Burnett, J. C., Bove, A. A. (1986). Effects of hypertonic saline infusion and water drinking on atrial peptide. *Am. J. Physiol.* **251**: R1091–4.

Sasaki, A., Kida, O., Kato, J., Nakamura, S., Kodama, K., Miyata, A., *et al.* (1987). Effects of anti-serum against α-rat atrial natriuretic peptide in anesthetized rats. *Hypertension* **10**: 308–12.

Schwab, T. R., Edwards, B. S., Heublein, D. M. & Burnett, J. C. (1986). Role of atrial natriuretic peptide is volume-expansion natriuresis. *Am. J. Physiol.* **251**: R310–3.

Seidman, C. E., Bloch, K. D., Klein, K. A. & Seidman, J. G. (1984). Nucleotide sequences of the human and mouse atrial natriuretic factor genes. *Science* **226**: 1206–9.

Seymour, A. A., Fennell, S. A. & Swerdel, J. N. (1989). Potentiation of renal effects of atrial natriuretic factor (99–126) by SQ 29072. *Hypertension* **14**: 87–97.

Singer, D. R., Shore, A. C., Markandu, N. D., Buckley, M. G., Sagnella, G. A. & MacGregor, G. A. (1987). Dissociation between plasma atrial natriuretic peptide levels and urinary sodium excretion after intravenous saline infusion in normal man. *Clin. Sci.* **73**: 285–9.

Smith, H. W. (1957). Salt and water volume receptors. *Am. J. Physiol.* **23**: 623–52.

Soejima, H., Grekin, R. J., Briggs, J. P. & Schnermann, J. (1988). Renal response of anesthetized rats to low-dose infusion of atrial natriuretic peptide. *Am. J. Physiol* **255**: R449–55.

Solomon, L. R., Atherton, J. C., Bobinski, H., Hillier, V. & Green, R. (1988). Effect of low dose infusion of atrial natriuretic peptide on renal function in man. *Clin. Sci.* **75**: 403–10.

Starling, E. H. (1909). The Fluids of the Body. (*The Herter Lectures*). Chicago: W. T. Keene and Co., p. 106.

Stasch, J.-P., Hirth, C., Kazda, S. & Wohlfeil, S. (1986). The elevation of cyclic GMP as a response to acute hypervolemia is blocked by monoclonal antibody directed against atrial natriuretic peptides. *Pharmacology* **129**: 165–8.

Thibault, G., Nemer, M., Drouin, J., Lavigne, J. P., Ding, J., Charbonneau, C., Garcia, R. *et al.* (1989). Ventricles as a major site of atrial natriuretic factor synthesis and release in cardiomyopathic hamsters with heart failure. *Circulation Res.* **65**: 71–82.

Trapani, A. J., Smits, G. J., McGraw, D. E., Spear, K. L., Koepke, J. P., Olins, G. M. & Blaine, E. H. (1989) Thiorphan, an inhibitor of endopeptidase 24.11, potentiates the natriuretic activity of atrial natriuretic peptide. *J. Cardiovasc. Pharmacol.* **14**: 419–24.

Tunny, T. J., Higgins, B. A. & Gordon, R. D. (1986). Plasma levels of atrial natriuretic peptide in man is primary aldosteronism, in Gordon's syndrome and in Bartter's syndrome. *Clin. Exp. Pharmacol. Physiol.* **13**: 341–5.

Verburg, K. M., Freeman, R., Davis, J. O., Villarreal, D. & Vari, R. C. (1986). Control of atrial natriuretic factor release in conscious dogs. *Am. J. Physiol.* **251**: R947–56.

Veress, A. T. & Sonnenberg, H. (1984). Right atrial appendectomy reduces the renal response to acute hypervolemia in the rat. *Am. J. Physiol.* **247**: R610–13.

Villarreal, D., Freeman, R. H., Davis, J. O., Verburg, K. M. & Vari, R. C. (1986). Effects of atrial appendectomy on circulating atrial natriuretic factor during volume expansion in the rat. *Proc. Soc. Exp. Biol. Med.* **183**: 54–8.

Wilkins, M. R., Settle, S. L. & Needleman, P. (1989). Augmentation of the natriuretic activity of exogenous and endogenous atriopeptin in rats by inhibition of cyclic GMP degradation. *J. Clin. Invest.* (in press).

Wilkins, M. R., Wood, J. A., Adu, D., Lote, C. J., Kendall, M. J. & Michael, J. (1986). Change in plasma immunoreactive atrial natriuretic peptide during sequential ultrafiltration and haemodialysis. *Clin. Sci.* **71**:157–60.

Wong, K. R., Xie, M.-H., Shi, L.-B., Liu, F.-Y., Huang, C.-L., Gardner, D. G. & Cogan, M. G. (1988). Urinary cGMP as biological marker of the renal activity of atrial natriuretic factor. *Am. J. Physiol.* **255**: F1220–4.

Yasue, H., Obata, K., Okumata, K., Kurose, M., Ogawa, H., Matsuyama, K., Jongasaki, M. *et al.* (1989). Increased secretion of atrial natriuretic polypeptide from the left ventricle in patients with dilated cardiomyopathy. *J. Clin. Invest.* **83**: 46–51.

Yasujima, M., Abe, K., Kohzuki, M., Tarro, M., Kasai, Y., Saro, M., Omata, K. *et al.* (1985). Atrial natriuretic factor inhibits the hypertension induced by chronic infusions of norepinephrine in conscious rats. *Circulation Res.* **57**: 470–4.

Chapter 4
The cardiovascular effects of atrial natriuretic factor

David B. Northridge and John McMurray

Introduction

This chapter reviews the vascular actions of atrial natriuretic factor (ANF). Particular emphasis has been placed on studies conducted in man.

This partly reflects our own interests and experience but also the human literature is less conflicting than that in animals. Furthermore most of our text relates to the effects of ANF in healthy animals and humans mainly because the vascular effects of ANF in pathophysiological conditions are discussed elsewhere in this volume.

Effects of ANF on isolated blood vessels

Conduit arteries

Strips or rings of preconstricted large arteries can be made to relax by the addition of ANF (Winquist, Faison & Nutt, 1984). However, this effect is complicated by apparent differences in the responses of arteries of different sizes and from different organs. The artery most sensitive to the vasorelaxant effects of ANF is the aorta in the rabbit and rat (Garcia *et al.*, 1984; Cohen & Schenck, 1985; Faison *et al.*, 1985). This preparation relaxes in response to ANF following preconstriction with serotonin, histamine, methoxamine, angiotensin II, noradrenaline or potassium (Garcia *et al.*, 1984; Faison *et al.*, 1985—see 'Cellular mechanisms of action'). The IC_{50} for ANF relaxation in these preparations is approximately 10^{-9} mol/l, with the exception of potassium where ANF is relatively ineffective, the IC_{50} being approximately 10^{-7} mol/l (Garcia *et al.*, 1984; Winquist *et al.*, 1984). ANF-induced relaxation of arterial rings *in vitro* is not dependent upon an intact endothelium (Winquist *et al.*, 1984; Ishihara *et al.*, 1985).

ANF also relaxes human arterial rings. Studies of brachial, pulmonary, coronary and uterine arteries have demonstrated a threshold ANF concentration for this effect of 10^{-9} mol/l (Rapoport *et al.*, 1986; Hughes *et al.*, 1988; Labat *et al.*, 1988). Half-maximal relaxation is seen at 10^{-8} mol/l, and no further response occurs at concentrations above 10^{-7} mol/l (Hughes *et al.*, 1988).

Important regional differences have been demonstrated in the sensitivity of large arteries to ANF. In the rat, the carotid artery is the most sensitive after the aorta, followed by the mesenteric artery (Cohen & Schenk, 1985). In the rabbit, ANF relaxes renal and mesenteric arteries as effectively as the aorta (Faison *et al.*, 1985). The carotid artery is slightly less sensitive, and the iliac, femoral, saphenous and basilar arteries are relatively insensitive. The renal artery of the dog is also significantly more sensitive to ANF than the coronary, femoral or basilar artery (Ishihara *et al.*, 1985).

Resistance arteries

The large arteries used in these organ bath experiments do not contribute significantly to vascular resistance in the intact organism. Studies of small resistance arteries with a lumen diameter of approximately 250 μm might be expected to predict better the actions of ANF *in vivo*. In an organ bath concentration up to 10^{-7} mol/l, ANF has no effect on resistance arteries taken from rat coronary, femoral, mesenteric or cerebral vasculature (Aalkjaer, Mulvany & Nyborg, 1985; Osol *et al.*, 1986; DeMey *et al.*, 1987). Similar observations have been made using human resistance vessels (Hughes *et al.*, 1987, 1988; Hughes, Nielsen & Sever, 1989). Arteries from subcutaneous fat failed to relax when exposed to ANF 10^{-9} to 10^{-6} mol/l. These investigators also found that ANF had no effect on omental arteries, in contrast to the findings of Bruschi *et al.* (1988).

Renal resistance arteries behave differently since they do appear to be sensitive to ANF with approximately 50% relaxation of rat arteries at an organ bath concentration of 10^{-8} mol/l (DeMey *et al.*, 1987). Rat renal resistance arteries dilate in response to ANF irrespective of the agent used to preconstrict the vessels (Aalkjaer *et al.*, 1985). This finding is supported by the observation that ANF infusion rapidly decreases the resistance to flow through the isolated perfused rat kidney, but has no effect on a perfused mesenteric arterial preparation (Garcia *et al.*, 1984). Although ANF has relatively little effect on vessels from other vascular beds, it does partially dilate skeletal muscle resistance arteries which have been preconstricted with angiotensin although not if preconstricted with noradrenaline, arginine vasopressin or α_2-agonists (Faber *et al.*, 1987; Proctor & Bealer, 1987).

Veins

In organ bath preparations it is much more difficult to demonstrate relaxation of venous smooth muscle with ANF as compared to arterial preparations. Pharmacological doses of ANF which relax arterial rings from rabbits are without effects on most venous preparations (Faison *et al.*, 1985). An exception to this rule is the rabbit facial vein, which is sensitive to the vasorelaxant effects of ANF (Winquist *et al.*, 1984). However, this is an unusual preparation which develops intrinsic tone on stretching and behaves differently from other veins (Winquist *et al.*, 1984). A similar lack of responsiveness in veins compared with arteries has been demonstrated in rat blood vessels. The concentration of ANF which produced 90% relaxation of large arterial rings caused only 10% relaxation of a jugular vein ring, and a plateau in the dose–response curve was seen after only 15% relaxation (Cohen & Schenck, 1985). The same jugular vein preparation has been shown to respond to other vasodilators including β-agonists and nitroglycerin (Cohen & Wiley, 1978). Similar experiments using human saphenous vein preparations have shown that ANF in concentrations between 10^{-9} and 10^{-6} mol/l has no effect on precontracted veins (Hughes *et al.*, 1987, 1988).

The large anatomical veins studied in these experiments do not contribute significantly to venous capacitance in the intact animal, and it is possible that small venules may be more sensitive to the effects of ANF *in vitro*. In a study of the microscopic responses of venules within sections of rat muscle ANF caused 70% relaxation following preconstriction with noradrenaline (Faber, Gettes & Gianturco, 1988). However these observations were not confirmed in a study of rat mesenteric venules (Smits *et al.*, 1987). Further *in vitro* studies, possibly using human tissue obtained from muscle biopsy, may help to elucidate the effects of ANF on venules.

In summary, these studies have shown that ANF in concentrations > 10^{-9} mol/l consistantly causes direct vasodilatation of preconstricted conduit arteries taken from animals or humans. However these concentrations are rarely if ever achieved in physiological or pathophysiological circumstances. Resistance arterioles from numerous tissues are insensitive to ANF *in vitro*, with the exception of rat renal vessels and skeletal muscle arteries preconstricted with angiotensin. Veins are generally insensitive to the effects of ANF *in vitro*, even with high organ bath concentrations of the peptide.

Effect of ANF on arterial pressure and heart rate

The effects of ANF on arterial blood pressure have been studied *in vivo* by administering the peptide, by bolus injection or short-term infusion, to a range of laboratory animals and humans.

Animal studies

ANF has reduced the systemic arterial blood pressure in almost every species studied so far. In rats, the fall in blood pressure is associated with no change, or a fall in heart rate (Lappe *et al.*, 1985; Gellai, Allen & Beeuwkes, 1986; Chien, Frohlich & Trippodo, 1987; Criscione et al., 1987). In dogs ANF has been infused over a wide dose range, and hypotensive effects have consistently occurred at doses of 100 ng/kg/min and above (Zimmerman *et al.*, 1987; Bie *et al.*, 1988; Iwanga *et al.*, 1988; Lee & Goldman, 1989). The fall in blood pressure is accompanied by an increase in heart rate (Zimmerman *et al.*, 1987; Bie *et al.*, 1988; Iwanga *et al.*, 1988; Lee & Goldman, 1989). ANF has also been infused into sheep at a rate of 300 ng/kg/min, causing a 9% fall in blood pressure and a

16% rise in heart rate (Breuhaus et al., 1985).

High-dose infusions, as employed in the short-term studies discussed above, produce plasma ANF levels well outside the pathophysiological range (Bie et al., 1988). The effects of lower doses on arterial blood pressure have been studied in rats, dogs and sheep during long-term administration of ANF. A low-dose infusion at 20 ng/kg/min produced plasma ANF levels within the physiological range and caused a progressive fall in blood pressure over 3 days in spontaneously hypertensive rats, but not in normotensive rats (DeMey et al., 1987). In dogs an infusion rate of 50 ng/kg/min produced slightly higher plasma levels, but still within the pathophysiological range, and reduced mean arterial pressure by 15 mmHg after 4 days (Granger et al., 1986). In sheep an even lower dose, 10 ng/kg/min for 5 days, had no hypotensive effect on the first day, but caused a progressive reduction in blood pressure over subsequent days (Parkes et al., 1988).

Human studies

Numerous studies have evaluated the effect of ANF on arterial pressure in man. ANF has usually been given intravenously either by bolus or infusion or both. In some cases the infusion has involved incremental doses of the peptide. Interpretation of these studies is hampered by the frequent lack of placebo controls (i.e. 'baseline', before, and after values have been compared), inconsistent method of blood pressure measurement (cuff v. intra-arterial cannula) and failure to control diet or maintain a given posture during the study. The threshold dose for reduction in arterial pressure by bolus injection appears to be 50 μg. Most infusion studies suggest that the threshold dose for reduction in arterial pressure is 50 ng/kg/min. Two studies, however, suggest that doses of ANF as low as 2–3 ng/kg/min may lower blood pressure (Richards et al., 1988b; Shenker, 1988). ANF appears to have no more consistent effect on systolic than diastolic blood pressure in man.

Sodium status

Weidmann and colleagues (1986a,b) have evaluated the effect of ANF on blood pressure during a low (17 mmol/day), normal (140 mmol/day) and high (310 mmol/day) dietary sodium intake. ANF 90 ng/kg/min for 45 min lowered arterial pressure to a comparable degree in all three groups, despite causing a greater reduction in plasma volume during the high-salt diet. Cuneo et al. (1987) reported that ANF 50 ng/kg/min had no significant effect on blood pressure in six male subjects whether studied on 10 mmol/day or 200 mmol/day sodium diets.

Posture

In many reported studies subjects have been studied supine and in others while seated (often standing intermittently). Some groups have, however, specifically evaluated the effect of posture on the blood pressure response to ANF administration. Cody *et al.* (1986) found that ANF 120 ng/kg/min lowered systolic arterial pressure (SBP) in seated volunteers but not in supine volunteers. Allen, Ang & Bennett (1989) found that ANF 200 ng/kg/min lowered SBP only during 80° passive head-up tilt and not when subjects were supine. By contrast, Williams *et al.* (1988) found that ANF 5 ng/kg/min had no effect on blood pressure in either the supine position or after 45° head-up tilt for 2 h. These findings suggest that high doses of ANF have more effect on arterial pressure when given to erect rather than supine subjects.

Effects of ANF on total vascular resistance

Early investigators attributed the hypotensive action of ANF to arterial vasodilatation (Kleinert, 1984; Winquist *et al.*, 1984; Garcia *et al.*, 1985). More recently this traditional view has been questioned and some doubt exists as to whether ANF lowers total vascular resistance when infused into intact experimental animals (Gellai, Allen & Beeuwkes, 1986) or human volunteers (Cody *et al.*, 1986).

In rats the fall in blood pressure following ANF administration is associated with an increase in systemic vascular resistance (SVR) (Lappe *et al.*, 1985; Gellai *et al.*, 1986; Chien *et al.*, 1987; Criscione *et al.*, 1987). Short-term infusion in sheep at a rate of 300 ng/kg/min, caused a 9% fall in blood pressure and a 13% rise in total peripheral resistance (Breuhaus *et al.*, 1985). Similarly in dogs, reduction of blood pressure by infusion of ANF is associated with an increase (Zimmerman *et al.*, 1987; Bie *et al.*, 1988; Iwanga *et al.*, 1988) or no change in SVR (Lee & Goldman, 1989). In normal human volunteers, Cody *et al.* (1986) found no change in SVR during ANF infusion on invasive haemodynamic assessment. Similarly Morice *et al.* (1988), using electrical bioimpedance cardiography, found no change in calculated SVR. By contrast Hynynen *et al.* (1988) and Allen *et al.* (1989) both found a fall in peripheral resistance using Doppler echocardiographic techniques.

Thus in experimental animals the fall in blood pressure during short-term infusions of ANF cannot be attributed to vasodilatation, and in man the evidence suggesting a fall in SVR is controversial and based on non-invasive haemodynamic monitoring. However the situation may be different if ANF is infused over a prolonged period. Parkes *et al.* (1988) administered a very low dose of 10 ng/kg/min over 5 days to five sheep. On the first day a fall in cardiac output was associated with a rise in SVR and little change in blood pressure. However over subsequent days SVR and blood pressure fell progressively. Thus the fall in blood pressure during long-term low-dose ANF infusion may be due to arterial vasodilatation, but controlled studies in animals and man will be necessary to confirm this.

Effects of ANF on ventricular function

Invasive haemodynamic studies of the short-term effects of ANF infusion in rats, rabbits, dogs and sheep have demonstrated a fall in cardiac output of between 14% and 39% (Breuhaus *et al.*, 1985; Lappe *et al.*, 1985; Almeida, Suzaki & Maack, 1986; Chien *et al.*, 1987; Criscione *et al.*, 1987; Zimmerman *et al.*, 1987; Iwanga *et al.*, 1988; Volpe *et al.*, 1988b; Lee & Goldman, 1989; Woods, Oliver & Korner, 1989). During a 5-day infusion of ANF at low dosage in conscious sheep, a fall in cardiac output was noted during the first 24 h, followed by a gradual return to the pre-infusion value (Parkes *et al.*, 1988). In an invasive haemodynamic study of normal human volunteers Cody *et al.* (1986) found no change in cardiac output following ANF. Non-invasive studies have demonstrated both falls (Morice *et al.*, 1988; Roy *et al.*, 1989), and increases (Allen *et al.*, 1988, 1989; Floras 1987; Hynynen *et al.*, 1988) in stroke volume and cardiac output following ANF.

The fall in blood pressure and cardiac output noted in these studies lead to the suggestion that ANF possessed either direct, or indirect negative inotropic properties. However a study of rat hearts, both *in vivo* and using isolated ventricular muscle strips, showed no depressant effect of ANF (Criscione *et al.*, 1987). Similarly in dogs infusion of ANF in doses from 100 to 300 ng/kg/min does not affect left ventricular contractility (Iwanga *et al.*, 1988; Lee & Goldman, 1989), and intracoronary infusion of ANF is also without effect (Iwanga *et al.*, 1988). The only detailed study in man was performed by Indolfi *et al.* (1989). ANF infusion at a rate of 50 ng/kg/min lowered mean blood pressure and ventricular dimensions, but did not affect indices of contractility. Therefore ANF appears to reduce cardiac output in animals, and possibly also in normal man, but this is not due to a negative inotropic effect.

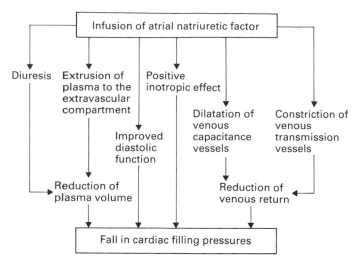

Fig. 4.1 Possible mechanisms to explain the fall in cardiac filling pressures produced by ANF.

Effects of ANF on cardiac filling pressures

Preload

One of the few consistent findings from studies of the effects of ANF *in vivo* is a reduction of cardiac filling pressures. The reduction of cardiac output during ANF infusion in the animal studies discussed above can be entirely explained by the simultaneous fall in cardiac preload. A fall in filling pressure has been demonstrated in rats (Lappe *et al.*, 1985; Almeida *et al.*, 1986; Trippodo *et al.*, 1986; Chien *et al.*, 1987; Criscione *et al.*, 1987), rabbits (Volpe *et al.*, 1988b; Woods *et al.*, 1989), dogs (Shapiro *et al.*, 1986; Zimmerman *et al.*, 1987; Bie *et al.*, 1988; Iwanga *et al.*, 1988; Lee & Goldman, 1989) and sheep (Breuhaus *et al.*, 1985). The dose of ANF administered to these experimental animals has varied from as little as 2.5 ng/kg/min to 4000 ng/kg/min. In a dose-ranging study in dogs, the minimum infusion rate required to reduce right atrial pressure significantly was 5 ng/kg/min, and increases in infusion rate beyond 10 ng/kg/min did not cause any further fall in filling pressure.

ANF infusion also reduces cardiac filling pressures in normal human subjects. Cody *et al.* (1986) reported that ANF 100 ng/kg/min reduced pulmonary capillary wedge pressure from 11 to 7 mmHg. This, and many other studies have shown that ANF also decreases central venous pressure (Takeshita *et al.*, 1987; Elbert *et al.*, 1988; Volpe *et al.*, 1988a; Groban *et al.*, 1989). The reduction in preload is accompanied by decreased ventricular volumes as measured by angiography (Indolfi *et al.*, 1989). Thus ANF infusion consistently reduces cardiac preload in animals and man, although the mechanism of this effect is not clear (see below).

Mechanism of reduction in preload

The possible causes of a reduction in cardiac filling pressures are summarized in Fig. 4.1. There is no evidence to support the concept that ANF has positive inotropic effects (Zimmerman *et al.*, 1987; Iwanga *et al.*, 1988; Indolfi *et al.*, 1989; Woods *et al.*, 1989). If improvement in left ventricular diastolic relaxation was an important mechanism then an increase in left ventricular end diastolic dimensions should be apparent during ANF infusion. This is not the case, in fact the opposite has been reported in animal experiments (Iwanga *et al.*, 1988; Lee & Goldman, 1989) and in man (Indolfi *et al.*, 1989; Roy *et al.*, 1989). Therefore, the fall in cardiac filling pressures induced by ANF infusion is not due to an improvement in left ventricular systolic or diastolic function. Two possibilities remain: either a reduction in plasma volume, or a direct effect on veins leading to reduced venous return to the heart. These will be considered in turn.

Reduction of plasma volume

The simplest way of measuring short-term changes in plasma volume is to monitor the haematocrit since acute removal of plasma from the intravascular compartment leads to a proportional increase in haematocrit. This method is relatively insensitive and assumes a constant circulating red cell volume, so it can be affected by sequestration of cells in the spleen. Despite these limitations it has proved a useful method of studying the effects of ANF on plasma volume. A rise in haematocrit has been a consistent finding in studies of rats, rabbits and dogs (Fluckeger *et al.*, 1986; Trippodo *et al.*, 1986; Zimmerman *et al.*, 1987; Lee & Goldman, 1989; Williamson *et al.*, 1989). The fall in plasma volume as estimated from haematocrit measurements has ranged from 4% to 16%, with a mean of 9%. In a recent study of rats direct measurements of blood volume were made by radioisotope dilution, and a mean reduction in blood volume of 2.2 ml/kg occurred 15 min after a bolus of 30 μg/kg ANF (Sugimoto *et al.*, 1989). In rats, the minimum infusion rate of ANF required to significantly reduce plasma volume is approximately 100 ng/kg/min, and the effect is seen after 5–10 min of infusion, reaching a plateau after 30 min (Williamson *et al.*, 1989).

In man many investigators have also shown that ANF increases haematocrit (usually 3–12%) and plasma protein concentration (Weidmann *et al.*, 1986a,b; Richards *et al.*, 1988a; Solomon *et al.*, 1988; Roy *et al.*, 1989). These changes suggest a reduction in plasma volume of

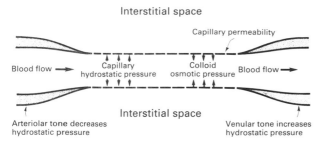

Fig. 4.2   Factors affecting flow of fluid in and out of capillaries.

approximately 10%, or net haemoconcentration (after allowing for urinary losses) of about 300 ml (Weidmann *et al.*, 1986b; Allen *et al.*, 1989). Reduction in plasma volume occurs within 15 min of initiation of ANF infusion, and has been described with doses as low as 4 ng/kg/min. A greater fall in plasma volume occurs when ANF is given to subjects on a high, as opposed to a low, salt diet and when subjects are seated or upright rather than supine (Cody *et al.*, 1986; Gnadinger *et al.*, 1986).

The mechanism through which ANF reduces plasma volume is poorly understood. The diuresis may contribute, but changes in plasma volume have been seen in studies where little or no diuresis was apparent (Richards *et al.*, 1988a; Allen *et al.*, 1989). Furthermore, a fall in plasma volume has been described in nephrectomized animals (Almeida *et al.*, 1986; Fluckeger *et al.*, 1986; Trippodo *et al.*, 1986; Volpe *et al.*, 1988b; Williamson *et al.*, 1989). Likewise splenectomy does not prevent this effect (Fluckeger *et al.*, 1986; Woods *et al.*, 1989). Therefore, the reduction in plasma volume is likely to be due to a shift of fluid from the intravascular to the extravascular compartment (Williamson *et al.*, 1989). The factors affecting the flow of fluid out of and back into capillaries are shown in Fig. 4.2. The net loss of fluid from the intravascular compartment depends upon the capillary hydrostatic pressure, capillary permeability and plasma oncotic pressure. Infusion of ANF could affect hydrostatic pressure at capillary level by dilating precapillary arterioles, or constricting the venous side of the capillary bed. Alternatively the peptide could directly increase capillary permeability to albumin, and this effect has been demonstrated *in vitro* (Huxley *et al.*, 1987).

The evidence from *in vivo* studies is somewhat conflicting. Two studies have shown no effect on capillary permeability in the rat mesentery or dog forelimb, despite infusion of high hypotensive doses of ANF (Smits *et al.*, 1987; Eliades *et al.*, 1989). On the other hand in rats the relative increase in plasma protein is less than the rise in haematocrit with ANF, indicating increased capillary permeability to plasma constituents (Valentin, Ribstein & Mimran, 1988; Sugimoto *et al.*, 1989). A recent well conducted study demonstrated   increased   vascular   permeability   in   multiple   tissues

(Williamson *et al.*, 1989). Important differences were seen in this study between the effects of ANF on different tissues. The peptide caused a two- to fivefold increase in the permeation of radiolabelled albumin in spleen, gut, kidney, skin and muscle, but had no effect on brain, lung and liver (Williamson *et al.*, 1989).

Venous effects of ANF

ANF has no direct effect on venous tone *in vitro* (see above). *In vivo* the relationship between venous tone and central cardiac filling pressures is complex. The rate of return of blood to the heart depends on both venous capacitance and the resistance to venous return which is a function of the tone of larger veins. ANF infusion has been shown not to increase venous capacitance in animal studies (Trippodo *et al.*, 1986; Lee & Goldman, 1989). However, it does appear to increase the resistance to venous return in rats and dogs, presumably via venoconstriction (Chien *et al.*, 1987; Lee & Goldman, 1989).

Unfortunately determination of resistance to venous return depends upon measurement of mean circulating filling pressure which in turn demands complete circulatory arrest. In animal studies this has been achieved by blowing up a balloon in the right atrium, so it is unlikely that these observations will be verified in human volunteers! However three groups have examined the effects of ANF on human veins by infusing it locally into a dosal hand vein. In doses up to 0.25 μg/min, ANF has no effect on resting tone, reflex venoconstriction or on serotonin, noradrenaline or phenylephrine preconstriction (Ford *et al.*, 1988; Webb *et al.*, 1988). In addition, Sato *et al.* (1988) reported, in a preliminary communication, that systemic infusion of ANF does not increase forearm venous capacitance.

In conclusion, ANF infusion has consistently been found to reduce cardiac filling pressures in all experimental animals studied so far and in normal human volunteers. Two effects of the peptide contribute to this observation. The first and probably most significant effect is a reduction in plasma volume primarily due to a shift of fluid from the intravascular to the extravascular space. The second is a direct effect on veins. ANF does not increase venous capacitance, but may increase the resistance to venous return from the peripheral circulation back to the heart.

Effect of ANF on regional vascular resistance

Although short-term infusion of ANF does not decrease total peripheral vascular resistance, the peptide could still cause vasodilatation of certain vascular beds. This effect could easily be disguised by reflex vaso- constriction in other vascular beds if only total peripheral resistance is considered. Therefore, the effects of ANF on regional blood flow have been studied in rats by central venous injection of radioactive microspheres, and in larger experimental animals by implantation of electromagnetic or Doppler flow probes. There is a limited amount of information available on the effect of ANF on regional blood flow in man. The techniques available to measure regional blood flow non-invasively are imprecise. In addition the posture and sodium–volume–hormonal status is not standardized between studies, making comparison difficult.

Skeletal muscle blood flow

Garcia *et al.* (1985) studied the effects of a 1-μg bolus of ANF on regional blood flow in rats using radioactive microspheres and found no change in muscle blood flow. In a second study using rats chronically instrumented with flow probes, infusion of ANF in doses from 250–4000 ng/kg/min reduced both total cardiac output and hindquarters blood flow to a similar degree (Lappe *et al.*, 1985). In dogs ANF infusion (300–10 000 ng/kg/min) has no effect on muscle blood flow measured by injection of microspheres (Shapiro *et al.*, 1986; Lee & Goldman, 1989). Bolus doses of the peptide (5 μg/kg) are similarly without effect on iliac blood flow measured with flow probes (Hintze, Currie & Needleman, 1985).

Infusion of ANF in man (15 ng/kg/min for first hour and 50 ng/kg/min for second hour, each preceded by a 50-μg bolus) has no effect on forearm vascular resistance (Roy *et al.*, 1989). However the effects of systemic infusions are difficult to interpret because cardiovascular reflexes (see below) may obscure any local actions of the peptide. Therefore four groups have studied the effects of brachial arterial infusion of ANF in man (Hughes *et al.*, 1987, 1988, 1989; Bolli *et al.*, 1987; Fujita *et al.*, 1987; Webb *et al.*, 1988). All of these studies have reported dose-dependent decreases in forearm vascular resistance and increases in forearm blood flow (between 150 and 340%). No tolerance to ANF was seen during 60 min of infusion. The threshold dose appears to be between 10 and 100 ng/min, with no further response occurring at doses in excess of 5000 ng/min (Fijita *et al.*, 1987; Webb *et al.*, 1988). Even the lowest doses infused (10 and 50 ng/min), associated with a marginal (10%) increase in forearm blood flow, resulted in plasma ANF concentrations above the physiological range (150–750 pg/ml, Webb *et al.*, 1988). Therefore, in contrast to the results of systemic infusion of the peptide, these studies suggest that ANF given locally into the human brachial artery acts as a direct vasodilator. However this effect is only prominent when supraphysiological plasma levels are obtained.

Skin blood flow

In rats Garcia *et al.* (1985) found that a 1-µg bolus of ANF increased skin blood flow measured by radioactive microspheres, but the change was not statistically significant. In a 15-min incremental dose-ranging study in man, ANF 2–40 µg/min caused a progressive increase in forearm skin blood flow as measured with a laser Doppler flowmeter (Biollaz *et al.*, 1986a). The rise in skin blood flow was coincident with a fall in arterial pressure and rise in heart rate. However, in a subsequent study the same group found that a 4-h constant rate infusion of ANF 1 µg/min initially increased skin blood flow as before, but this declined again after 1 h, eventually falling below baseline levels by the end of the infusion (Biollaz *et al.*, 1988). Interestingly, Webb *et al.* (1988) also found that forearm skin blood flow, measured in a similar way, increased during brachial arterial infusion of ANF.

Hepatic blood flow

ANF does not increase total mesenteric or hepatic blood flow in rats (Garcia *et al.*, 1985; Lappe *et al.*, 1985). In dogs, infusion of the peptide in a dose of 300–10000 ng/kg/min has no effect on hepatic blood flow measured by radioactive microspheres (Shapiro *et al.*, 1986; Lee & Goldman, 1989). In a study of human volunteers ANF infused at 7.5 ng/kg/min for 2 h caused a 21 % reduction in apparent hepatic blood flow as measured by clearance of indocyanine green (Biollaz *et al.*, 1986b). Blood pressure remained constant during this study and the circulating concentrations of angiotensin II and arginine vasopressin were unchanged (noradrenaline was not measured).

Renal blood flow

Early experiments in rats with bolus doses of ANF suggested an increase in renal blood flow (Garcia *et al.*, 1985; Wakitani *et al.*, 1985). However, subsequent studies using a range of infusion rates from 30 to 4000 ng/kg/min and incorporating direct measurements of renal blood flow have failed to confirm this, and in fact demonstrated significant falls in flow to the kidneys of rats (Lappe *et al.*, 1985; Gellai *et al.*, 1986; Criscione *et al.*, 1987). Different results have been obtained when dogs have been studied. Relatively high dose systemic infusions of ANF (300 ng/kg/min) increase renal blood flow, even though total peripheral resistance rises or does not change (Hintze *et al.*, 1985; Ishihara *et al.*, 1985; Zimmerman *et al.*, 1987; Lee & Goldman, 1989).

On the other hand, ANF consistently reduces PAH clearance in man. Janssen *et al.* (1989) have recently demonstrated that ANF does not change the renal extraction of PAH in man and that the decline in PAH clearance usually reported reflects a true reduction in renal blood flow. This effect has been observed with doses as low as 6 ng/kg/min (Richards *et al.*, 1988) which generally have no effect on arterial pressure or vasoconstrictor hormones. This regional circulatory effect would be consistent with the known action of ANF to cause afferent glomerular arteriolar dilatation and efferent arteriolar constriction.

Coronary blood flow

The effect of ANF on the coronary circulation has been studied by local administration of the peptide in dogs (Bach *et al.*, 1988; Iwanga *et al.*, 1988; Adachi *et al.*, 1989). Large intracoronary bolus doses of ANF reduce coronary vascular resistance by up to 27%, but infusion of the peptide has no effect (Bach *et al.*, 1988; Iwanga *et al.*, 1988; Adachi *et al.*, 1989).

Cerebral blood flow

ANF has no effect on cerebral blood flow when administered as a bolus dose to conscious rats or anaesthetized dogs (Garcia *et al.*, 1985; Ishihara *et al.*, 1985). Biollaz *et al.* (1986b) also found that carotid blood flow in normal subjects did not change after a 2-h infusion of ANF 2 μg/min.

Retinal arterial circulation

Mann *et al.* (1987) have used fluorescein photography to report on the *in vivo* effects of ANF (1 μg/kg bolus given over 60 s) on the retinal arterial tree. ANF, given in this way, had a variable effect on vessel calibre. The largest retinal arteries (first-order arteries) uniformly increased in diameter. A high proportion of second- and third-order arteries also dilated. By contrast, fourth-order arteries generally showed a reduction in calibre. This latter observation is interesting as the dose of ANF used had no effect on arterial pressure and retinal vessels are poorly innervated by comparison to other regional circulations.

Mechanisms of ANF-induced vasodilatation

In attempting to understand the vascular effects of ANF, interactions with other vasoconstrictor and vasodilator mechanisms must be considered. Obviously the effects of ANF could be mediated solely by antagonizing one or more of the former or by promotion of the latter. Most evidence, however, would suggest that ANF has direct actions of its own possibly mediated through a second messenger, though these actions may be modulated by other neuroendocrine effects.

Cyclic guanyl monophosphate (cGMP)

cGMP is widely accepted as the active second messenger of ANF (see cellular mechanisms of action in vascular smooth muscle). Several studies have examined the effect of local and systemic ANF infusion on plasma cGMP in man. Fujita *et al.* (1987) reported that ANF (20, 100, 500 ng/min incremental doses) given intra-arterially (brachial) produced a significant increase in cGMP in the ipsilateral forearm venous effluent (which was partially inhibited by coinfusion of calcium chloride). Intravenous infusion of ANF, even at a low non-hypotensive dose, elevates plasma and urinary cGMP levels (Gerzer *et al.*, 1985; Ohashi *et al.*, 1986b; Cusson *et al.*, 1987, 1988, 1989; Miyamori *et al.*, 1987; Richards *et al.*, 1988a; Roy *et al.*, 1989). The rise in plasma cGMP appears to persist for some time after ANF levels have returned to normal (Gertzer *et al.*, 1985; Ohashi *et al.*, 1986b). Non-steroidal anti-inflammatory drugs do not appear to inhibit the plasma increment in cGMP and ACE inhibitors do not attenuate the increase in urinary cGMP (Miyamori *et al.*, 1987; Wambach *et al.*, 1989). The precise role of cGMP is considered in more detail in the following section on cellular action of ANF in vascular smooth muscle.

Role of calcium

Calcium is essential for muscular contraction (see cellular mechanism of action) and may therefore influence the vascular response to ANF. Fujita *et al.* (1987) reported that arterial coinfusion of iso-osmolar calcium chloride blunted the forearm vasodilator response to ANF (incremental doses of 20, 100 and 500 ng/min). This diminished vascular effect was associated with a reduced efflux of cGMP. No studies employing a hypotensive dose of ANF during calcium channel blockade have been reported in normal human subjects.

Renin–angiotensin system

The potential interaction between ANF and the renin–angiotensin system (RAS) has been examined by many groups. The most common approach has been to coinfuse angiotensin II (ANGII) and ANF. Anderson *et al.* (1986b) administered ANF up to 40 ng/kg/min or placebo, followed by a pressor infusion of ANGII (10 ng/kg/min). Absolute blood pressure following ANGII was lower in the presence of ANF than placebo. The increment in diastolic blood pressure with ANGII was also significantly less with ANF (14 mmHg) than with placebo (21 mmHg). In this study, it is worth noting that the aldosterone response to ANGII was totally abolished by ANF whereas the vascular response to ANGII was only reduced by about 30%. However, subsequent studies have also shown that ANF blunts both the absolute and incremental pressor responses to ANGII infusion (Vierhapper, Nowotony & Waldhausl, 1986; Oelkers, Kleiner & Bahr, 1988).

Two groups have employed the opposite experimental format. Uehlinger et al. (1986) found that ANF (10, 40 and 75 μg intravenous boluses) had only a marginal effect on DBP in subjects preinfused with ANGII to elevate MAP by 20 mmHg (mean dose 15 ng/kg/min). Rakugi and colleagues (1989) administered ANF 100 ng/kg/min during coinfusion of ANGII 10 ng/kg/min or placebo. ANF caused a similar percentage reduction in BP in both circumstances.

These studies do not support a specific interaction but suggest that ANF and ANGII probably have opposite but independent effects on blood pressure. If a sufficient dose of ANF is given it seems that the pressor effect of ANGII can be completely inhibited and vice versa. However, in all these studies pharmacological responses have been investigated and physiological doses of both peptides may have no effect on blood pressure, either alone or in combination, at least in the short term (Cuneo et al., 1987).

A second approach to the study of an interaction between ANF and the RAS has been to employ ACE inhibitors. The peptide has been administered to rabbits following 'total neurohormonal blockade' with a cocktail of drugs including a ganglion blocker, muscarinic receptor blocker, converting enzyme inhibitor and vasopressin antagonist along with an infusion of noradrenaline and ANGII to maintain the blood pressure. ANF retained its haemodynamic effects, with a fall in blood pressure and cardiac output despite this elaborate pharmacological intervention (Woods et al., 1989). The effects of ANF following ACE inhibition have also been investigated in normal human subjects, however these studies have not been designed primarily to examine vascular effects. In some of these studies ANF alone did not affect arterial pressure (Gaillard, Koomans & Dorhout-Mees, 1988; Gaillard et al., 1989; Richards et al., 1989). In the report of Wilkins and colleagues (1987) ANF 35 ng/kg/min appeared to significantly lower blood pressure after pretreatment with captopril 25 mg compared to pretreatment with placebo. Rakugi et al. (1989) found that blood pressure fell after enalapril 20 mg pretreatment in subjects given ANF 100 ng/kg/min for 60 min. ANF without pretreatment reduced MAP to 86% of baseline and to 92% of a lower baseline following enalapril pretreatment. Of greater interest, Hughes et al. (1988) demonstrated that captopril 50 mg did not affect the forearm vascular response to intra-arterial (brachial) infusion of ANF 0.1–10 μg/min.

These findings are hard to interpret but suggest overall that ANF continues to have a hypotensive and vasodilator effect even when systemic

ANGII levels have been reduced acutely by ACE inhibition. More definitive studies need to be conducted in this area.

Sympathetic nervous system

Various pharmacological manoeuvres have been used in an attempt to separate the direct cardiovascular effects of ANF from those secondary to interaction with the sympathetic nervous system. Partial ganglionic blockade with trimethaphan camsylate was employed to prevent reflex sympathetic neuronal responses in conscious sheep. Ganglionic blockade did not affect the ANF-induced fall in cardiac output, but by preventing the reflex increase in peripheral resistance it potentiated (threefold) the fall in systemic arterial pressure. Uehlinger et al. (1986) infused noradrenaline (NA) at a dose (mean 153 ng/kg/min) sufficient to increase MAP by 20 mmHg in normal volunteers. Successive bolus injections of ANF 10, 40 and 75 μg progressively lowered both SBP and DBP. However, in another study noradrenaline 50 ng/kg/min appeared to prevent the reduction in MAP seen with ANF 1 μg/min given for 6 h (Vierhapper & Nowotny, 1987).

Intra-arterial infusion of noradrenaline 0.3, 0.6, 1.2, 3, 8 and 20 ng dose dependently antagonizes the forearm vasodilator effect of ANF 0.0375–1.5 μg (Bolli et al., 1986). Conversely Takeshita et al. (1987) found that intravenous infusion of ANF 30 μg/kg/min did not significantly affect the forearm vasoconstrictor response to intra-arterial (brachial) noradrenaline 100, 200 and 500 ng/min. While it is appealing to propose that these findings suggest that noradrenaline can antagonize the vascular effects of ANF the truth of the matter is that sufficiently good data are lacking to draw any firm conclusions. As with ANGII properly controlled dose–response studies are still needed.

Arginine vasopressin

There is even less information available on the potential vascular interactions between ANF and arginine vasopressin (AVP). Brown & Corr (1987) reported that ANF 40 ng/kg/min caused a fall in arterial pressure despite coincident infusion of AVP 5.5×10^{-7} i.u./kg/min though no non-AVP control day was included. There have been no reports of local arterial infusion of ANF and AVP.

Prostaglandins

Brown et al. (1987) reported that immediate pretreatment with intravenous indomethacin did not affect the hypotensive response to ANF 40 ng/kg/min. However, Miyamori et al. (1987) reported that treatment with indomethacin 150 mg 3 times daily for 1 week attenuated the hypotensive response to ANF infused at 12.5, 25, 50 and 100 ng/kg/min, 20 min for each increment. Clearly in this area too, more work is needed.

Dopamine

Dopamine and ANF, superficially, seem to share similar properties. Consequently several groups have looked for an interaction between ANF and dopamine. Allen et al. (1988) reported that 60 mg of domperidone, a DA_2-specific dopamine antagonist, raised baseline arterial pressure but did not appear to affect the hypotensive effect of subsequently infused ANF 5 μg/min. The effects of DA_1-receptor antagonism and dopamine decarboxylase inhibition on the hypotensive response to ANF have not been reported. Hughes et al. (1988) found that coadministration of intra-arterial (brachial) (R)-sulpiride (a DA_1-specific antagonist) 100 μg/min did not affect the forearm vasodilator response to ANF 0.01–1.0 μg/min.

Thus the limited information available from systemic and local administration studies suggests that the vascular and haemodynamic effects of ANF are not dependent on stimulation of dopamine production, or facilitation of its actions.

Influence of ANF on baroreflexes

ANF may also exert an effect on vascular tone and responsiveness by modulating baroreflexes. Such an action could arise from the effect of circulating ANF or local production of the peptide; the latter is suggested by the expression of the ANF gene in the aortic arch (Gardner, Deschepper & Baxter, 1987).

Lower body negative pressure

Four groups have examined the effects of ANF on the vascular and haemodynamic responses to activation of the low-pressure (or cardio-pulmonary) baroreceptors using the technique of lower body negative pressure (LBNP). Takeshita et al. (1987) found that ANF 30 μg/kg/min attenuated the reflex increase in forearm vascular resistance (FVR) after −10, −20 and −40 mmHg of LBNP. These observations have been supported by Iman et al. (1989) but contradicted by Volpe and colleagues (1988a). The latter workers performed LBNP at −20 mmHg for 15 min. ANF (0.5 μg/kg bolus plus 50 ng/kg/min) in this study augmented the increase in FVR compared to placebo infusion. Another study has recently found that ANF (50-μg bolus plus 50 ng/kg/min for 20 min) does not affect the FVR response to −40 mmHg LBNP (Floras et al., 1988).

There are no explanations immediately apparent in these reports to account for the discrepancy between their findings. All four studies do, however, agree on one interesting point. In each, preinfusion of ANF prior to LBNP did not appear to change FVR; yet in the two studies where it was measured, ANF caused a decrease in central venous pressure similar to that seen with LBNP at -10 to -20 mmHg. This degree of LBNP on the control days was sufficient to cause a significant reflex increase in FVR. This also highlights a deficiency common to all three studies in that starting CVP, prior to LBNP, was very different on the control and ANF study days and thus fell to very different nadirs on these days. The weight of evidence here seems to suggest that ANF infusion results in a relatively lower basal forearm vascular tone for a given CVP. This could result from either a local vasodilator effect of ANF (which is possible at the doses used), or inhibition of reflex vasoconstrictor outflow.

Carotid baroreceptors and heart rate response

The increase in total peripheral resistance during high-dose ANF infusion in experimental animals is probably due to baroreceptor-mediated increases in sympathetic nervous activity (Goetz, 1988). However ANF infusion does not cause a tachycardia in rats, rabbits or dogs despite a significant fall in blood pressure (Chien et al., 1987; Zimmerman et al., 1987; Lee & Goldman, 1989; Woods et al., 1989). This may be explained by the observation of Ferrari et al. (1988) that ANF selectively inhibits the tachycardic response to hypotension in the rat, without affecting the pressor response to carotid occlusion. In other words, ANF-induced hypotension in experimental animals leads to a baroreceptor-mediated increase in total peripheral resistance, whilst simultaneously inhibiting the baroreceptor-mediated heart rate response.

In man, ANF blunts the reflex tachycardia obtained by applying $+20$ mmHg neck pressure, and tends to augment the reflex bradycardia associated with -40 mmHg neck suction (Elbert & Cowley, 1988). These findings could reflect an effect of ANF on afferent, efferent or both reflex pathways (see reflex sympathetic activation below).

Head-up tilt

Williams et al. (1988a) examined the effect of ANF 3.75 ng/kg/min on the reflex haemodynamic responses to 2 h 45° head-up tilt. DBP and HR increased and these responses were unchanged by ANF infusion. ANF did not affect the rise in noradrenaline seen with tilt but did inhibit the reflex increases in plasma renin activity and arginine vasopressin; this occurred despite the additional hypovolaemic stimulus of ANF (7% fall in plasma volume with tilt: 18% fall with tilt plus ANF). There was no attentuation of the reflex tachycardia caused by upright tilt; indeed there was a trend for the increase in heart rate to be enhanced. This study shows that ANF can inhibit some of the reflex mechanisms which affect vascular tone.

Reflex sympathetic action

In man, sufficiently hypotensive doses of ANF can increase circulating noradrenaline though this is an insensitive marker of sympathetic neural activity. Elbert *et al.* (1988) have also shown that reduction in CVP alone, by ANF 1500 ng/kg/min, can increase reflex sympathetic outflow, as measured by direct recording of peroneal nerve activity (PNA). Restoration of CVP, by head-down tilt or lower body positive pressure, abolished this adrenergic activation.

The key question is, however, whether the magnitude of the adrenergic response is appropriate for the magnitude of the haemodynamic stimulus. Floras and colleagues (1988) have addressed this. In a preliminary report, these authors confirmed that ANF (50-μg bolus plus 50 ng/kg/min) lowered CVP and DBP, whilst increasing peroneal nerve activity. However, the increase in peroneal nerve activity (and in plasma noradrenaline) was less than that seen with a dose of sodium nitroprusside (SNP) having similar haemodynamic effects. This dose of ANF also reduced the sympathetic response to a cold pressor test. This study, if confirmed, would support the view that ANF can relatively attenuate sympathetic outflow in man.

Vascular distribution of ANF receptors

Binding sites for ANF are present in many tissues including the kidney, adrenal, liver, small intestine, colon, lung and blood vessels (Bianchi *et al.*, 1985; Von Schroeder *et al.*, 1985). A high concentration of binding sites can be demonstrated in rat vascular tissues, particularly the aorta, large and small renal arteries and veins. The vascular binding sites are localized to endothelial and smooth muscle cells (Bianchi *et al.*, 1985; Von Schroeder *et al.*, 1985).

A study of the binding of ANF to its receptor in crude tissue extracts from rat blood vessels demonstrated a single high-affinity receptor with a K_D of 0.1 nmol/l (Schiffrin *et al.*, 1985). A single high-affinity ANF receptor with a similar K_D has also been demonstrated on cultured endothelial cells (Vlasuk *et al.*, 1986). Since ANF-mediated vasodilatation of large arteries *in vitro* is not dependent upon an intact endothelium (Winquist *et al.*, 1984b; Ishihara *et al.*, 1985) it is interesting to speculate upon the role of the endothelial ANF receptor. This could represent a 'clearance' receptor, whose role is to remove ANF from the circulation once it has produced the desired effect (Maack *et al.*, 1987). It is also possible that ANF-induced peripheral vasodilatation *in vivo* is mediated

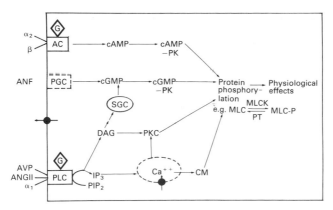

Fig. 4.3   Mechanisms regulating vascular tone. ---, smooth endoplasmic reticulum; -●-, calcium ATPase; AC, adenylate cyclase; PLC, phospholipase C; G, guanylate cyclase regulatory subunit; PGC, particulate guanylate cyclase; SGC, soluble guanylate cyclase; IP_3, inositol 1,4,5-triphosphate; PIP_2, phosphoinositol 4,5-biphosphate; -PK, phosphokinase; CM, calmodulin; PKC, phosphokinase C; PT, phosphatase; MLC, myosin light chain; MLC-P, phosphorylated myosin light chain; MLCK, myosin light chain kinase; DAG, diacylglycerol.

through endothelial mechanisms: either stimulation of EDRF production or inhibition of endothelin release (Parkes *et al.*, 1988). Finally, this receptor may be involved in the control of capillary permeability and thereby mediate the fall in plasma volume during ANF infusion (Vlasuk *et al.*, 1986; Valentin *et al.*, 1988).

Cellular action of ANF in vascular smooth muscle

cGMP stimulation

It is now widely believed that the vasodilator effect of ANF is mediated by cGMP (Fig. 4.3). ANF causes a rise in intracellular cGMP which bears a temporal relationship to the development of vasodilatation, and there is a proportional relationship between the magnitude of cytoplasmic cGMP production and the degree of vasorelaxation. The rise in cGMP occurs because of stimulation of particulate rather than soluble guanylate cyclase (GC) activity and not through inhibition of cGMP degradation.

Mechanism of vascular smooth muscle contraction

To understand how ANF causes vasorelaxation some explanation of the mechanisms regulating vascular tone is necessary (Fig. 4.3). Vascular smooth muscle (VSM) contraction is primarily determined by the concentration of intracellular calcium (Ca_i^{2+}). This in turn is determined by stimulation of receptor-operated, or opening of potential sensitive, calcium channels in the cell membrane promoting extracellular calcium uptake. Cytosolic Ca^{2+} may also rise because of release of Ca^{2+} from intracellular stores. This may be brought about by hydrolysis of membrane phosphatidylinositol. Breakdown of phosphoinositol 4,5-biphosphate (PIP_2) by phospholipase C (PL_C) produces inositol 1,4,5-triphosphate (IP_3) which releases Ca^{2+} from smooth endoplasmic reticulum into the cytosol. Through activation of protein kinase C (PKC) and calmodulin, protein phosphorylation is initiated, ultimately resulting in myocyte contraction. One important step in the contractile process is calcium–calmodulin activation of the enzyme myosin light chain kinase (MLCK) which phosphorylates myosin light chain (MLC). This account of VSM contraction is necessarily much simplified but serves as a model for examining the effects of ANF and cGMP.

How does cGMP cause vasorelaxation?

Possible mechanisms to reduce vascular tone could include inhibition of uptake of extracellular Ca^{2+}, inhibition of Ca^{2+} release from intracellular stores and extrusion of calcium from the cytosol. There is some evidence that ANF may operate through all of these mechanisms (Fig. 4.3.). Several groups have reported that ANF reduces agonist-induced extracellular Ca^{2+} uptake (Hassid, 1986; Taylor & Meisheri, 1986; Takeuchi & Abe, 1989) though this has not been a universal finding (Capponi et al., 1986; Hirata et al., 1988b). Intracellular calcium mobilization takes place as a consequence of the production and action of IP_3. Fujii, Ishimatsu & Kuriyama (1986) and Rapoport (1986) have reported that ANF can inhibit hydrolysis of membrane phosphatidyl inositol (PI). However, Meyer-Helnert et al. (1988) found that ANF (and 8-bromo cGMP) inhibited the increase in Ca_i^{2+}, but IP_3 levels were not reduced (though IP_1, a metabolite of IP_3, was reduced). This is in keeping with the findings of Rapoport et al. (1986). Chiu, Tetzhoff & Sybertz (1986), Fujii et al. (1986) and Meisheri, Taylor & Saneii (1986), have, however, produced evidence that ANF inhibits intracellular liberation of Ca^{2+} whether through inhibition of IP_3 production or antagonism of its effect on the SER. By activation of Ca^{2+} ATPase cytosolic Ca^{2+} can be extruded from the cell or sequestrated into the SER. Popescu et al. (1985) have reported that Ca^{2+} ATPase can be activated by a cGMP-dependent protein kinase.

Myosin light chain phosphorylation

Reduction in cytosolic Ca^{2+} will ultimately decrease MLC phosphorylation, a critical step in myocyte contraction. ANF could also inhibit contraction by encouraging phosphorylation of MLC through an increase in the activity of one or more phosphatases acting at this site.

Rapoport, Draznin & Murad (1982) found that cGMP causes dephosphorylation of protein in rat aorta which is thought to be MLC. Similarly Hirata *et al.* (1989b) have reported that ANF inhibits MLC phosphorylation, though whether this occurs through inhibition of kinase activity or augmentation of phosphatase(s) activity is not known. Interestingly ANF has little if any effect on basal Ca^{2+}, which may explain why its vasodilator effects are mainly seen in preconstricted tissues.

Interaction with other hormones at the cellular level

Much of the above work on cellular Ca^{2+} fluxes has employed agonists such as ANGII and AVP. Several interesting observations on the interaction between ANF and these vasoconstrictors can be made. While ANF may inhibit accumulation of Ca^{2+} caused by ANGII and AVP, some reports suggest that these hormones can reduce ANF-evoked cGMP production (Bingham-Smith & Lincoln, 1987). Bingham-Smith and Lincoln (1987) have suggested that these and other calcium-mobilizing stimuli inhibit cGMP production by activating cyclic nucelotide phospho-diesterase but current evidence is against this (Otsuka *et al.*, 1988; Nakumara *et al.*, 1989). This appears to offer a mechanism by which functional antagonism can exist between ANF and these other vaso-constrictor hormones. These observations also concur with the *in vivo* findings of Fujita *et al.* (1987) (see 'role of calcium in the forearm vascular response to ANF').

It is also of interest that ANF appears to inhibit noradrenaline-induced PI hydrolysis in the rat aorta and rabbit renal artery (Fujii *et al.*, 1986; Rapoport, 1986) but not ANGII- or AVP-mediated PI metabolism in cultured VSM cells from rat aorta (Hirata *et al.*, 1989). This could mean that ANF preferentially inhibits phospholipase C coupled to adrenergic receptors and there is some evidence, *in vitro*, that ANF may preferentially interact with α_1 and not α_2 vasoconstrictor pathways (Faber *et al.*, 1988; Hirata *et al.*, 1989). This suggests the further possibility of selective or specific interactions between ANF and other hormones. It is also of interest that ANF is less effective in inhibiting the rise in Ca^{2+} due to extracellular potassium exposure than it is in attenuating that due to hormonal agonists. This parallels its anti-vasoconstrictor potency *in vitro* (see above).

Role of endothelium

ANF receptors are present on the vascular endothelium (see above) and ANF stimulates cGMP production in these cells (this is the likely origin of circulating cGMP). An intact endothelium is, however, not essential for ANF-induced VSM relaxation *in vitro*. Bonhomme, Cantin & Garcia

(1989) have recently shown that a pharmacological dose of ANF can antagonize the vasoconstrictive effect of endothelin in rabbit mesenteric and aortic strips. The role of the endothelium in the *in vivo* vascular response to ANF is unknown but this recent report from Montreal suggests that this is worthy of further investigation.

Other mechanisms by which ANF could cause smooth muscle relaxation

The best-known cyclic nucleotide second messenger mechanism is the adenylate cyclase–cAMP system which may be involved in vasoconstrictor pathways. Anand-Srivastava *et al.* (1984) found that ANF inhibited both basal and hormonal stimulated adenylate cyclase in vascular tissue. Two other groups, however, have reported that ANF had no effect on adenylate cyclase activity in the rabbit aorta (Winquist *et al.*, 1984; Ohlstein & Berkowitz 1985).

There is also a recent report that ANF may partially mediate its VSM-relaxing effect through activation of the electrogenic Na, K pump (Sato *et al.*, 1988). This mechanism has been previously supported by some (Sybertz & Desideno, 1985) and dismissed by others (Mulvany, 1988). Hegde, DeFeo & Jandhyala (1989) have shown that suppression of Na^+, K^+-ATPase does not affect ANF-induced cGMP production in VSM, suggesting that this mechanism, if it exists, is cGMP-independent.

Just cGMP?—a note of caution

Though most evidence supports the cGMP theory of the vascular effects of ANF, there are several disconcerting reports at variance with this consensus. Budzik *et al.* (1987) have used modified peptide analogues of ANF to separate the cGMP stimulating effect from the vasorelaxant action. Tyrosine replacement of phenylalanine in position 106 of ANF 103–125 resulted in loss of cGMP stimulation yet the peptide retained potent vasorelaxant activity. This finding, and the general observation that 5–10 nM concentrations of ANF are needed to augment cGMP synthesis, require reconciliation before the cGMP theory of action can be fully accepted.

Conclusion

Any discussion of the cardiovascular effects of ANF is complicated by the different doses and modes of administration of the peptide used by various investigators. This probably accounts for some, but not all, of the differences in results and conclusions drawn from different studies. Another important factor is species variability, and in particular cardiovascular responses to ANF in the rat are very different to those in man. Dogs and more especially sheep provide much closer models of human responses.

Despite these problems some fairly certain conclusions can be drawn from the present literature. First, the effects of ANF on large arteries in organ bath experiments are of little value in predicting *in vivo* effects. ANF does not consistently reduce peripheral vascular resistance during systemic infusion, but the predicted baroreceptor-mediated reflex rise in heart rate and peripheral resistance may be attenuated. Regional vascular effects include a reduction of renal blood flow in man and some experimental animals, but not in dogs. The hypotensive effect of ANF is not primarily due to vasodilatation or to a direct negative inotropic effect. Rather it is due to a reduction in cardiac output which is secondary to a decrease in preload and hence also a decrease in cardiac filling pressures. The precise cause of this remains uncertain and further research is required. The diuresis certainly contributes, as does a reduction in plasma volume of approximately 10% due to a shift of fluid from the intravascular to the extravascular compartment. ANF may also increase the resistance to the return of blood from the peripheral circulation to the heart by a direct effect on veins. Despite a vast literature on the cardiovascular effects of ANF, many fundamental questions remain to be answered.

References

Aalkjaer, C., Mulvany, M. J. & Nyborg, N. C. B. (1985). Atrial natriuretic factor causes specific relaxation of rat renal arcuate arteries. *Br. J. Pharmacol.* **86**: 447–53.

Adachi, H., Tomoika, H., Nishijima, H., Egashira, S. & Nakamura, M. (1989). Sustained dilatation of large coronary artery by alpha-human atrial natriuretic peptide in conscious dogs: a comparison with nitroglycerin. *Eur. J. Pharmacol.* **161**: 189–96.

Allen, M. J., Ang, V. T. Y. & Bennett, E. D. (1988). Domperidone, a Da₂-specific dopamine antagonist, has no effect on the renal or haemodynamic response to atrial natriuretic peptide in man. *Clin. Sci.* **75**: 569–75.

Allen, M. J., Ang, V. T. Y. & Bennett, E. D. (1989). A comparison of head-down tilt with low-dose infusion of atrial natriuretic peptide in man. *J. Physiol.* **410**: 341–50.

Allen, M. J., Gilmour, S. M., Singer, M. & Bennett, E. D. (1989). Effects of atrial natriuretic peptide on systemic haemodynamics and cardiac function in normal man. *Cardiovasc. Res.* **23**: 70–5.

Almeida, F. A., Suzaki, M. & Maack, T. (1986). Atrial natriuretic factor increases hematocrit and decreases plasma volume in nephrectomized rats. *Life Sci.* **39**: 1193–9.

Anand-Srivastava, M. B., Franks, D. J., Cantin, M. & Genest, J. (1984). Atrial natriuretic factor inhibits adenylate cyclase activity. *Biochem. Biophys. Res. Commun.* **121**: 855–62.

Anderson, J., Struthers, A., Christofides, N. & Bloom, S. (1986a). Atrial natriuretic peptide: an endogenous factor enhancing sodium excretion in man. *Clin. Sci.* **70**: 327–31.

Anderson, J. V., Donckier, J., Payne, N. N., Beacham, J., Slater, J. D. H. & Bloom, S. R. (1987). Atrial natriuretic peptide: evidence of action as a natriuretic hormone at physiological plasma concentrations in man. *Clin. Sci.* **72**: 305–12.

Anderson, J. V., Struthers, A. D., Payne, N. N., Slater, J. D. H. & Bloom, S. R. (1986b). Atrial natriuretic peptide inhibits the aldosterone response to angiotensin II in man. *Clin. Sci.* **70**: 507–12.

Bach, R. J., Dai, X. Z., Schwartz, J. S. & Chen, D. G. (1988). Effects of atrial natriuretic peptide in the canine coronary circulation. *Circulation Res.* **62**: 178–83.

Bianchi, C., Gutkowska, J., Thibault, G., Garcia, R., Genest, J. & Cantin, M. (1985). Radiographic localization of ¹²⁵I- atrial natriuretic factor in rat tissues. *Histochemistry* **82**: 441–52.

Bie, P., Wang, B. C., Leadley, R. J. & Goetz, K. L. (1988). Haemodynamic and renal effects of low-dose infusions of atrial peptide in awake dogs. *Am. J. Physiol.* **254**: R161–9.

Bingham-Smith, J. & Lincoln, T. M. (1987). Angiotension decreases cyclic GMP accumulation produced by atrial natriuretic factor. *Am. J. Physiol.* **253**: C147–50.

Biollaz, J., Nussberger, J., Porchet, M., Brunner-Ferber, F., Otterbein, E. S., Gomez, H., Waeber, B. *et al.* (1986a). Four hour infusions of synthetic atrial natriuretic peptide in normal volunteers. *Hypertension* **8** (Suppl. II): 96–105.

Biollaz, J., Nussberger, J., Waeber, B. & Brunner, H. R. (1986b). Clinical pharmacology of atrial natriuretic (3–28) eicosahexapeptide. *J. Hypertension* **4** (Suppl. 2): S101–8.

Biollaz, J., Waeber, B., Nussberger, J., Porchet, M., Brunner-Ferber, F., Otterbein, E. S., Gomex, H. J. *et al.* (1986c). Atrial natriuretic peptides: Reproducibility of renal effects and response of liver blood flow. *Eur. J. Clin. Pharmacol.* **31**: 1–8.

Bolli, P., Muller, F. B., Linder, L., Raine, A. E. G., Resink, T. J., Erne, P., Kiowski, W. *et al.* (1987). The vasodilator potency of atrial natriuretic peptide in man. *Circulation* **75**: 221–8.

Bolli, P., Muller, F. B., Raine, A. E. G., Erne, P., Resink, T. J., Linder, L. & Buhler, F. R. (1986). Atrial natriuretic peptide induces potent vasodilatation in the human forearm and this is antagonised by noradrenaline. *Blood Vessels* **23**: 60.

Bonhomme, M.-C., Cantin, M. & Garcia, R. (1989). Relaxing effect of atrial natriuretic factor on endothelin-precontracted vascular strips. *Proc. Soc. Exp. Biol. Med.* 309–14.

Breuhaus, B. A., Saneii, H. H., Brandt, M. A. & Chimoskey, J. E. (1985). Atriopeptin II lowers cardiac output in conscious sheep. *Am. J. Physiol.* **249**: R776–80.

Brown, J., Dollery, C. T., Ritter, J. & Valdes, G. (1987). Prostaglandins do not mediate the hypotensive effect of human α-atrial natriuretic peptide in man. *Proceedings of the British Pharmacological Society, December 1987, P24.*

Bruschi, G., Bruschi, M. E., Orlandini, G., Banchini, E. & Borghetti, A. (1988). The vasodilator effect of human atrial natriuretic factor (99–126) on human omental arteries. *J. Hypertension* **6** (Suppl. 4): S333–5.

Budzik, G. P., Firestone, S. L., Bush, E. N., Connolly, P. J., Rockway, T. W., Sarin, K. K. & Holleman, W. H. (1987). Divergence of ANF analogs in smooth muscle cell cGMP response and aorta vasorelaxation: evidence for receptor subtypes. *Biochem. Biophys. Res. Commun.* **144**: 422–31.

Bussien, J. P., Biollaz, J., Waeber, B., Nussberger, J., Turini, G. A., Brunner, H. R., Brunner-Ferber, F. *et al.* (1986). Dose dependent effect of atrial natriuretic peptide on blood pressure, heart rate and skin blood flow of normal volunteers. *J. Cardiovasc. Pharmacol.* **8**: 216–20.

Capponi, A. M., Lew, P. D., Wuthrich, R. & Wallotton, M. B. (1986). Effects of synthetic atrial natriuretic peptide on the stimulation by angiotensin II of various target cells. *J. Hypertension* **4** (Suppl. 2): S61–5.

Chien, Y. W., Frohlich, E. D. & Trippodo, N. C. (1987). Atrial natriuretic peptide increases resistance to venous return in rats. *Am. J. Physiol.* **252**: H894–9.

Chiu, P. J. S., Tetzloff, G. & Sybertz, J. (1986). The effects of atriopeptin II on calcium fluxes in rabbit aorta. *Eur. J. Pharmacol.* **124**: 277–84.

Cody, R. J., Atlas, S. A., Laragh, J. H., Kubo, S. H., Covit, A. B., Ryman, K. S., Shaknovich, A. *et al.* (1986). Atrial natriuretic factor in normal subjects and heart failure patients. *J. Clin. Invest.* **78**: 1362–74.

Cohen, M. L. & Schenck, K. W. (1985). Atriopeptin II: Differential sensitivity of arteries and veins from the rat. *Eur. J. Pharmacol.* **108**: 103–4.

Cohen, M. L. & Wiley, K. S. (1978). Rat jugular vein relaxes to norepinephrine, phenylephrine and histamine. *J. Pharmacol. Exp. Therapeut.* **205**: 400–9.

Criscione, L., Burdet, R., Hanni, H., Kamber, B., Truog, A. & Hofbauer, K. G. (1987). Systemic and regional hemodynamic effects of atriopeptin II in anaesthetized rats. *J. Cardiovasc. Pharmacol.* **9**: 135–41.

Cuneo, R. C., Espiner, E. A., Nicholls, M. G., Yandle, T. G. & Livesey, (1987). Effect of physiological levels of atrial natriuretic peptide on hormone secretion: inhibition of angiotensin-induced aldosterone secretion and renin release in normal man. *J. Clin. Endocrinol. Metab.* **65**: 765–72.

Cunew, R. C., Espiner, E. A., Nicholls, M. G., Yandle, T. G., Joyce, S. L. & Gilchrist, N. L. (1986). Renal, haemodynamic and hormonal responses to atrial natriuretic peptide infusions in normal man and effect of sodium intake. *J. Clin. Endocrinol. Metab.* **63**: 946–53.

Cusson, J. R., DuSouich, P., Hamet, P., Schiffrin, E. L., Kuchel, O., Tremblay, K. J., Cantin, M. *et al.* (1988). Effects and pharmacokinetics of bolus injections of atrial natriuretic factor in normal volunteers. *J. Cardiovasc. Pharmacol.* **11**: 635–42.

Cusson, J. R., Hamet, P., Gutkowska, J., Kuchel, O., Genest, J., Genest, J., Cantin, M. &

Larochelle, P. (1987). Effects of atrial natriuretic factor on natriuresis and cGMP in patients with essential hypertension. **5**: 435–43.

Cusson, J. R., Thibault, G., Kuchel, O., Hamet, P., Cantin, M. & Larochelle, P. (1989). Cardiovascular, renal and endocrine responses to low doses of atrial natriuretic factor in mild essential hypertension. *J. Human Hypertension* **3**: 89–96.

DeMey, J. G., Defreyn, G., Lenaers, A., Calderon, P. & Roba, J. (1987). Arterial reactivity, blood pressure and plasma levels of atrial natriuretic peptide in normotensive and hypertensive rats: Effects of acute and chronic administration of atriopeptin III. *J. Cardiovasc. Pharmacol.* **9**: 525–35.

Elbert, T. J. (1988). Reflex activation of sympathetic nervous system with ANF in humans. *Am. J. Physiol.* **255**: H685–9.

Elbert, T. J. & Cowley, A. W. (1988). Atrial natriuretic factor attenuates carotid baroreflex-mediated cardioacceleration in humans. *Am. J. Physiol.* **254**: R590–4.

Eliades, D., Swindall, B., Johnston, J., Pamnam, M. & Haddy, F. J. (1989). Effects of atrial natriuretic peptide on various pressures and microvascular protein permeability in dog prelimb. *Am. J. Physiol.* **257**: H272–9.

Faber, J. E., Gettes, D. R. & Gianturco, D. P. (1988). Microvascular effects of atrial natriuretic factor: Interaction with α_1- and α_2-adrenoceptors. *Circulation Res.* **63**: 415–28.

Faison, E. P., Siegl, P. K. S., Morgan, G. & Winquist, R. J. (1985). Regional vasorelaxant selectivity of atrial natriuretic factor in isolated rabbit vessels. *Life Sci.* **37**: 1073–9.

Ferrari, A. U., Daffonchio, A., Cavallazzi, A., Gerosa, S., Napoletano, G. & Mancia, G. (1988). Effect of atrial natriuretic factor on arterial baroreceptor control of heart rate and blood pressure in conscious rats. *J. Hypertension* **6** (Suppl. 4): S284–6.

Floras, J. S. (1987). Effect of atrial natriuretic peptide on sympathetic nerve activity in humans. *Circulation* **76** (Suppl. IV): IV-320.

Fluckeger, J. P., Waeber, B., Matsueda, G., Delaloye, B., Nussberger, J. & Brunner, H. R. (1986). Effect of atriopeptin III on hematocrit and volemia of nephrectomized rats. *Am. J. Physiol.* **251**: H880–3.

Ford, G. A., Eichler, H. G., Hoffman, B. B. & Blaschke, T. F. (1988). Venous responsiveness to atrial natriuretic factor in man. *Br. J. Clin. Pharmacol.* **26**: 797–9.

Fujii, K., Ishimatsu, T. & Kuriyama, H. (1986). Mechanism of vasodilatation induced by α-human atrial natriuretic polypeptide in rabbit and guinea pig renal arteries. *J. Physiol.* **377**: 315–22.

Fujio, N., Ohashi, M., Nawata, H., Kato, K. I., Matsuo, H. & Ibayashi, H. (1989). Cardiovascular, renal and endocrine effects of α-human atrial natriuretic peptide in patients with Cushings syndrome and primary aldosteronism. *J. Hypertension* **7**: 653–9.

Fujita, T., Ito, Y., Noda, H., Sato, Y., Ando, K., Kangawa, K. & Matsuo, H. (1987). Vasodilatory actions of α-human atrial natriuretic peptide and high Ca^{2+} effects in normal man. *J. Clin. Invest.* **80**: 832–40.

Gaillard, C. A., Koomans, H. A. & Dorhout-Mees, E. J. (1988). Enalapril attenuates natriuresis of atrial natriuretic factor in humans. *Hypertension* **11**: 160–5.

Gaillard, C. A., Koomans, H. A., Rebelink, T. J., Boer, P. & Dorhout-Mees, E. J. (1989). Opposite effects of enalapril and nitrendipine on natriuretic response to atrial natriuretic factor. *Hypertension* **13**: 173–80.

Garcia, R., Thibault, G., Cantin, M. & Genest, J. (1984). Effect of a purified atrial natriuretic factor on rat and rabbit vascular strips and vascular beds. *Am. J. Physiol.* **247**: R34–9.

Garcia, R., Thibault, G., Gutkowska, J., Cantin, M. & Genest, J. (1985). Changes of regional blood flow induced by atrial natriuretic factor in conscious rats. *Life Sci.* **36**: 1687–92.

Gardner, D. G., Deschepper, C. F. & Baxter, J. D. (1987). The gene for atrial natriuretic factor is expressed in the aortic arch. *Hypertension* **9**: 103–6.

Gellai, M., Allen, D. E. & Beeuwkes, R. (1986). Contrasting views on the action of atrial natriuretic peptide: lessons from studies of conscious animals. *Fed. Proc.* **45**: 2387–91.

Gerzer, R. *et al.* (1985). Rapid increase in plasma urinary cyclic GMP after bolus injection of atrial natriuretic factor in man. *J. Clin. Endocrinol. Metab.* **61**: 1217–19.

Gnadinger, M. P., Weidman, P., Rascher, W., Lang, R. E., Hellmuller, B. & Vehlinger, D. E. (1986). Plasma arginine vasopressin levels during infusion of synthetic atrial natriuretic peptide on different sodium intakes in man. *J. Hypertens.* **4**: 623–9.

Granger, J. P., Opgenorth, T. J., Salazar, J., Romero, J. C. & Burnett, J. C. (1986). Long-term hypotensive and renal effects of atrial natriuretic peptide. *Hypertension* **8** (Suppl. 2): 112–16.

Groban, L., Ebert, T. J., Kreis, D. U., Skelton, M. M., van Wynserghe, D. M. & Cowley, A. W. (1989). Haemodynamic, renal and hormonal responses to incremental ANF infusions in humans. *Am. J. Physiol.* **256**: F780–6.

Hassid, A. (1986). Atriopeptin II decreases cytosolic free Ca in cultured vascular smooth muscle cells. *Am. J. Physiol.* **251**: C681–6.

Hegde, S. S., DeFeo, M. L. & Jandhyala, B. S. (1989). Effects of atrial natriuretic factor on cyclic GMP content in the rat aortic smooth muscle: studies on the role of membrane Na$^+$, K$^+$-ATPase. *Clin. Exp. Pharmacol. Physiol.* **16**: 623–9.

Hintze, T. H., Currie, M. G. & Needleman, P. (1985). Atriopeptins: renal-specific vasodilators in conscious dogs. *Am. J. Physiol.* **248**: H587–91.

Hirata, Y., Ishii, M., Sugimoto, T., Matsuoka, H., Fukui, K., Sugimoto, T., Yamakado, M. *et al.* (1988a). Hormonal and renal effects of atrial natriuretic peptide in patients with secondary hypertension. *Circulation* **78**: 1401–10.

Hirata, Y., Shoichiro, T., Kawahara, Y., Takai, Y., Chino, N., Kimura, T., Sakakibara, S. (1988b). Molecular mechanism of action of atrial peptide in rat vascular smooth muscle cells. *Jap. Circulation J.* **52**: 1430–5.

Hughes, A., Thom, S., Goldberg, P., Martin, G. & Sever, P. (1988). Direct effect of α-human atrial natriuretic peptide on human vasculature *in vivo* and *in vitro*. *Clin. Sci.* **74**: 207–11.

Hughes, A. D., Nielsen, H. & Sever, P. S. (1989). The effect of atrial natriuretic peptide on human isolated resistance arteries. *Br. J. Pharmacol.* **97**: 1027–30.

Hughes, A. D., Nielsen, H., Thom, S., Martin, G. N. & Sever, P. S. (1987). The effect of atrial natriuretic peptide on human blood vessels. *J. Hypertension* **5** (Suppl. 5): 551–3.

Huxley, V. H., Tucker, V. L., Verburg, K. M. & Freeman, R. H. (1987). Increased capillary hydraulic conductivity induced by atrial natriuretic peptide. *Circulation Res.* **60**: 304–7.

Hynynen, M., Kupari, M., Salmenpera, M., Tikkanen, I., Heinonen, J., Fyhrquist, F. & Totterman, K. J. (1988). Haemodynamic effects of α-human atrial natriuretic peptide in healthy volunteers. *J. Cardiovasc. Pharmacol.* **11**: 711–15.

Iman, K., Maddens, M., Mohanty, P. K., Felicetta, J. V. & Sowers, J. R. (1989). Atrial natriuretic peptide attenuates the reflex sympathetic responses to lower body negative pressure. *Am. J. Med. Sci.* **298**: 1–7.

Indolfi, C., Piscione, F., Volpe, M., Focaccio, A., Lembo, G., Trimarco, B., Condorelli, M., Chiariallo, M. (1989). Cardiac effects of atrial natriuretic peptide in subjects with normal left ventricular function. *Am. J. Cardiol.* **63**: 353–7.

Ishihara, T., Aisaka, K., Hattori, K., Hamasaki, S., Morita, M., Noguchi, T., Kanjawa, K. & Matsuo, H. (1985). Vasodilatory and diuretic actions of α-human ANP. *Life Sci.* **36**: 1205–15.

Iwanga, R., Hori, S., Suzuki, H., Nakajima, S., Saruta, T., Kojima, S., Fukuda, K. *et al.* (1988). Cardiovascular effects of intravenous and intracoronary administration of atrial natriuretic peptide in halothane anaesthetised dogs. *Life Sci.* **42**: 179–86.

Janssen, W. M. T., deZeeuw, D., van der Hem, G. K. & deJong, P. E. (1989). Atrial natriuretic peptide-induced decreases in renal blood flow in man: implications for the natriuretic mechanism. *Clin. Sci.* **77**: 55–60.

Kleinert, H. D., Maack, T., Atlas, S. A., Januszewicz, A., Sealey, J. E. & Laragh, J. H. (1984). Atrial natriuretic factor inhibits angiotensin, norepinephrine and potassium induced vascular contractility. *Hypertension* **6** (Suppl. I): 143–7.

Labat, C., Norel, X., Benveniste, J. & Brink, C. (1988). Vasorelaxant effects of atriopeptid II on isolated human pulmonary musclepreparations. *Eur. J. Pharmacol.* **150**: 397–400.

Lappe, R. W., Smits, J. F. M., Todt, J. A., Debets, J. M. & Wendt, R. L. (1985). Failure of atriopeptin II to cause arterial vasodilation in the conscious rat. *Circulation Res.* **56**: 606–12.

Laxson, D. D., Dai, X. Z., Schwartz, J. S. & Bache, R. J. (1988). Effects of atrial natriuretic peptide on coronary vascular resistance in the intact awake dog. *J. Am. Coll. Cardiol.* **11**: 624–9.

Lee, R. W. & Goldman, S. (1989). Mechanism for decrease in cardiac output with atrial natriuretic peptide in dogs. *Am. J. Physiol.* **256**: H760–5.

Maack, T., Suzuki, M., Almeida, F. A., Nussenzveig, D., Scarborough, R. M., McEnroe, G. A. & Lewicki, J. A. (1987). Physiological role of silent receptors of atrial natriuretic factor. *Science* **238**: 675–7.

Mann, J. F. E., Gallasch, G., Zeier, M., Karcher D., Bergbreiter, R. & Ritz, E. (1987). Size dependent differential response of human retinal arteries to atrial natriuretic factor (102–126) *in vivo*. *J. Hypertension* **5** (Suppl. 5): S49–50.

Mantero, F., Rocco, S., Pertile, F., Carpene, G., Fallo, F. & Menegus, A. (1987). α-h-ANP injection in normals, low renin hypertension and primary aldosteronism. *J. Ster. Biochem.* **27**: 935–40.

Meisheri, K. D., Taylor, C. J. & Saneii, H. (1986). Synthetic atrial peptide inhibits intracellular calcium release in smooth muscle. *Am. J. Physiol.* **250**: C171–4.

Meyer-Helnert, H., Caramelo, C., Tsai, P. & Schrier, R. W. (1988). Interaction of atriopeptin III and vasopressin on calcium kinetics and contraction of aortic smooth muscle cells. *J. Clin. Invest.* **82**: 1407–14.

Miyamori, I., Ikeda, M., Matsubara, T., Okamoto, S., Koshida, H., Yasuhara, S., Morise, T., Takeda, R. (1987). The renal, cardiovascular and hormonal actions of human atrial natriuretic peptide in man; effects of indomethacin. *Br. J. Clin. Pharmacol.* **23**: 425–31.

Morice, A., Pepke-Zaba, J., Loysen, E., Lapworth, R., Ashby, M., Higenbottam, T. & Brown, M. (1988). Low dose infusion of atrial natriuretic peptide causes salt and water excretion in normal man. *Clin. Sci.* **74**: 359–63.

Mulvany, M. J. (1988). Vascular actions of atrial natriuretic peptide. *Pharmacol. Res. Commun.* **20** (Suppl. III): 23–34.

Nakamura, M., Hatori, N., Nakamura, A., Fine, B. P. & Aviv, A. (1989a). Cytosolic Ca^{2+} attenuates ANF-induced cyclic GMP response in vascular smooth muscle cells. *J. Hypertension* **7**: 51–6.

Nakamura, M., Nakamura, A., Hatori, N., Fine, B. P. & Aviv, A. (1989b). Cytosolic Ca^{2+} regulation attenuates ANP-induced cGMP response in vascular smooth muscle cells of the SHR. *Am. J. Hypertension* **2**: 111–13.

Nambi, P., Whitman, M., Gessner, G., Aiyar, N. & Crooke, S. T. (1986). Vasopressin-mediated inhibition of atrial natriuretic factor stimulated cGMP accumulation in an established smooth muscle cell line. *Proc. Nat. Acad. Sci.* **83**: 8492–5.

Oelkers, W., Kleiner, S. & Bahr, V. (1988). Effects of incremental infusions of atrial natriuretic factor on aldosterone, renin and blood pressure in humans. *Hypertension* **12**: 462–7.

Ohashi, M., Fujio, N., Kato, K., Nawata, H., Ibayashi, H. & Matsuo, H. (1986a). Effect of human α-atrial natriuretic polypeptide on adrenocortical function in man. *J. Endocrinol.* **110**: 287–92.

Ohashi, M. *et al.* (1986b). Human atrial natriuretic polypeptide induced rise of plasma and urinary cyclic 3′5′-guanosine monophosphate concentration in human subjects. *Clin. Exp. Hypertension: Part A. Theory Pract.* **A8**: 67–73.

Ohlstein, E. H. & Berkowitz, B. A. (1985). Cyclic guanosine monophosphate mediates vascular relaxation induced by atrial natriuretic factor. *Hypertension* **7**: 306–10.

Osol, G., Halpern, W., Tesfamariam, B., Nakayama, K. & Weinberg, D. (1986). Synthetic atrial natriuretic factor does not dilate resistance-sized arteries. *Hypertension* **8**: 606–10.

Otsuka, Y. *et al.* (1988). Vascular relaxation and cGMP in hypertension. *Am. J. Physiol.* **254**: H163–9.

Parkes, D. G., Coghlan, J. P., McDougall, J. G. & Scoggins, B. A. (1988). Long-term hemodynamic actions of atrial natriuretic factor in conscious sheep. *Am. J. Physiol.* **254**: H811–15.

Pedrinelli, R., Panarace, G., Spessot, M., Taddei, S., Favilla, S., Gradiadei, L., Lucarini, A. *et al.* (1989). Low dose atrial natriuretic factor in primary aldosteronism: renal haemodynamic and vascular effects. *Hypertension* **14**: 156–63.

Popescu, L. M., Panoiu, C., Hinescu, M., Nutu, O. (1985). The mechanism of cGMP-induced relaxation in vascular smooth muscle. *Eur. J. Pharmacol.* **107**: 393– .

Proctor, K. G. & Bealer, S. L. (1987). Selective antagonism of hormone-induced vasoconstriction by synthetic atrial natriuretic factor in the rat microcirculation. *Circulation Res.* **61**: 42–9.

Rakugi, H., Ogihara, T., Nakamaru, M., Saito, H., Shimu, J., Sakaguchi, K., Kumahara, Y. (1989). Renal interaction of atrial natriuretic peptide with angiotensin II: glomerular and tubular effects. *Clin. Exp. Pharmacol. Phys.* **16**: 97–107.

Rapoport, R. M. (1986). Cyclic guanosine monophosphate inhibition of contraction may be mediated through inhibition of phosphatidylinositol hydrolysis in rat aorta. *Circulation Res.* **58**: 407–10.

Rapoport, R. M., Draznin, M. B. & Murad, F. (1982). Sodium nitroprusside-induced phosphorylation in intact rat aorta is mimicked by 8-bromocyclic GMP. *Proc. Nat. Acad. Sci. USA* **79**: 6470–4.

Rapoport, R. M., Ginsburg, R., Waldman, S. A. & Murad, F. (1986). Effects of atriopeptins on relaxation and cyclic GMP levels in human coronary artery *in vitro*. *Eur. J. Pharmacol.* **124**: 193–6.

Richards, A. M., McDonald, D., Fitzpatrick, M. A., Nicholls, M. G., Espiner, E. A., Ikram, H., Jans, S. *et al.* (1988a). Atrial natriuretic hormone has biological effects in man at physiological plasma concentrations. *J. Clin. Endocrinol. Metab.* **67**: 1134–9.

Richards, A. M., Nicholls, M. G., Ikram, H., Webster, M. W. I., Yandle, T. G. & Espiner, E. A. (1985). Renal haemodynamic and hormonal effects of human alpha atrial natriuretic peptide in healthy volunteers. *Lancet* **i**: 545–8.

Richards, A. M., Rao, G., Espiner, E. A. & Yandle, T. (1989). Interaction of angiotensin converting enzyme inhibition and atrial natriuretic factor. *Hypertension* **13**: 193–9.

Richards, A. M., Tonolo, G., Montorsi, P., Finlayson, J., Fraser, R., Inglis, G., Towrie, A. & Morton, J. J. (1988b). Low dose infusions of 26- and 28-amino acid human atrial natriuretic peptides in normal man. *J. Clin. Endocrinol. Metab.* **66**: 465–72.

Richards, A. M., Tonolo, G., Polonia, J. & Montorsi, P. (1988). Contrasting plasma atrial natriuretic factor concentrations during comparable natriuresis with infusions of atrial natriuretic factor and saline in normal man. *Clin. Sci.* **75**: 455–62.

Roy, L. F., Ogilvie, R. I., Larochelle, P., Hamet, P. & Leenen, F. H. H. (1989). Cardiac and vascular effects of atrial natriuretic factor and sodium nitroprusside in healthy men. *Circulation* **79**: 383–92.

Sato, H., Rector, T. S., Heifetz, S. M. & Kubo, S. H. (1988a). Atrial natriuretic factor decreased forearm vascular capacitance and changes in blood flow distribution in man. *Clin. Res.* **36**: 827A.

Sato, K., Murakami, K., Nishimura, K., Ito, K., Kangawa, K. & Matsuo, H. (1988b). Possible involvement of sodium pump in the relaxation of rat aorta induced by α-human atrial natriuretic polypeptide. *Jap. J. Physiol.* **38**: 187–98.

Schiffrin, E. L., Chartier, L., Thibault, G., St-Louis, J., Cantin, M. & Genest, J. (1985). Vascular and adrenal receptors for atrial natriuretic factor in the rat. *Circulation Res.* **56**: 801–7.

Shapiro, J. T., DeLeonardi, M., Needleman, P. & Hintze, T. H. (1986). Integrated cardiac and peripheral vascular response to atriopeptin 24 in conscious dogs. *Am. J. Physiol.* **251**: H1292–7.

Shenker, Y. (1988). Atrial natriuretic hormone effect on renal function and aldosterone secretion in sodium depletion. *Am. J. Physiol.* **255**: R867–73.

Smits, J. F. M., le Noble, J. L. M. L., van Essen, H. & Slaaf, D. W. (1987). Synthetic atrial natriuretic peptide does not increase protein extraction in rat mesentery. *J. Hypertension* **5** (Suppl. 5): S45–7.

Solomon, L. R., Atherton, J., Bobinski, H., Hillier, V. & Green, R. (1988). Effect of low dose infusion of atrial natriuretic peptide on renal function in man. *Clin. Sci.* **75**: 403–10.

Sugimoto, E., Shigemi, K., Okuno, T., Yawata, T. & Morimoto, T. (1989). Effect of atrial natriuretic peptide on circulating blood volume. *Am. J. Physiol.* **257**: R127–31.

Sybertz, E. J. & Desiderio, D. M. (1985). The role of Na⁺–K⁺-ATPase in the vasorelaxant actions of synthetic atrial natriuretic factor. *Arch. Int. Pharmacodynam. Therapeut.* **278**: 142–9.

Takeshita, A., Imaizumi, T., Nakamura, N., Higashi, H., Sasaki, T., Nakamura, M., Kangawa, K. *et al.* (1987). Attenuation of reflex forearm vasoconstriction by α-human atrial natriuretic peptide in men. *Circulation Res.* **61**: 555–9.

Taylor, C. J. & Meisheri, K. D. (1986). Inhibitory effects of a synthetic atrial peptide on contractions and $^{45}Ca^{2+}$ fluxes in vascular smooth muscle. *J. Pharmacol. Exp. Therapeut.* **237**: 803–8.

Torikai, S. (1988). Factors influencing vascular and natriuretic responses to atrial natriuretic factor. *Jap. Circulation J.* **52**: 1450–2.

Trippodo, N. C., Cole, F. E., Frohlich, E. D. & MacPhee, A. A. (1986). Atrial natriuretic peptide decreases circulatory capacitance in areflexic rats. *Circulation Res.* **59**: 291–6.

Uehlinger, D. E., Weidmann, P., Gnaedinger, M. P., Shaw, S. & Lang, R. E. (1986). Depressor effects and release of atrial natriuretic peptide during norepinephrine or angiotensin II infusion in man. *J. Clin. Endocrinol. Metab.* **63**: 669–74.

Valentin, J. P., Ribstein, J. & Mimran, A. (1988). Nicardipine and atrial natriuretic factor increase whole body vascular permeability in rats. *J. Hypertension* **6** (Suppl. 4): S303–5.

Vierhapper, H. & Nowotny, P. (1987). Prolonged administration of human atrial natriuretic peptide in healthy men: evanescent effect on diuresis in spite of simultaneous infusion of norepinephrine. *Eur. J. Clin. Invest.* **17**: 544–7.

Vierhapper, H., Nowotny, P. & Waldhausl, W. (1986). Prolonged administration of human atrial natriuretic peptide in healthy men. *Hypertension* **8**: 1040–3.

Vlasuk, G. P., Babilon, R. W., Nutt, R. F., Ciccarone, T. M. & Winquist, R. J. (1986). The actions of atrial natriuretic factor on the vascular wall. *Canad. J. Physiol. Pharmacol.* **65**: 1684–9.

Volpe, M., deLuca, N., Bigazzi, M., Vecchione, F., Lembo, G., Condorelli, M. & Trimarco, B. (1988a). Atrial natriuretic factor potentiates forearm reflex vasoconstriction induced by cardiopulmonary receptor deactivation in man. *Circulation* **77**: 849–55.

Volpe, M., Vecchiore, F., Cuocolo, A., Lenbo, G., Pignalosa, S., Condorelli, M. & Trimarco, B. (1988b). Hemodynamic responses to atrial natriuretic factor in nephrectomized rabbits:

attentuation of the circulatory consequences of acute volume expansion. *Circulation Res.* **63**: 322–9.

Von Schroeder, H. P., Nishimura, E., McIntosh, C. H. S., Buchanan, A. M. J., Wilson, N. & Ledsome, J. R.(1985). Autoradiographic localisation of binding sites for atrial natriuretic factor. *Canad. J. Physiol. Pharmacol.* **63**: 1373–7.

Wakitam, K., Oshima, T., Loewy, A. D., Holmberg, S. W., Cole, B. R., Adams, S. P., Fok, K. F., Currie, M. G. & Needleman, P. (1985). Comparative vascular pharmacology of the atriopeptins. *Circulation Res.* **56**: 621–7.

Waldhausl, W., Vierhapper, H. & Nowotny, P. (1986). Prolonged administration of human atrial natriuretic peptide in healthy men: evanescent effects on diuresis and natriuresis. *J. Clin. Endocrinol. Metab.* **62**: 956–9.

Wambach, G., Schittenhelm, U., Stimpel, M., Bonner, G. & Kaufmann, W. (1989). Natriuretic action of ANP is blunted by ACE inhibition in humans. *J. Cardiovasc. Pharmacol.* **13**: 748–53.

Webb, D. J., Benjamin, N., Allen, M. J., Brown, J., O'Flynn, M. & Cockcroft, J. R. (1988). Vascular responses to local atrial natriuretic peptide infusion in man. *Br. J. Clin. Pharmacol.* **26**: 245–51.

Weidmann, P., Hasler, L., Gnadinger, M. P., Lang, R. E., Uehlinger, D. E., Shaw, S., Rascher, W. & Reubi, F. C. (1986a). Blood vessels and renal effects of atrial natriuretic peptide in normal man. *J. Clin. Invest.* **77**: 734–42.

Weidmann, P., Hellmueller, B., Uehlinger, D. E., Lang, R. E., Gnaedinger, M. P., Hasler, L., Shaw, S. & Bachman, C. (1986b). Plasma levels and cardiovascular, endocrine and excretory effects of atrial natriuretic peptide during different sodium intakes in man. *J. Clin. Endocrinol. Metab.* **62**: 1027–36.

Wilkins, M. R., Lewis, H. M., West, M. J., Kendall, M. J. & Lote, C. J. (1987). Captopril reduces the renal response to intravenous atrial natriuretic peptide in normotensives. *J. Human Hypertension* **1**: 47–51.

Williams, T. D. M., Walsh, K. P., Lightman, S. L. & Sutton, R. (1988a). Atrial natriuretic peptide inhibits postural release of renin and vasopressin in humans. *Am. J. Physiol.* **255**: R368–72.

Williams, T. D. M., Walsh, K. P., Pitts, E., Sutton, E. & Lightman, S. L. (1988b). Rebound increase in plasma renin and vasopressin following graded infusions of atrial natriuretic peptide in man. *J. Endocrinol. Invest.* **11**: 31–5.

Williamson, J. R., Holmberg, S. W., Chang, K., Marvel, J., Sutera, S. & Needleman, P. (1989). Mechanisms underlying atriopeptin-induced increases in hematocrit and vascular permeation in rats. *Circulation Res.* **64**: 890–9.

Winquist, R. J., Faison, E. P. & Nutt, R. F. (1984a). Vasodilator profile of synthetic atrial natriuretic factor. *Eur. J. Pharmacol.* **102**: 169–73.

Winquist, R. J., Faison, E. P., Waldman, S. A., Schwartz, K., Murad, F. & Rapoport, R. M. (1984b). Atrial natriuretic factor elicits an endothelium-independent relaxation and activates particulate guanylate cyclase in vascular smooth muscle. *Proc. Nat. Acad. Sci. USA* **81**: 7661–4.

Woods, R. L., Oliver, J. R. & Korner, P. I. (1989). Direct and neurohumoral cardiovascular effects of atrial natriuretic peptide. *J. Cardiovasc. Pharmacol.* **13**: 177–85.

Zimmerman, R. S., Schirger, J. A., Edwards, B. S., Schwab, T. R., Heublein, D. M. & Barnett, J. C. (1987). Cardio-renal-endocrine dynamics during stepwise infusion of physiologic and pharmacologic concentrations of atrial natriuretic factor in the dog. *Circulation Res.* **60**: 63–9.

Chapter 5
Renal actions of atrial natriuretic factor

R. Green

Introduction

Ever since the classical experiments of de Wardener and his co-workers (1961), investigators have searched for a natriuretic hormone. With the reports that extracts of atria caused a natriuresis (de Bold *et al.*, 1981) it was concluded that such a hormone had been discovered; it now seems unlikely that this is the only natriuretic factor, if indeed natriuresis is the major action of the substance. Other chapters deal with the isolation, characterization, alternative sites of production and receptors for what is now known as atrial natriuretic factor (ANF), but here we are concerned with the actions of this factor or putative hormone. Although the number of target sites which are being discovered are increasing, it is generally accepted that the major sites of action are in the kidney and the vascular system. This chapter deals with the renal effects, while Chapter 4 is devoted to cardiovascular responses.

One problem which has bedevilled investigators and made coherent interpretation of data difficult is the lack of clear knowledge about the physiological range of plasma ANF concentrations. It will be obvious from the following account that many early studies used injections or infusions of ANF which elevated plasma concentrations far above those found in healthy individuals or animals. These data may be important when the role of ANF in hypertension (see Chapter 7), congestive heart failure (see Chapter 8), or supraventricular tachycardia is being considered, but not in what might be termed 'normal' life. This chapter tries to distinguish between the physiological and pharmacological effects of ANF.

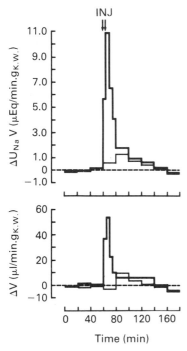

Fig. 5.1 Time-course of the increase in sodium excretion ($\Delta U_{Na}V$) and urine flow rate (ΔV) in rats receiving an injection of atrial extract (heavy lines) or vehicle alone (light lines). Redrawn (with permission) from de Bold *et al.* (1981).

Effects on salt and water excretion

Initial experiments (de Bold *et al.*, 1981) showed that bolus injection of crude atrial extracts in rats caused a large increase in urine flow rate and a marked natriuresis which reached peak values in 5–10 min (Fig. 5.1). Since that time many workers have shown that in *rats* with both atrial extracts, and latterly with purified or manufacturered ANF, there is a natriuresis and a diuresis with, at higher doses, a kaliuresis and a fall in blood pressure (Briggs *et al.*, 1982; Sonnenberg, 1986, 1987; Soejima *et al.*, 1988; van de Stolpe & Jamison, 1988). The natriuresis occurred in both anaesthetized and conscious animals (Pollock & Banks, 1983). Effects of ANF, at least, in anaesthetized rats, could be blocked by a monoclonal antibody (Naruse *et al.*, 1985; Hirth *et al.*, 1986, 1987; Fried *et al.*, 1987). Although, as will become obvious later, there is much disagreement about the mechanisms which cause this diuresis and natriuresis, the results in rats are very consistent.

The same cannot be said about the data from *dogs*. In spite of early reports which confirmed that, as in rats, infusion of ANF increased sodium and water output (Burnett, Granger & Opgenorth, 1984; Maack *et al.*, 1984; Sosa *et al.*, 1986), Goetz and his co-workers (1988) go so far as to deny a role for ANF in the natriuresis following atrial distension or volume expansion. In conscious dogs acute increases of left atrial pressure caused by partial mitral stenosis resulted in a two- to fourfold increase of plasma ANF concentration but only a small natriuresis; denervation of the heart had no effect on the plasma ANF concentration but prevented the natriuresis. Infusion of synthetic peptide to raise plasma concentrations by 10–15-fold was not associated with a natriuresis in conscious dogs (Goetz et al., 1986) nor was long-term administration (Granger et al., 1986). On the other hand, Cernacek et al. (1988) showed that infusion of graded amounts of synthetic ANF gave a linear increase in natriuresis. Doses of ANF injected directly into the renal artery although rather high also caused natriuresis (Burnett, Opgenorth & Granger, 1986). In later experiments where plasma ANF concentration was measured, infusion rates which increased plasma concentrations by 40- to 50-fold in 20 min in conscious dogs did change sodium excretion but lower ones did not; infusion of lower doses over an hour however, which only raised plasma concentration by 10-fold also increased sodium excretion (Bie et al., 1988). However, in anaesthetized dogs very much lower doses enhanced sodium excretion by over 400%. If this were not enough, it has recently been reported that rapid pacing of the right ventricle, while raising plasma concentrations of ANF, did not cause natriuresis but resulted in a marked diuresis (Walsh et al., 1988).

Much more information, and more consistency, is available in studies in man. There is also more information about the range of values elicited by physiological stimuli, such as ingestion of a high salt diet (Solomon et al., 1987) head-up water immersion (Anderson et al., 1986) and assumption of supine posture (Solomon et al., 1986). Even though these experiments do not constitute evidence for the action of ANF, they do indicate the physiological range within which it is necessary to work. A number of early studies used doses of ANF which resulted in frankly pathological plasma concentrations of ANF (Richards et al., 1985; Tikkanen et al., 1985; Biollaz et al., 1986b; Cuneo et al., 1986; Brown & Corr, 1987; Singer et al., 1989), but even low dose infusions (1–2 pmol/kg/min) had an effect (Biollaz et al., 1986a; Anderson et al., 1987; Solomon et al., 1988). Fig. 5.2 is representative of these results and it can be be seen that as the plasma concentration of ANF rose, so did the fractional excretion of sodium and water. At the end of the infusion the plasma concentration rapidly fell towards control values. Baboons give similar responses to man (Bourgoignie, 1987); in other primates the response to ANF was potentiated by barbiturate anaesthesia while destruction of the renal nerves attenuated the effect (Peterson et al., 1989).

Overall, then, apart from some experiments in dogs, there is consistent evidence that ANF at both physiological and pharmacological doses results in a natriuresis and a diuresis. Sonnenberg (1987) suggests that the

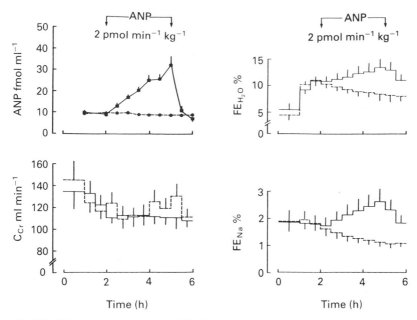

Fig. 5.2   Time-course of changes of ANF concentrations in plasma, clearance of creatinine (C_{Cr}) and the fractional excretion of water (FE_{H_2O}) and sodium (FE_{Na}) during an infusion of ANF (solid lines ■) or a control solution (dashed lines, ●). Values are mean ± SEM. Significant differences between ANF and control are given: *, $P < 0.05$; **, $P < 0.01$; ***, $P < 0.001$. The period of ANF infusion is indicated. Redrawn (with permission) from Solomon *et al.* (1988).

reason some, at least, of the dog experiments are different might be explained as follows. Vagotomy, and/or cooling of the vagi often causes denervation of the heart (Knapp *et al.*, 1986) and therefore interrupts a number of cardiovascular reflexes which would normally potentiate the efects of ANF. Left atrial stretch causes a specific cardiorenal vasodilatory reflex. (Weaver, 1977) which would be additive to the vasorelaxation caused by ANF. Denervation of the heart would remove this potentiating effect. In addition, it might be expected that vasodilatation caused by ANF would result in reflex vasoconstriction. If this does not occur, renal perfusion pressure would fall, and a reduction in renal perfusion pressure alters the responsiveness to ANF (Sosa *et al.*, 1986; Firth, Raine & Ledingham, 1988). If indeed this really is the explanation then one would expect that the response to ANF would be greater in anaesthetized than in conscious animals; this has been observed (Maack *et al.*, 1984).

Accepting that ANF can cause a natriuresis still leaves the intriguing question of how this is achieved. Is the primary renal effect on the blood vessels or the tubules? Most investigators have taken up entrenched positions; the evidence needs to be evaluated.

Haemodynamic effects

Renal blood flow

Since ANF has a major action on blood vessels (see Chapter 4) it is not surprising that many authors have suggested that the renal effects of the peptide are primarily due to changes in glomerular function. Many changes in glomerular dynamics depend directly or indirectly on changes in renal plasma flow (Baylis & Brenner, 1978). The picture is not clear however because, first, renal plasma (or blood) flow has been measured much less frequently than glomerular filtration rate (GFR), and secondly, because many studies have not reported plasma ANF concentrations, although the amounts infused lead one to suspect that the resulting plasma concentrations may have been in the pharmacological range.

Even with large doses of ANF it is unusual to get an increase in renal blood flow in the absence of other stimuli; flow resistance either remains constant or increases. Probably of more importance is the ability of ANF to cause relaxation of previously constricted renal vessels (Baines, de Bold & Sonnenberg, 1983; Camargo et al., 1984; Murray et al., 1985). Some studies have shown that in dogs there is a transient rise in renal plasma flow on infusion of ANF, which rapidly returns to control values (Burnett et al., 1984; Maack et al., 1984). The data are confused however. Falls in effective renal plasma flow (ERPF), generally measured by clearance techniques, have been reported in humans (Biollaz et al., 1986a; Cottier et al., 1988; Solomon et al., 1988; Janssen et al., 1989), in dogs (Banks, 1988), in rats (Pollock & Arendhost, 1986; Gellai, Allen & Beeuwkes, 1986), and in isolated rat kidneys (Baines et al., 1983; Camargo et al., 1984; Murray et al., 1985). Because most investigators showed that haematocrit changes on infusion of ANF, and few monitored extraction ratios by the kidney, ERPF might not accurately reflect renal blood flow. Janssen et al. (1989), however, have showed that even taking this into account there is still a true fall in blood flow to the kidney. In contrast, other workers have reported that there is no change in renal plasma flow (Huang et al., 1985; Weidmann et al., 1986; Brown & Corr, 1987; Cernacek et al., 1988; Méndez et al., 1988). Finally, two separate groups of workers have reported that while renal blood flow does not change at 'physiological' doses, at higher 'pharmacological' doses there is an increased renal plasma flow in rats (Gardiner, Compton & Bennett, 1988) and in dogs (Murphy, Bass & Goldberg, 1988). This is consistent with previously reported increases in renal plasma flow in anaesthetized rats (Dunn et al., 1986) and conscious dogs (Hintze, Currie & Needleman, 1985) and probably reflects an effect on partially constricted vessels.

Thus we are left with inconsistent evidence. It may be that differences not so far considered, such as the amount of salt in the diet, or the concentration of circulating vasoconstrictor hormones or changes in the glomerular capillary perfusion pressure, have an important effect and thus modulate the effects of administered ANF.

It might be expected that more consistent results would be forthcoming on preparations of isolated arteries derived from the kidney, but such is not the case. Aalkjaer, Mulvaney & Nyberg (1985) showed that ANF caused a specific relaxation of rat renal arcuate arteries and caused relaxation of arteries previously constricted by noradrenaline. Using a preparation involving split hydronephrotic rat kidneys (which may not be ideal for 'physiological' studies), it was shown that there was generalized dilatation of arteries and arterioles prior to the glomerulus but vasoconstriction of the efferent vessels (Marin-Grez, Fleming & Steinhausen, 1986; Fig. 5.3). While not acting to cause vasoconstriction of efferent arterioles *per se* it has been shown that ANF potentiates vasoconstriction caused by noradrenaline (Loutzenhiser, Hayashi & Epstein, 1988). These preliminary observations would accord with much of what is known. In rabbits, however, atriopeptin II (a smaller fragment of ANF corresponding to ANF 102–125 compared to 'true' ANF which is ANF 99–126) used in doses of 10^{-12}–10^{-7} M failed to have any effect on single dissected afferent or efferent arterioles (Edwards & Weidley, 1987). In addition, there was no effect on arterioles which were constricted by noradrenaline, even though ANF 103–125 was able to increase the production of cGMP, which is thought to be the intracellular mediator (Leitman & Murad, 1987). In isolated afferent arterioles derived from the superficial renal cortex of dogs, however, ANF caused vasodilatation when added alone and attenuated the constriction caused by noradrenaline in doses of 10^{-10}–10^{-6} M (Ohishi, Hishida & Hendo, 1988); again there was an increase in cGMP. In the light of the previous results the role of cGMP in vasodilation may have to be reassessed. The results of Ohishi *et al.* (1988) are consistent with those reported on isolated dog glomeruli where ANF 103–125 was shown either to vasodilate afferent or to vasoconstrict efferent arterioles (Fried *et al.*, 1986).

Finally, videometric analysis of *in vitro* blood-perfused juxtamedullary vessels showed that atriopeptin III (ANF 103–126) caused vasodilation of arcuate arteries and efferent arterioles when superfused at concentrations of 3×10^{-9} M. At 3×10^{-10} M only arcuate arteries were dilated and less than at the higher dose; 3×10^{-11} M was without effect. None of the doses used affected the efferent arterioles (Veldkamp *et al.*, 1988). Whether the differences reported depend on the different species used or the different preparations of ANF is not yet clear.

Nor is it certain how these changes in vascular resistance in isolated arterioles relate to the overall kidney responses given above. The simplest story, given the concomitant changes in GFR (see below) is that there is dilatation of the afferent arteriole and probably arcuate artery with

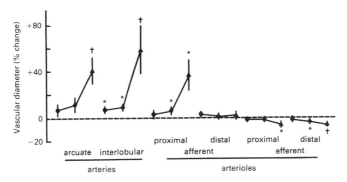

Fig. 5.3 Percentage change in the vascular diameter at different levels of the renal vasculature. Control measurements were made at the end of a 20-min i.v. infusion of buffer at 10 or 100 μl/min. Semipurified ANF was infused for 20 min at rates of 1, (●), 10 (◆) and 100 (▲) μl/min. Statistically significant differences are indicated: *, $P < 0.05$; †, $P < 0.02$. From Marin-Grez et al. (1986) (with permission), Nature **324**: 437–76. Copyright Macmillan Magazines Ltd.

vasoconstriction of the efferent arteriole; the extent of the changes depends on pre-existing conditions at the time that ANF is given. Direct evidence for vasoconstriction of efferent vessels is lacking, but must follow if there is dilatation of the afferent vasculature without an increase in total renal blood flow.

The mechanism of the vasodilation of afferent vessels is not clear. It was suggested that it might be mediated by dopamine (Baines & Drangova, 1986) and drugs that block the dopamine receptor DA-1 appear to block the effects of infused ANF (Marin-Grez et al., 1987); blockers of the DA-2 receptor have no effect (Allen, Ang & Bennett, 1988). An alternative pathway for ANF to cause vasodilatation might be by activation of particulate guanylate cyclase (Winquist, 1986; Leitman & Murad, 1987); the cGMP produced then would activate a Ca^{2+} ATPase and thereby increase calcium extrusion from the cells. This would, in turn, decrease cytosolic calcium activity and reduce muscular contraction (Popescu, Panouiu & Hinescu, 1985). There are no direct measurements of intracellular calcium in glomerular endothelial cells, but in mesangial cells ANF is able to inhibit the rise caused by vasopressin and other vasoconstrictors and also to reduce the constriction of the cells (Meyer-Lehnert et al., 1988). They also suggested that there were mediators other than cGMP involved. Exactly how these changes might be translated into vasodilatation is not yet clear. The relaxation of afferent arterioles does not seem to be mediated by endothelium-derived relaxing factor (Winquist, 1986).

The renal vasoconstriction effect might, theoretically, be due to direct efferent arteriolar constriction, perhaps due to subtle changes in mesangial cell contractibility or to increases in cortical intestitial pressure which would compress postglomerular blood vessels (Atlas & Maack, 1987). Of these, the latter seems unlikely since direct measurement of cortical pressure shows that ANF has no effect (Burnett et al., 1984). The second also seems unlikely since ANF reduces mesangial cell contractility (Meyer-Lehnert et al., 1988), so we are left with a direct effect of ANF on the efferent arteriole. The vasoconstriction effect is calcium-dependent.

Regional blood flow

There is evidence, not only that total renal blood flow might be altered, but also that the blood flow may be redistributed so that more goes to juxtamedullary rather than to superficial cortical nephrons. Early, indirect measurements of vasa recta blood flow suggested a marked increase (Borenstein et al., 1983), a moderate increase (Fujioka et al., 1985) or even no change (Hintze et al., 1985). Later results showed that infusion of 30 pmol/kg/min of ANF 103–126 into rats increased medullary blood flow by 15 % (Takezawa et al., 1987); even higher doses have been shown to cause an increase in pressure in the vasa recta within 90 s (Méndez et al., 1988). Whether this can be related to the natriuresis is uncertain however. Using fluorescent videomicroscopic techniques in Munich–Wister rats, Kiberd et al. (1987) showed that 67 pmol/kg/min of ANF increased urine flow and sodium excretion within 2 min, but there was no corresponding increase in flow in the vasa recta. After 45 min, however, the urine flow rate and sodium excretion had increased further but now there was a significant increase in vasa recta flow. Clearly, increased medullary blood flow would result in washout of solutes from the renal medulla and hence increase the excretion of fluid; it would also have an effect on sodium excretion (see later). Davis & Briggs (1987b) showed that indeed the gradient in the medulla was dissipated, but presented evidence to show that some of the solute, particularly urea, was lost in the urine. Recent evidence suggests that the osmolality and sodium concentration both *rise* in the papilla in conscious animals after ANF infusion (Ashworth et al., 1989), but the reason for this and the differences between the conscious and anaesthetized animals are obscure. Using rats in which the papilla was destroyed by bromoethylamine hydrobromide it was possible to show that, in any case, washout of medullary solute was not essential for the natriuresis following ANF (Torikai, 1986) a conclusion supported by Awazu, Granger & Knox (1988) in a study of diabetes insipidus rats.

Glomerular filtration rate

Apart from isolated reports (Cottier et al., 1988) investigators have found either no change or an increase in glomerular filtration rate (GFR) when ANF has been given. There is no consistency as to whether a change occurs and even investigators from the same laboratories have obtained different results. The first experiments (de Bold *et al.*, 1981) showed that *in vivo* there was no increase in GFR, but shortly afterwards it was reported that infusion of atrial extract into an isolated perfused kidney preparation dramatically increased GFR (Kleinert *et al.*, 1982). Thereafter there has been protracted debate about the presence or absence of an increase in GFR and about its significance in the natriuresis. In general, higher rates of infusion of ANF have been used when an increase in GFR has been noted in man (Weidmann *et al.*, 1986), dogs (Burnett *et al.*, 1986) and rats (Huang *et al.*, 1985; Cogan, 1986; Méndez *et al.*, 1988).

Where an increase in GFR does occur it should be noted that there is a rise in glomerular capillary pressure as would be expected if there is vasodilatation of the afferent arteriole with vasoconstriction of the efferent arteriole as discussed above (Ichikawa *et al.*, 1985; Fried *et al.*, 1986; Schnermann, Marin-Grez & Briggs, 1986). There is also evidence that the filtration coefficient (K_f) might increase.

More recent data, some from the same laboratories however, indicate that with small doses of ANF there is little or no increase in GFR in rats (Gellai *et al.*, 1986; Pollock & Arendshorst, 1986; Fried, Osgood & Stein, 1988; Soejima *et al.*, 1988), dogs (Banks, 1988; Cernacek *et al.*, 1988) and man (Biollaz *et al.*, 1986b; Brown & Corr, 1987; Anderson *et al.*, 1987; Solomon *et al.*, 1988).

It is not certain whether an increased GFR is essential for the natriuresis. When the aorta was partially clamped to reduce the GFR back to normal, some workers (Burnett *et al.*, 1986) found that a natriuresis still occurred, while others found that natriuresis had been abolished (Cogan, 1986; Davis & Briggs, 1987a). In isolated perfused kidneys the action of ANF 103–126 seems to be on both GFR and on tubular function (Itabashi *et al.*, 1987). It is not certain whether the altered differences are due to species differences or to other factors such as changes in angiotensin II (ANGII) levels. Siragy *et al.* (1988), worked at low doses of ANF and still found an effect of ANF on GFR; this could be blocked by giving ANGII at the same time. In dogs also, infusion of angiotensin altered the response to ANF, attenuating the rise in GFR (Showalter *et al.*, 1988). However, after the renin–angiotensin system was blocked by enalaprilat, ANF alone had no effect. Infusion of ANGII directly into the renal artery enhanced the effect of ANF and a diuresis ensued (Seymour & Mazack, 1988). There then seems to be a dual effect of ANG II first to maintain pressure and secondly to interact directly with ANF.

One example of how pressure and ANF interact has been described in isolated perfused kidneys (Firth *et al.*, 1988). Huge concentrations of ANF (1000 pmol/l) were unable to produce an increase in GFR or a natriuresis when the mean renal perfusion pressure was 90 mmHg or less.

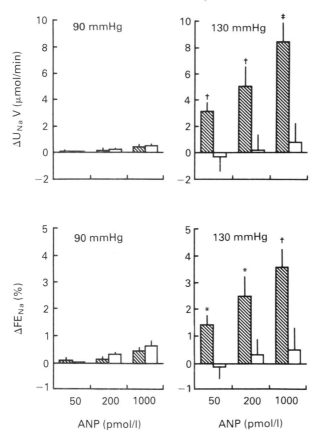

Fig. 5.4   Changes in absolute sodium excretion ($U_{Na}V$) and fractional sodium excretion (FE_{Na}) in isolated kidneys perfused at 90 and 130 mmHg and exposed to either 50, 200 or 1000 pmol/l ANF (hatched bars) and in controls at equivalent times (open bars). Statistically significant differences between ANF and controls are indicated: *, $P < 0.05$; †, $P < 0.02$; ‡, $P < 0.01$ on unpaired 't' tests. From Firth *et al.* (1988) (with permission).

Very much smaller concentrations (50 pmol/l) gave a marked increase in sodium excretion and GFR if the mean perfusion pressure was 130 mmHg (see Fig. 5.4).

The balance of evidence seems to suggest that only at higher plasma concentrations of ANF is there a consistent increase in GFR. Whether this occurs at physiological concentrations is open to doubt and depends on the background condition.

Some of the differences may be due to the use of different species or even strains of animals. One underlying reason for this may be explained in the following way. If the oncotic pressure of plasma proteins balances the hydrostatic pressure for filtration at the end of the glomerular capillary, or at some point before the end (pressure equilibrium), then the major determinant of GFR is the glomerular plasma flow (Baylis & Brenner, 1978). This is the case in rats, particularly Munich–Wistar rats. If on the other hand there is pressure disequilibrium the major determinant is the glomerular capillary pressure; this occurs particularly in dogs and isolated kidney preparations. Thus, if there is pressure disequilibrium, and vasodilatation of the afferent arteriole occurs with constriction of the efferent (giving no increase in flow but an increase in pressure) an increase in GFR would occur with ANF; conversely, if there is pressure equilibrium then little increase would occur since there is no increase in flow (Schnermann & Briggs, 1987). For factors which might produce disequilibrium readers should consult Baylis & Brenner (1978). Unfortunately, there is no information as to whether pressure equilibrium occurs or not in man, so those data cannot be used to test this hypothesis.

Tubular actions of ANF

So far we have considered only indirect evidence that there is a tubular action for ANF, i.e. that a natriuresis occurred without a change in GFR. It must be acknowledged, however, that small changes in GFR, which are undetectable by methods currently in use could account for the increased natriuresis. For example an increase in GFR of 2 ml/min on top of a normal GFR of 125 ml/min in man could, if tubular reabsorption of sodium remained constant, result in a fourfold rise in excretion. It is pertinent, therefore, to consider more direct evidence. ANF has been proposed to affect transport in most parts of the nephron and we will examine these in turn.

Proximal tubule

Classical clearance techniques such as free water clearance in diuretic animals or free water absorption in dehydrated animals (Hropot et al., 1986; Shimizu & Nakamura, 1986) indicate a proximal site of action for ANF. An effect of ANF on reabsorption of ions such as phosphate, which is predominantly reabsorbed in the proximal tubule by cotransport with sodium, strengthens this contention (Ortola, Bannerman & Brenner, 1988). Support for the inhibition of sodium cotransport in the proximal tubule was provided by Hammond et al. (1985) who demonstrated an increase in sodium excretion induced by ANF together with increased fractional excretion of bicarbonate and phosphate. Brush border membrane vesicles prepared from the same animals showed inhibition of sodium transport linked to either phosphate or bicarbonate and direct inhibition of the sodium phosphate cotransporter and the sodium hydrogen antiporter was proposed. The dose of ANF used was quite high—the maximal natriuretic dose without producing hypotension, and vesicles were treated at a concentration of about 1000 pmol/l. The physiological significance of these observations is not clear.

Direct micropuncture evidence does not confirm these suppositions. A number of workers have shown that fractional reabsorption by the proximal tubule is not altered (Briggs *et al.*, 1982; Sonnenberg *et al.*, 1982; Huang *et al.*, 1985; Cogan, 1986). It should be remembered however, that even if fractional reabsorption does not alter, an increased GFR would result in increased delivery of sodium and fluid to the loop of Henle. The lack of a direct effect on the proximal tubule has been confirmed in isolated perfused rat tubules (Baum & Toto, 1986).

All the evidence available from studies in man is indirect. Much of it is derived from a consideration of the clearance of lithium—a technique introduced by Thomsen (1984) for estimation of proximal tubular reabsorption. The evidence is inconsistent; some authors using physiological doses of ANF found little effect on lithium clearance (Solomon *et al.*, 1988) while others giving pharmacological doses found a marked effect (McMurray, Seidelin & Struthers, 1989). Lithium clearance has also been used to study proximal tubular reabsorption in animals; in conscious animals there are few other methods. Early work showed that in dogs ANF inhibited proximal tubular reabsorption. Although much of this could be attributed to the change in GFR, clamping the aorta to bring GFR to normal still left an increased fractional excretion of lithium after ANF (Burnett *et al.*, 1986). ANF has also been shown to increase the fractional excretion of lithium in Brattleboro (Awazu, Granger & Knox, 1986) and Long Evans rats (Awazu *et al.*, 1988; Haris, Skinner & Zhou, 1989). The problem underlying all these studies is the following. It is undoubtedly true that lithium clearance is the best method available for estimating proximal and distal tubular function in conscious animals and man, but it is still not sufficiently accurate to detect small changes. A major advantage is that it measures reabsorption from all proximal tubules, whereas micropuncture studies sample only from superficial nephrons. On the other hand, there is evidence (summarized in Atherton *et al.*, 1989) that with low sodium intake there is significant reabsorption of lithium beyond the proximal tubule; even with raised sodium intakes, furosemide and bumetanide were able to increase lithium clearance. If one believes that the action of these diuretics is on the loop of Henle (Greger & Wangemann, 1987) then it can be seen that some lithium may be absorbed by the loop and interpretation of changes in the clearance of lithium becomes much more complicated than originally thought (Thomsen, 1984). Other markers of proximal tubular function, which are not nearly as specific as the imperfect lithium, have given very variable results (Biollaz *et al.*, 1986b; Anderson *et al.*, 1987; Solomon *et al.*, 1988).

Thus there is little hard evidence that ANF at physiological concentrations exerts a direct effect on the proximal tubule. Indeed, it might be surprising if it did since the proximal tubule lacks receptors with a high affinity for ANF (Biachi et al., 1985; Murphy et al., 1985;Chai et al., 1986; Healey & Fanestil, 1986; Butlen, Mistaoui & Morel, 1987) even though there are a number of tubular endopeptidases which break down ANF (Olins et al., 1987). In addition, the proximal tubule does not generate cGMP in response to ANF either in vivo (Huang et al., 1985) or in vitro (Tremblay et al., 1985; Stokes, McConkey & Martin, 1986; Charbardes et al., 1987; Nonoguchi, Knepper & Manganiello, 1987).

However, experiments by Harris, Thomas & Morgan (1987), showed that ANF was able to antagonize the stimulatory effect of ANGII even though ANF by itself had no effect on reabsorption from split drops (Fig. 5.5). Effects of ANF would therefore depend on the animal preparation and local levels of angiotensin. The results would fit with many observations of functional antagonism between ANF and ANGII (e.g. McMurray & Struthers, 1988). Others workers (Liu & Cogan, 1987, 1988) have demonstrated the effects of ANGII and confirmed that there was no effect of ANF directly on basal transport of water, bicarbonate or chloride. They did not, however, find any antagonism of the ANGII effect by ANF (Liu & Cogan, 1988). The difference cannot be easily reconciled. It might be methodological since while Harris et al. (1987) used split drop or stationary perfusion of the tubules, Liu & Cogan (1988) used continuous perfusion; it is known that there are a number of inherent difficulties with the split drop method (Nakajima, Clapp & Robinson, 1970). Harris et al. (1987) infused the angiotensin and ANF directly into peritubular capillaries while Liu & Cogan (1988) infused the peptides into the animal. It may even be the strain of rat used, Sprague–Dawley vs. Munich–Wister but no further evidence is available at this time.

Another way of influencing proximal reabsorption of sodium and fluid has been proposed (Harris, Skinner & Zhou, 1988; Harris et al., 1989). It is suggested that ANF inhibits the glomerular–tubular feedback mechanism. Thus while normally increasing the filtered load to the proximal tubule increases the reabsorption from that segment (Orloff & Burg, 1971) ANF reduces this feedback (Harris et al., 1988, 1989). Unfortunately, proximal reabsorption has been measured using lithium clearances and as explained above this is less than ideal. Thus, although interesting, this must await further verification.

Taking into consideration all the evidence reviewed it is hard to accept that ANF has a major action on sodium reabsorption from the proximal tubule at physiological concentrations. It may act as one of a multitude of factors with interrelating actions, but much more work needs to be done to disentangle this.

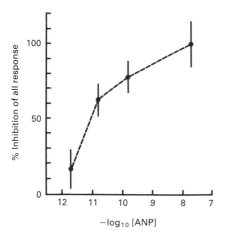

Fig. 5.5 Dose responses of inhibition of angiotensin-stimulated proximal fluid reabsorption by addition of ANF to peritubular infusion fluid containing ANGII $(1.1 \times 10^{-12}\text{ M})$. Values are mean $\pm$ SEM. Reproduced from Harris *et al.* (1987) (with permission), *Nature* **326**: 697–8. Copyright Macmillan Magazines Ltd.

Loop of Henle and distal tubule

The data about reabsorption from the loop of Henle and the different divisions of the distal tubules are fragmentary. All direct evidence has to be derived from micropuncture or microperfusion data. Use of the lithium clearance technique gives data but its interpretation (see above) is difficult and usually amenable to more than one explanation.

Early micropuncture studies showed that delivery of chloride ions (and by inference sodium ions) and fluid into the distal tubule was increased by ANF even when GFR was not altered (Briggs *et al.*, 1982; Sonnenberg *et al.*, 1982); this was in spite of no change in reabsorption from the proximal tubules and implied decreased reabsorption by the loop of Henle. These conclusions seem to have been confirmed (Schnermann & Briggs, 1987) by reports that perfusion of short loops of Henle in rats showed reduced fluid and chloride reabsorption by about 15% after a bolus injection of ANF.

The papillae of young rats protrude into the pelvis of the ureter and it is possible to perform micropuncture experiments directly on the long loops of Henle. Using young Munich–Wistar rats, Roy (1986) showed that there was increased delivery of sodium and water to the tip of the loops of Henle. This was in spite of a *reduced* GFR, a very odd finding compared with most other investigators; it may be attributable to the strain or age of rats used. The implication from these experiments is that reabsorption from either the descending limb of the loop of Henle or the proximal tubule was reduced. It must be borne in mind that these were juxtamedullary nephrons. Previous micropuncture data on proximal nephrons (Briggs *et al.*, 1982; Sonnenberg *et al.*, 1982; Huang *et al.*, 1985; Cogan, 1986) and even data presented in the same paper (Roy, 1986) on proximal reabsorption are not necessarily comparable since only *superficial* proximal tubules can be studied directly.

In spite of these data purporting to show a decreased reabsorption by the loop of Henle it seems unlikely that the transport or permeability characteristics of the loop had altered. In isolated perfused segments of rabbit nephron, ANF even in concentrations as high as 10^{-6} M in the bath had no effect on transepithelial voltage or chloride flux in the thick part of the ascending limb (diluting segment), no effect on the isotopically measured chloride flux in the thin part of the ascending limb (so permeability, at least to chloride, was not changed) and no effect on the osmotic water permeability in the descending limb (Kondo *et al.*, 1986).

These differences may be reconciled when one remembers that one action of ANF may be wash-out of solutes from the medulla consequent on altered redistribution of blood flow (see above). The consequence of this will be decreased water abstraction from the descending limb of Henle's loop and a decreased chloride concentration at the tip of the loop. This would reduce passive movement of chloride, and presumably sodium, from the thin ascending limb of the loop of Henle even though there was no change in the permeability of the epithelium. It might even reduce reabsorption in the thick ascending limb.

There have been few direct investigations of the effect of ANF on the distal tubule, partly because of the difficulty of perfusing this segment and partly because of difficulties in interpretation. Data from humans which demonstrate a 'distal' effect using lithium clearance techniques (Solomon *et al.*, 1988; McMurray, Seidelen & Struthers, 1989) are difficult to interpret because the so-called 'distal' effect could be an effect in the loop of Henle, distal tubule proper, or collecting ducts. Thus, the evidence may be interpreted in the light of known effects on collecting ducts rather than segment and not in the true distal tubule.

Collecting duct

Micropuncture and microcatheterization studies of the effect of ANF of sodium handling in the collecting duct all agree in a number of important areas. There is an increase in delivery of fluid and sodium to those parts of the collecting ducts in the inner medulla (IMCD) and there is marked inhibition of reabsorption from the IMCD and the papillary collecting duct.

Early experiments established these basic findings (Briggs *et al.*, 1982; Sonnenberg *et al.*, 1982) and subsequent work has not necessitated changing this view. Normally, increasing delivery of sodium and fluid to the IMCD results in an increased reabsorption. The reabsorption is

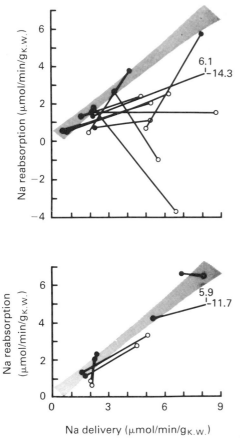

Fig. 5.6   Relationship between absolute delivery of sodium to inner medullary collecting duct and sodium reabsorption along the duct. Solid circles represent control data and open circles represent experimental data. In the upper panel the experimental period was for ANF infusion. In the lower panel the experimental period was induction of a water diuresis. The shaded area represents 99% confidence limits for the linear relationship between sodium delivery and reabsorption when sodium delivery was increased by infusion of KCl. It can be seen that for ANF infusion the normal relationship is disrupted. Modified from Sonnenberg *et al.* (1986) (with permission).

mainly active and inhibitable by amiloride in the tubular lumen (Diezi *et al.*, 1973; Ullrich & Papavassiliou, 1979; Rocha & Kudo, 1982). This normal response to increasing the load delivered to IMCD is abolished by ANF (Sonnenberg *et al.*, 1986); increasing the load to IMCD by other means such as KCl infusion had no effect on fractional reabsorption (see Fig. 5.6). Similar results were obtained by Fried *et al.* (1988) who measured chloride rather than sodium and used a synthetic analogue (Wy47663) of ANF. While they found no difference from controls in late distal delivery of solute, measured by micropuncture of surface nephrons, nevertheless there was an increased delivery to the base of the papillary collecting duct. Further inhibition of fluid reabsorption within the terminal collecting duct also occurred. Similar results were reported in young Munich–Wistar rats with increased delivery of sodium chloride to the base of the papilla and inhibition of reabsorption, which was specific to sodium with no effect on calcium and magnesium, following ANF (van de Stolpe & Jamison, 1988). This degree of unanimity seems unique in the whole field of ANF!

There are two further questions that these results raise. How is the increased delivery to the beginning of the IMCD achieved? How is the sodium reabsorptive mechanism disrupted?

Increased delivery

Theoretically there are two reasons why increased delivery to the IMCD could be achieved. It is possible, but there is no evidence, that sodium reabsorption in outer medullary portions of the collecting ducts is reduced so that a similar mechanism might obtain as occurs in the IMCD. Alternatively it might arise because of redistribution of blood to juxtamedullary nephrons by ANF. There is much evidence (see e.g. Jacobson & Kokko, 1976) that juxtamedullary and superficial nephrons have different rates of reabsorption and different characteristics; for example the ratios of the permeabilities of sodium and chloride is very different in the two populations. It might be that ANF has different actions on juxtamedullary than superficial nephrons and this leads to increased delivery of sodium and water into the collecting duct below the renal surface. Since data on distal delivery (Briggs *et al.*, 1982; Sonnenberg *et al.*, 1982) can only be derived from superficial cortical nephrons this hidden effect may play a part. Again, there is no direct evidence.

Altered sodium reabsorption

The mechanism whereby sodium reabsorption is inhibited has been worked out in some detail in cultured cells. Some of the cells used are derived from established lines of pig kidney cells (LLC-PK) but much of the more recent work is from primary cultures of cells from rabbit IMCD. The origin of these latter cells is well established although there is some doubt about the origin of the former and there is always the possibility, with established lines, of de-differentiation. Nevertheless, the results are generally similar to those from rabbit IMCDs.

The earliest studies showed that oxygen consumption, which was used as an indirect meaurement of metabolic activity, was reduced by ANF (Zeidel *et al.*, 1986). Further study showed that this was not a direct effect of ANF on the Na/K ATPase, but was secondary to decreased sodium entry via an amiloride-sensitive channel (Cantiello & Ausiello, 1986; Zeidel *et al.*, 1988). ANF acts through a specific receptor (Murphy *et al.*,

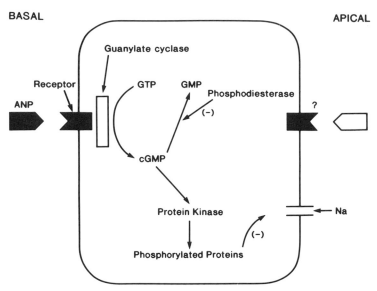

Fig. 5.7 Diagrammatic representation of events following attachment of ANF to receptors in the collecting ducts. GMP, guanosine monophosphate; cGMP, cyclic guanosine monophosphate; GTP, guanosine triphosphate. The receptor at the apical membrane has not been positively identified.

1985; Chai *et al.*, 1986; Healey & Fanestil, 1986; Koseki *et al.*, 1986) which is linked to particulate guanylate cyclase (Gunning *et al.*, 1989) for signal transduction (Fig. 5.7). In support of this scheme it has been shown that cGMP accumulates in suspensions of IMCD cells exposed to ANF (Zeidel, 1988), mediates the inhibition of sodium-dependent transport (Zeidel *et al.*, 1988) and oxygen consumption (Zeidel *et al.*, 1986), and mimics the action of ANF when applied to isolated perfused IMCD (Zeidel *et al.*, 1987; Nonoguchi *et al.*, 1987). It has recently been shown to reduce the open time of sodium channels in the apical membrane of IMCD cells (Light *et al.*, 1989).

While this is a convincing and coherent story in isolated and cultivated cells there are some discordant results. In anaesthetized rabbits amiloride has been reported to attenuate the effects of ANF on potassium excretion but to *increase* the natriuresis (Nushiro *et al.*, 1988) in spite of reducing the filtered load of sodium. Thus, as regards the natriuresis, the effects were additive and would argue against an effect of ANF on sodium channels unless submaximal doses had been used. Perfusing medullary collecting ducts *in situ* indicated that amiloride and ANF in the luminal fluid both inhibited the flux of ^{22}Na to the same extent. However, when ANF was given systemically, it had other effects (Sonnenberg, Honrath & Wilson, 1989). It may be, then, that ANF has multiple actions on the two sides of the cell and this may give rise to some of the conflict.

Using isolated perfused terminal IMCDs, ANF at 10^{-7} M in the bath inhibited the isotopically measured chloride permeability but not the sodium permeability (Sands, Nonoguchi & Knepper, 1988). It is difficult to relate this finding to the natriuresis. The same group have also reported that while ANF had no direct effect on water permeability it did inhibit the increase in permeability induced by arginine vasopressin (Nonoguchi, Sands & Knepper, 1988). Again, the concentration was relatively high so the significance is not clear.

In summary then, there is more agreement about actions of ANF on the collecting duct than elsewhere in the kidney. ANF increases cGMP which inhibits an amiloride-sensitive sodium channel so reducing sodium entry into cells and resulting in increased excretion.

General summary

Clearly the extensive literature, of which only a fraction has been quoted in this review, indicates the explosion of interest in ANF in the past 8 years. Any summary obviously reflects the prejudices and reading of the author. Nevertheless, it seems safe to conclude that there is strong evidence for an effect of ANF on collecting ducts, inhibiting sodium entry to the cells through a sodium channel. Even acting alone this could cause a natriuresis.

However, such an effect would be magnified by any mechanism which increased delivery of sodium and water to the collecting ducts. The evidence that sodium and water reabsorption is reduced in the proximal tubule is not sufficiently strong to warrant drawing firm conclusions. It must be recognized that it is always difficult to prove a negative assertion. ANF may be one of a number of factors, each of which has a fairly minor role on proximal reabsorption. Manipulating experimental conditions or giving massive doses will highlight actions of ANF even though it may have little importance as a physiological action.

Evidence for an effect on the glomerulus also falls into this category. The evidence that ANF at physiological concentrations has a primary action on glomerular vessels is not convincing. Nevertheless, even minor changes, perhaps undetectable with current methodology could enhance the effect of ANF on the collecting ducts. There also seems to be an effect of ANF on redistribution of blood flow which alters reabsorption by the loop of Henle.

Much more work is needed. One thing is certain, the subtle interplay between ANF and the host of other agents which affect, or are reported to affect, sodium reabsorption by the kidney will provide employment for years to come—at least, until the discovery of another 'salt-losing hormone'!

Acknowledgements

It is a pleasure to acknowledge the contribution of colleagues in experiments and discussions. Especial thanks to Dr J. C. Atherton for reading this manuscript critically, and to my secretary, Joan Clark, for transcribing my illegible handwriting.

References

Aalkjaer, C., Mulvany, M. J. & Nyborg, N.C.B. (1985). Atrial natriuretic factor causes specific relaxation of rat renal arcuate arteries. *Br. J. Pharmacol.* **86**: 447–53.

Allen, M. J., Ang, V. T. Y. & Bennett, E. D. (1988). Domperidone, a DA_2-specific dopamine antagonist, has no effect on the renal or haemodynamic response to atrial natriuretic peptide in man. *Clin. Sci.* **75**: 569–75.

Anderson, J. V., Donckier, J., Payne, N. N., Beacham, J., Slater, J. D. H. & Bloom, S. R. (1987). Atrial natriuretic peptide: evidence of action as a natriuretic hormone at physiological concentration in man. *Clin. Sci.* **72**: 305–12.

Anderson, J. V., Miller, N., O'Hare, J. P., McKenzie, J. C., Corroll, R. J. C. & Bloom, S. R. (1986). Atrial natriuretic peptide; physiological release associated with natriuresis during head-out water immersion in man. *Clin. Sci.* **71**: 319–22.

Ashworth, R., Lote, C. J., Thewles, A. & Wood, J. A. (1989). Increased renal papillary solute concentrations in response to atrial natriuretic factor (ANF) infusion in rats. *J. Physiol.* **417**: 167.

Atherton, J. C., Green, R., Higgins, A., Large, A., McNicholas, C., Parker, D., Pempkowiak, L. *et al.* (1989). Lithium clearance in healthy humans: effects of sodium intake and diuresis. *Kidney Int.* (in press).

Atlas, S. A. & Maack, T. (1987). Effects of atrial natriuretic factor on the kidney and the renin–angiotensin–aldosterone system. *Endocrinol. Metabol. Clin. N. Am.* **16**: 107–13.

Awazu, M., Granger, J. & Knox, F. G. (1986). Natriuretic effects of atrial natriuretic peptide (ANP) in diabetes insipidus rats. *Kidney Int.* **29**: 390A.

Awazu, M., Granger, J. P. & Knox, F. G. (1988). Natriuretic effect of atrial natriuretic peptide in diabetes insipidus rats. *Proc. Soc. Exp. Biol. Med.* **187**: 165–8.

Baines, A. D. & Drangova, R. (1986). Neural and tubular dopamine increases glomerular filtration rate in perfused rat kidneys. *Am. J. Physiol.* **250**: F674–9.

Baines, A. D., de Bold, A. J. & Sonnenberg, H. (1983). Natriuretic effect of atrial extract on isolated rat kidney. *Canad. J. Physiol. Pharmacol.* **61**: 1462–6.

Banks, R. O. (1988). Effects of a physiological dose of ANP on renal function in dogs. *Am. J. Physiol.* **255**: F907–10.

Baum, M. & Toto, R. (1986). Lack of direct effect of atrial natriuretic factor in the rat proximal tubule. *Am. J. Physiol.* **250**: F66–9.

Baylis, C. & Brenner, B. M. (1978). The physiological determinants of glomerular ultrafiltration. *Rev. Physiol. Pharmacol. Biochem.* **80**: 1–46.

Biachi, G., Gutkowska, G. Thibault, G., Garcia, R., Genest, J. & Cantin, M. (1985). Radioautographic localisation of ^{125}I—atrial natriuretic factor ANF in rat tissues. *Histochemistry* **82**: 441–52.

Bie, P., Wang, B. C., Leadley, R. J. & Goetz, K. L. (1988). Haemodynamic and renal effects of low dose infusion of atrial peptide in awake dogs. *Am. J. Physiol.* **254**: R161–9.

Biollaz, J., Nussberger, J., Perchet, M., Brunner-Ferber, F., Otterbein, E. S., Gomez, H. *et al.* (1986a). Four-hour infusions of synthetic atrial natriuretic peptide in normal volunteers. *Hypertension* (Dallas) **8** (Suppl. II): II96–105.

Biollaz, J., Nussberger, J., Waeber, B. & Brunner, H. R. (1986b). Clinical pharmacology of atrial natriuretic (3–28) eicosahexapeptide. *J. Hypertension* (Suppl. 2): S101–8.

Borenstein, H. B., Cupples, W. A., Sonnenberg, H. & Veress, A. T. (1983). The effect of a natriuretic atrial extract on renal haemodynamics and urinary excretion in anaesthetized rats. *J. Physiol.* **334**: 133–40.

Bourgoignie, J. J. (1987). Natriuretic hormones: comparison of renal effects. *Klin. Wochensch.* **65**: (Suppl. VIII): 14–20.

Briggs, J. P., Steipe, B., Schubert, G. & Schnermann, J. (1982). Micropuncture studies of the renal effects of atrial natriuretic substance. *Pflügers Arch.* **395**: 271–6.

Brown, J. & Corr, L. (1987). Renal mechanisms of human α-atrial natriuretic peptide in man. *J. Physiol.* **387**: 31–46.

Burnett, J. C., Granger, J. P. & Opgennorth, T. J. (1984). Effects of synthetic atrial natriuretic factor on renal function and renin release. *Am. J. Physiol.* **247**: F863–6.

Burnett, J. C., Opgenorth, T. J. & Granger, J. P. (1986). The renal action of atrial natriuretic peptide during control of glomerular filtration. *Kidney Int.* **30**: 16–19.

Butlen, D., Mistaoui, M. & Morel, F. (1987). Atrial natriuretic peptide receptors along the rat and rabbit nephrons: [^{125}I] alpha—rat atrial natriuretic peptide binding in microdissected glomeruli and tubules. *Pflügers Arch.* **408**: 356–65.

Camargo, M. J. F., Kleinert, H. D., Atlas, S. A., Sealey, J. E., Laragh, J. H. & Maack, T. (1984). Ca dependent haemodynamic and natriuretic effects of atrial extract in isolated rat kidney. *Am. J. Physiol.* **246**: F447–56.

Cantiello, H. F. & Ausiello, D. (1986). Atrial natriuretic factor and cGMP inhibit amiloride-sensitive Na$^+$ transport in the cultured renal epithelial line, LLC-PK1. *Biochem. Biophys. Res. Commun.* **134**: 852–60.

Cernacek, P., Maher, E., Crawhall, J. C. & Levy, M. (1988). Renal dose response and pharmacokinetics of atrial natriuretic factor in dogs. *Am. J. Physiol.* **255**: R929–35.

Chai, S. Y., Sexton, P. M., Allen, A. M., Figdor, R. & Mendelsohn, F. A. O. (1986). *In vitro* autoradiographic localisation of ANP receptors in rat kidney and adrenal gland. *Am. J. Physiol.* **250**: F753–7.

Charbardes, D., Montegut, M., Mistaoui, M., Butlen, D. & Morel, F. (1987). Atrial natriuretic peptide effects on cGMP and cAMP contents in microdissected glomeruli and segments of the rat and rabbit nephrons. *Pflügers Arch.* **408**: 366–72.

Cogan, M. G. (1986). Atrial natriuretic factor can increase renal solute excretion primarily by raising glomerular filtration. *Am. J. Physiol.* **250**: F710–14.

Cottier, C., Matter, L., Weidmann, P., Shaw, S. & Gnädinger, M. P. (1988). Renal response to low dose infusion of atrial natriuretic peptide in normal man. *Kidney Int.* **34** (Suppl. 25): S72–8.

Cuneo, R. C., Espiner, E. A., Nicholls, G., Yandle, T.G., Joyce, S. L. & Gilchrist, N. L. (1986). Renal, haemodynamic and hormonal responses to atrial natriuretic peptide infusions in normal man, and effects of sodium intake. *J. Clin. Endocrinol. Metab.* **63**: 946–53.

Davis, C. L. & Briggs, J. P. (1987a). Effect of reduction in renal artery pressure on atrial natriuretic peptide-induced natriuresis. *Am. J. Physiol.* **252**: F146–53.

Davis, C. L. & Briggs, J. P. (1987b). Effect of atrial natriuretic peptides on renal medullary solute gradients. *Am. J. Physiol.* **253**: F679–84.

de Bold, A. J., Borenstein, H. B., Veress, A. T. & Sonnenberg, H. (1981). A rapid and potent natriuretic response to intravenous injection of atrial myocardial extract in rats. *Life Sci.* **28**: 94–8.

de Wardener, H. E., Mills, I. H., Clapham, W. F. & Hayter, C. J. (1961). Studies on the efferent mechanism of the sodium diuresis which follows the administration of saline in the dog. *Clin. Sci.* **21**: 249–58.

Diezi, J., Michoud, P., Aceves, J. & Giebisch, G. (1973). Micropuncture study of electrolyte transport across papillary collecting ducts of the rat. *Am. J. Physiol.* **224**: 623–34.

Dunn, B. R., Ichikawa, I., Pfeffer, J., Troy, J. L. & Brenner, B. M. (1986). Renal and systemic hemodynamic effects of synthetic atrial natriuretic peptide in the anesthetized rat. *Clin. Res.* **59**: 237–46.

Edwards, R. M. & Weidley, E. F. (1987). Lack of effect of atriopeptin II on rabbit glomerular arterioles *in vitro*. *Am. J. Physiol.* **252**: F317–21.

Firth, J. D., Raine, A. E. G. & Ledingham, J. G. G. (1988). Low concentration of ANP cause pressure-dependent natriuresis in the isolated kidney. *Am. J. Physiol.* **255**: F391–96.

Fried, T. A., Ayon, M. A., McDonald, G., Lau, A., Inagami, T. & Stein, J. H. (1987). Atrial natriuretic peptide, right atrial pressure and sodium excretion in the rat. *Am. J. Physiol.* **253**: F969–75.

Fried, T. A., McCoy, R. N., Osgood, R. W. & Stein, J. H. (1986). Effects of atriopeptin II on determinants of glomerular filtration rate in the *in vitro* perfused dog glomerulus. *Am. J. Physiol.* **250**: F1119–22.

Fried, T. A., Osgood, R. W. & Stein, J. H. (1988). Tubular sites of action of atrial natriuretic peptide in the rat. *Am. J. Physiol.* **255**: F313–6.

Fujioka, S., Tamaki, T., Fukui, K., Okahara, T. & Abe, Y. (1985). Effects of a synthetic human atrial natriuretic polypeptide on regional blood flow in rats. *Eur. J. Pharmacol.* **109**: 301–4.

Gardiner, S. M., Compton, A. M. & Bennett, T. (1988). Regional hemodynamic effects of atrial natriuretic peptide or captopril in Brattleboro rats. *Am. J. Physiol.* **255**: R737–43.

Gellai, M., Allen, D. E. & Beeuwkes, R. (1986). Contrasting views on the action of atrial peptides: lessons from studies of conscious animals. *Fed. Proc.* **45**: 2387–91.

Goetz, K. L., Wang, B. C., Bie, P., Leadley, R. J. & Greer, P. G. (1988). Natriuresis during atrial distension and a concurrent decline in plasma atriopeptin. *Am. J. Physiol.* **255**: R259–67.

Goetz, K. L., Wang, B. C., Greer, P. G., Leadley, R. J. & Reinhardt, H. W. (1986). Atrial stretch increases sodium excretion independently of release of atrial peptides. *Am. J. Physiol.* **250**: R946–50.

Granger, J. P., Opgenorth, T. J., Salazar, J., Romero, J. C. & Burnett, J. C. (1986). Long term hypotensive and renal effects of atrial natriuretic peptide. *Hypertension* (Dallas) **8** (Suppl. II): II112–16.

Greger, R. & Wangemann, P. (1987). Loop diuretics. *Renal Physiol.* **10**: 174–83.

Gunning, M., Silva, P., Brenner, B. M. & Zeidel, M. L. (1989). Characteristics of ANP-sensitive guanylate cyclase in inner medullary collecting duct cells. *Am. J. Physiol.* **256**: F766–75.

Hammond, T. G., Yusufi, A. N., Knox, F. G. & Dousa, T. P. (1985). Administration of atrial natriuretic factor inhibits sodium-coupled transport in proximal tubules. *J. Clin. Invest.* **75**: 1983–9.

Harris, P. J., Skinner, S. L. & Zhou, J. (1988). The effect of atrial natriuretic peptide and glucagon on proximal glomerulo-tubular balance in anaesthetised rats. *J. Physiol.* **402**: 29–42.

Harris, P. J., Skinner, S. L. & Zhou, J. (1989). Haemodynamics and renal tubular responses to low dose infusion or bolus injection of the peptide ANF in anaesthetised rats. *J. Physiol.* **412**: 309–20.

Harris, P. J., Thomas, D. & Morgan, T. O. (1987). Atrial natriuretic peptide inhibits angiotensin-stimulated proximal tubular sodium and water reabsorption. *Nature* **326**: 697–8.

Healy, E. P. & Fanestil, D. D. (1986). Localisation of atrial natriuretic peptide binding sites within the rat kidney. *Am. J. Physiol.* **250**: F573–8.

Hintze, T. H., Currie, M. G. & Needleman, P. (1985). Atriopeptins: renal specific vasodilators in conscious dogs. *Am. J. Physiol.* **248**: H587–91.

Hintze, T. H., Maude, D. L., Deleonardis, V. M., Shapiro, J. T. & Needleman, P. (1985). Possible mechanisms of natriuresis and diuresis following atriopeptin III infusion in conscious dogs. *Clin. Res.* **33**: 194A.

Hirth, C., Stasch, J. P., John, A., Kazda, S., Morich, F., Neuser, D. & Wohlfiel, S. (1986). The renal response to acute hypervolaemia is caused by atrial natriuretic peptides. *J. Cardiovasc. Pharmacol.* **8**: 268–75.

Hirth, C., Stasch, J. P., John, A., Kazda, S., Morich, F., Neuser, D. & Wohlfiel, S. (1987). Blockade of the response to volume expansion by monoclonal antibodies against atrial natriuretic peptides. *Klin. Wochenschr.* **65** (Suppl. VIII): 87–91.

Hropot, M., Klaus, E., Knolle, J., Koning, W. & Scholz, W. (1986). Effect of rat atriopeptin III on renal function in dogs during water diuresis and hydropenia. *Klin. Wochenschr.* **64** (Suppl. 6): 58–63.

Huang, C. L., Lewicki, J., Johnson, L. K. & Cogan, M. G. (1985). Renal mechanism of action of rat atrial natriuretic factor. *J. Clin. Invest.* **75**: 769–73.

Ichikawa, I., Dunn, B. R., Troy, J. L., Maack, T. & Brenner, B. M. (1985). Influence of atrial natriuretic peptide on glomerular microcirculation *in vivo. Clin. Res.* **33**: 487A.

Itabashi, A., Chan, L., Shapiro, J. I., Cheung, C. & Schrier, R. W. (1987). Comparison of the natriuretic response to atriopeptin III and loop diuretics in the isolated perfused rat kidney. *Clin. Sci.* **73**: 143–50.

Jacobson, H. R. & Kokko, J. P. (1976). Intrinsic differences in various segments of the proximal tubule. *J. Clin. Invest.* **57**: 818–25.

Janssen, W. M. T., de Zeeuw, D., van der Hem, G. K. & de Jong, P. E. (1989). Atrial natriuretic peptide-induced decreases in renal blood flow in man: implications for the natriuretic mechanism. *Clin. Sci.* **77**: 55–60.

Kiberd, B. A., Larson, T. S., Robertson, C. R. & Jamison, R. L. (1987). Effects of atrial natriuretic peptide on vasa recta blood flow in the rat *Am. J. Physiol.* **252**: F1112–17.

Kleinert, H. D., Camargo, M. J. F., Sealey, J. E., Laragh, J. H. & Maack, T. (1982). Hemodynamic and natriuretic effects of atrial extracts in the isolated perfused rat kidney. *Physiologist* **25**: 298.

Knapp, M. F., Hicks, M. N., Linden, R. J. & Mary, D. A. S. G. (1986). Evidence against ANP as a natriuretic hormone during atrial distension. *J. Endocrinol.* **109**: R5–8.

Kondo, Y., Imai, M., Kangawa, K. & Matsuo, H. (1986). Lack of direct action of α-human atrial natriuretic polypeptide on the *in vitro* perfused segments of Henle's loop isolated from rabbit kidney. *Pflügers Arch.* **406**: 273–8.

Koseki, C., Hayashi, Y., Toriyaki, S., Furoja, M., Ohnuma, N. & Imai, M. (1986). Localization of binding sites of α-rat atrial natriuretic polypeptide in rat kidney. *Am. J. Physiol.* **250**: F210–16.

Leitman, D. C. & Murad, F. (1987). Atrial natriuretic factor receptor heterogeneity and stimulation of particulate guanylate cyclase and cyclic GMP accumulation. *Endocrinol. Metab. Clin. N. Am.* **16**: 79–106.

Light, D. B., Schwiebert, E. M., Karlson, K. H. & Stanton, B. A. (1989). Atrial natriuretic peptide inhibits a cation channel in renal inner medullary collecting duct cells. *Science* **243**: 383–8.

Liu, F. Y. & Cogan, M. G. (1987). Angiotensin II: a potent regulator of acidification in the rat early proximal convoluted tubule. *J. Clin. Invest.* **80**: 272–5.

Liu, F. Y. & Cogan, M. G. (1988). Atrial natriuretic factor does not inhibit basal or angiotensin II-stimulated proximal transport. *Am. J. Physiol.* **255**: F434–7.

Loutzenhiser, R., Hayashi, K. & Epstein, M. (1988). Atrial natriuretic peptide reverses afferent arteriolar vasoconstriction and potentiates efferent arteriolar vasoconstriction in the isolated perfused rat kidney. *J. Pharmacol. Exp. Therapeut.* **246**: 522–8.

McMurray, J. & Struthers, A. D. (1988). Effects of angiotensin II and atrial natriuretic peptide alone and in combination on urinary water and electrolyte excretion in man. *Clin. Sci.* **74**: 419–25.

McMurray, J., Seidelin, P. H. & Struthers, A. D. (1989). Evidence for a proximal and distal nephron action of atrial natriuretic factor in man. *Nephron* **51**: 39–43.

Maack, T., Marion, D. N., Camargo, M. J. F., Kleinert, H. D., Vaughan, E. D. & Atlas, S. A. (1984). Effects of auriculin (atrial natriuretic factor) on blood pressure, renal function and the renin–aldosterone system in dogs. *Am. J. Med.* **77**: 1069–75.

Marin-Grez, M., Angchanpen, P., Gambaro, G., Schnermann, J. Schubert, G. & Briggs, J. P. (1987). Evidence for involvement of dopamine receptors in the natriuretic response to atrial natriuretic peptide. *Klin. Wochenschr.* **65** (Suppl. VIII): 97–102.

Marin-Grez, M., Fleming, J. T. & Steinhausen, M. (1986). Atrial natriuretic peptide causes preglomerular vasodilatation and post glomerular vasoconstriction in rat kidney. *Nature* **324**: 473–6.

Méndez, R. E., Dunn, B. R., Troy, J. L. & Brenner, B. M. (1988). Atrial natriuretic peptide and furosemide effects on hydraulic pressures in the renal papilla. *Kidney Int.*, **34**: 36–42.

Meyer-Lehnert, H., Tsai, P., Caramelo, C. & Schrier, R. W. (1988). ANF inhibits vasopressin induced Ca^{2+} mobilisation and contraction in glomerular mesangial cells. *Am. J. Physiol.* **255**: F771–80.

Murphy, K. M. M., McLaughlin, L. L., Michener, M. L. & Needleman, P. (1985). Autoradiographic localisation of atriopeptin III receptors in rat kidney. *Eur. J. Pharmacol.* **111**: 291–2.

Murphy, M. B., Bass, A. S. & Goldberg, L. I. (1988). Renal effects of atrial natriuretic factor are independent of dopamine receptors. *Am. J. Physiol.* **255**: F494–9.

Murray, R. D., Itoh, S., Inagami, T., Misono, K., Seto, S., Scicli, G. & Carretero, O. A. (1985). Effects of synthetic atrial natriuretic factor in the isolated perfused rat kidney. *Am. J. Physiol.* **249**: F603–9.

Nakajima, K., Clapp, J. R. & Robinson, R. R. (1970). Limitations of the shrinking-drop micropuncture technique. *Am. J. Physiol.* **219**: 345–51.

Naruse, M., Obana, K., Naruse, K., Sugino, N., Demura, H., Shizume, K. & Inagami, T. (1985). Antisera to atrial natriuretic factor reduces urinary sodium excretion and increases plasma renin activity in rats. *Biochem. Biophys. Res. Commun.* **132**: 954–60.

Nonoguchi, H., Knepper, M. A. & Manganiello, V. C. (1987). Effects of atrial natriuretic factor on cyclic guanosine monophosphate accumulation in microdissected nephron segments from rats. *J. Clin. Invest.* **79**: 500–7.

Nonoguchi, H., Sands, J. M. & Knepper, M. A. (1988). Atrial natriuretic factor inhibits vasopressin-stimulated osmotic water permeability in rat inner medullary collecting duct. *J. Clin. Invest.* **82**: 1383–90.

Nushiro, N., Abe, K., Seino, M. & Yoshinaga, K. (1988). Interaction between ANP and amiloride in renal tubular sodium handling in anesthetized rabbits. *Am. J. Physiol.* **254**: F521–6.

Ohishi, K., Hishida, A. & Hondo, N. (1988). Direct vasodilatory action of atrial natriuretic factor on canine glomerular afferent arterioles. *Am. J. Physiol.* **255**: F415–20.

Olins, G. M., Spear, K. L., Siegel, N. R., Reinhard, E. J. & Zurcher-Neely, H. A. (1987). Atrial peptide inactivation by rabbit-kidney brush-border membrane. *Eur. J. Biochem.* **170**: 432–4.

Orloff, J. & Burg, M. B. (1971). Kidney. *Ann. Rev. Physiol.* **33**: 83–130.

Ortola, F. Y., Bannerman, B. J. & Brenner, B. M. (1988). Endogenous ANP augments fractional excretion of Pi Ca and Na in rats with reduced renal mass. *Am. J. Physiol.* **255**: F1090–7.

Peterson, T., Benjamin, B., Metzler, C., Hurst, N. & Euler, C. (1989). Renal effects of ANP in non human primates are potentiated by pentobarbital anesthesia. In: *XXXIth International Congress Of Physical Science*, Helsinki, p. 272.

Pollock, D. M. & Arendshorst, W. J. (1986). Effect of atrial natriuretic factor on renal hemodynamics in the rat. *Am. J. Physiol.* **251**: F795–801.

Pollock, D. M. & Banks, R. O. (1983). Effect of atrial extract on renal failure in the rat. *Clin. Sci.* **65**: 47–55.

Popescu, L. M., Panouiu, C. & Hinescu, M. (1985). The mechanisms of cGMP induced relaxation in vascular smooth muscle. *Eur. J. Pharmacol.* **107**: 393–4.

Richards, A. M., Nicholls, M. G., Ikram, H., Webster, M. W. I., Yandle, T. G. & Espiner, E. A. (1985). Renal, haemodynamic and hormonal effects of human alpha atrial natriuretic peptide in healthy volunteers. *Lancet* **i**: 545–8.

Rocha, A. S. & Kudo, L. H. (1982). Water, urea, sodium, chloride and potassium transport in the *in vitro* isolated perfused papillary collecting duct. *Kidney Int.* **22**: 485–91.

Roy, D. R. (1986). Effect of synthetic ANP on renal and loop of Henle functions in the young rat. *Am. J. Physiol.* **251**: F220–5.

Sands, J. M., Nonoguchi, H. & Knepper, M. A. (1988). Hormone effects on NaCl permeability of rat inner medullary collecting duct. *Am. J. Physiol.* **255**: F421–8.

Schnermann, J. & Briggs, J. P. (1987). Renal effects of atrial natriuretic peptides. *Klin. Wochenschr.* **65** (Suppl. VIII): 92–96.

Schnermann, J., Marin-Grez, M. & Briggs, J. P. (1986). Filtration pressure response to infusion of atrial natriuretic peptides. *Pflügers Arch.* **406**: 237–9.

Seymour, A. A. & Mazack, E. K. (1988). Renal effects of atrial natriuretic factor during control of the renin–angiotensin system in anesthetised dogs. *Circulation Res.* **62**: 506–14.

Shimizu, T. & Nakamura, M. (1986). Renal effects of atrial natriuretic polypeptide: comparison with standard saliuretics. *Eur. J. Pharmacol.* **127**: 249–59.

Showalter, C. J., Zimmerman, R. S., Schwab, T. R., Edwards, B. S., Opgenorth, T. J. & Burnett, J. C. Jr. (1988). Renal response to atrial natriuretic factor is modulated by intrarenal angiotensin II. *Am. J. Physiol.* **254**: R453–6.

Singer, D. R. J., Markandu, N. D., Buckley, M. G., Miller, M. A., Sugden, A. L., Sagnella, G. A. & MacGregor, G. A. (1989). Prolonged decrease in blood pressure after atrial natriuretic peptide infusion in essential hypertension: a new anti-pressor mechanism? *Clin. Sci.* **77**: 253–8.

Siragy, H. M., Lamb, N. E., Rose, C. E., Peach, M. J. & Carey, R. M. (1988). Angiotensin II modulates the intrarenal effects of atrial natriuretic peptide. *Am. J. Physiol.* **255**: F545–51.

Soejima, H., Grekin, R. J., Briggs, J. P. & Schnermann, J. (1988). Renal responses of anesthetised rats to low dose infusion of atrial natriuretic peptide. *Am. J. Physiol.* **255**: R449–55.

Solomon, L. R., Atherton, J. C., Bobinski, H. & Green, R. (1986). Effect of posture on plasma immunoreactive atrial natriuretic peptide in man. *Clin. Sci.* **71**: 299–305.

Solomon, L. R., Atherton, J. C., Bobinski, H. & Green, R. (1987). Effect of dietary sodium chloride and posture on plasma immunoreactive atrial natriuretic peptide concentrations in man. *Clin. Sci.* **72**: 201–8.

Solomon, L. R., Atherton, J. C., Bobinski, H., Hillier, V. & Green, R. (1988). Effect of low dose infusion of atrial natriuretic peptide on renal function in man. *Clin. Sci.* **75**: 403–10.

Sonnenberg, H. (1986). Mechanisms of release and renal tubular actions of atrial natriuretic factor. *Fed. Proc.* **45**: 2106–10.

Sonnenberg, H. (1987). On the physiological role of atrial natriuretic factor. *Klin. Wochenschr.* **65** (Suppl. VIII): 8–13.

Sonnenberg, H., Cupples, W. A., de Bold, A. J. & Veress, A. T. (1982). Intrarenal localisation of the natriuretic effect of cardiac atrial extract. *Canad. J. Physiol. Pharmacol.* **60**: 1149–52.

Sonnenberg, H., Honrath, U., Chong, C. K. & Wilson, D. R. (1986). Atrial natriuretic factor inhibits sodium transport in medullary collecting duct. *Am. J. Physiol.* **250**: F963–6.

Sonnenberg, H., Honrath, U. & Wilson, D. R. (1989). Effects of luminal amiloride or ANF on ^{22}Na efflux from the medullary collecting duct *in vivo*. *Kidney Int.* **35**: 288(A).

Sosa, R. E., Volpe, M., Marion, D. N., Atlas, S. A., Laragh, J. H., Vaughan, E. D. & Maack, T. (1986). Relationship between renal hemodynamic and natriuretic effects of atrial natriuretic factor. *Am. J. Physiol.* **250**: F520–4.

Stokes, T. J., McConkey, C. & Martin, K. J. (1986). Atriopeptin III increases cGMP in glomeruli but not in proximal tubules of dog kidney. *Am. J. Physiol.* **250**: F27–31.

Takezawa, K., Cowley, A. W., Skelton, M. & Roman, R. J. (1987). Atriopeptin III alters renal medullary haemodynamics and the pressure-diuresis response in rats. *Am. J. Physiol.* **252**: F992–1002.

Thomsen, K. (1984). Lithium clearance: a new method for determining proximal and distal tubular reabsorption of sodium and water. *Nephron* **31**: 217–23.

Tikkanen, I., Metsarinne, K., Fyhrquist, F. & Leidenlus, R. (1985). Plasma atrial natriuretic peptide in cardiac diseases and during infusion in healthy volunteers. *Lancet* **ii**: 66–9.

Torikai, S. (1986). Renal response to atrial natriuretic factor in rats without intact papillae. *Clin. Sci.* **71**: 277–82.

Tremblay, J., Gerzer, R., Vinay, P., Pany, S. C., Beliveau, R. & Hamet, P. (1985). The increase of cGMP by atrial natriuretic factor (ANF) correlates with the distribution of particulate guanylate cyclase. *FEBS Lett.* **181**: 17–22.

Ullrich, K. J. & Papavassiliou, F. (1979). Sodium reabsorption in the papillary collecting duct of rats. Effect of adrenalectony, low Na^+ diet, acetazolamide, HCO_3 free solutions and of amiloride. *Pflügers Arch.* **379**: 49–52.

van de Stolpe, A. & Jamison, R. L. (1988). Micropuncture study of the effect of ANP on the papillary collecting duct of the rat. *Am. J. Physiol.* **254**: F477–83.

Veldkamp, P. J., Carmines, P. K., Inscho, E. W. & Navar, L. G. (1988). Direct evaluation of the microvascular actions of ANP in juxtamedullary nephrons. *Am. J. Physiol.* **254**: F440–4.

Walsh, K. P., Williams, T. D. M., Canepa-Anson, R., Roe, P., Pitts, E., Lightman, S.L. & Sutton, R. (1988). Atrial natriuretic peptide released by rapid ventricular pacing in dogs does not cause a natriuresis. *Clin. Sci.* **74**: 571–6.

Weaver, L. C. (1977). Cardiopulmonary sympathetic afferent influences on renal nerve activity. *Am. J. Physiol.* **233**: H592–9.

Weidmann, P., Hasler, L., Gnädinger, M. P., Lang, R. E., Uehlinger, D. E., Shaw, S., Rascher, W. & Reubi, F. C. (1986). Blood levels and renal effects of atrial natriuretic peptide in normal man. *J. Clin. Invest.* **77**: 734–42.

Winquist, R. J. (1986). Possible mechanisms underlying the vasorelaxant response to atrial natriuretic factor. *Fed. Proc.* **45**: 2371–5.

Zeidel, M. L. (1988). Regulation of inner medullary collecting duct sodium transport by atrial natriuretic peptide. In: *Nephrology*, (Davison, ed.) London: Balliere Tindall, 145–56.

Zeidel, M. L., Kikeri, D., Silva, P., Burrowes, M. & Brenner, B. M. (1988). Atrial natriuretic peptide inhibits conductive sodium uptake by rabbit inner medullary collecting duct cells. *J. Clin. Invest.* **82**: 1067–74.

Zeidel, M. L., Silva, P., Brenner, B. M. & Seiftet, J. (1987). cGMP mediates effects of atrial peptides on medullary collecting duct cells. *Am. J. Physiol.* **222**: F551–9.

Zeidel, M. L., Seifter, J. L., Lear, S. & Silva, P. (1986). Atrial peptides inhibit oxygen consumption in kidney medullary collecting duct cells. *Am. J. Physiol.* **251**: F379–83.

Chapter 6
Effects of atrial natriuretic factor on the renin–angiotensin–aldosterone system

C. C. Lang and A. D. Struthers

Introduction

The homeostatic mechanisms maintaining salt balance in man are complex, with the renin–angiotensin–aldosterone system (RAAS), the sympathetic nervous system, the renal dopaminergic system and now atrial natriuretic factor (ANF) playing important roles. There is now an increasing body of evidence from both human and animal studies to show that several interactions between the RAAS and ANF take place in the finer control of sodium balance. The purpose of this chapter is to review these interactions and to consider the cellular mechanisms involved. An emphasis is placed on the effects of circulating ANF although the effects of intracerebral ANF will also be considered briefly.

Historical aspects

In early studies atrial extracts were found to inhibit angiotensin II-mediated vasoconstriction in the preconstricted rabbit aorta and in the isolated rat kidney (Camargo *et al.*, 1984; Kleinert *et al.*, 1984). These findings led various workers to consider whether ANF might antagonize other known actions of angiotensin II (ANGII), and, it was logical to initially focus on its possible effect on aldosterone. In early studies with rat adrenal glomerulosa cell suspensions, rat atrial extracts lowered basal aldosterone release as well as the aldosterone response to ACTH and ANGII (Atarashi *et al.*, 1984; Kudo & Baird, 1984). Other workers employing partially purified or synthetic ANF also demonstrated similar inhibitory effects on aldosterone biosynthesis by isolated bovine zona glomerulosa cells (Goodfriend, Elliot & Atlas, 1984) and a decrease in plasma aldosterone levels in intact dogs (Maack *et al.*, 1984) and in rats with experimentally induced renovascular hypertension (Volpe, Odell & Kleinert, 1984a). With regard to renin, ANF was also found to decrease plasma renin activity in the dog and this was then shown to be due to inhibition of renin release by the kidney. These early observations led to the proposal that ANF was a naturally occurring antagonist of the renin–angiotensin–aldosterone system and this has been aptly confirmed by subsequent studies both in animals and humans.

Effects on renin release

A growing body of evidence suggests that ANF inhibits renin release although as will be discussed below, this was not originally a universal finding. Furthermore the mechanisms involved remain unclear.

In vivo animal studies

An inhibitory effect on renin release was first demonstrated in intact anaesthetized dogs receiving constant intravenous or intrarenal infusions of ANF (Burnett, Granger & Opgenorth, 1984; Maack *et al.*, 1984). This was a particularly striking finding because ANF caused a concurrent fall in arterial pressure in both studies which would normally stimulate the baroreflex and cause a rise rather than a fall in renin secretion. These investigators proceeded to suggest that since ANF increased GFR during steady state conditions, the inhibition of renin release might have resulted from the increased delivery of sodium (and other ions including chloride) to the distal nephron where the cells of the macula densa lie close to the juxtaglomerular apparatus. A similar reduction of renin release was observed in conscious dogs hence negating the complicating influence of anaesthesia (Freeman, Davis & Vari, 1985).

However, a similar ANF-induced inhibition in plasma renin activity (PRA) has been less consistently found in rats. A constant infusion of ANF failed to inhibit renin release in chronic two-kidney, one-clip renovascular rats, but instead caused a slight but significant further rise in the already high level of PRA (Volpe, Odell & Kleinert, 1984b). Furthermore, only a transient and modest reduction in PRA was observed in anaesthetized rats receiving a large bolus dose of ANF (Obana *et al.*, 1985). Nevertheless, other workers have since been able to demonstrate an ANF-induced decrease in renin. Chronically administered ANF in two-kidney, one-clip hypertenisve rats resulted in a significant reduction in PRA (Garcia *et al.*, 1986). In another study investigating the effects of ANF on rats with markedly different levels of salt intake, ANF inhibited renin release in rats on normal sodium diet as well as in rats following chronic sodium restriction (Vari *et al.*, 1986).

Human studies

An ANF-induced decrease in PRA has been demonstrated in most studies in man. In initial studies incorporating intravenous bolus injections of ANF in humans, PRA did not rise despite concomitant hypotension (Richards *et al.*, 1985; Tikkanen *et al.*, 1985). Subsequent studies in humans, employing constant infusions of ANF have yielded mixed results with PRA falling (Anderson *et al.*, 1987), remaining stable (Biollaz *et al.*, 1986) and even rising (Weidmann *et al.*, 1986). There may be several explanations for these initial discrepancies. Firstly, in subjects who are supine and sodium-replete, renin is already relatively suppressed and hence any further suppression by ANF may not be readily evident. Secondly, the control of posture is essential in such studies because of the marked stimulatory effect of upright posture on renin release. Finally and probably most importantly, many of the early studies employed pharmacological rather than physiological doses of ANF. Hence a tonic inhibitory effect on renin release at physiological ANF levels may be overcome by high doses of ANF, which cause decreases in arterial pressure and baroreflex activation. In recent studies in which some of these factors have been carefully controlled, constant infusions of ANF even at low-dose infusions (producing plasma levels close to the physiological range) have been shown to decrease PRA in supine, resting, salt-deplete volunteers and in seated healthy salt-replete subjects undergoing water diuresis (Struthers *et al.*, 1986; Anderson *et al.*, 1987; Cuneo *et al.*, 1987; Richards *et al.*, 1988a).

In recent years, a number of workers have studied the effect of ANF on stimulated renin release in man. These studies extend previous animal *in vitro* work whereby ANF has been shown to inhibit the renin response to a number of secretagogues in animal studies (Obana *et al.*, 1985; Henrich, Needleman & Campbell, 1986; Scheur *et al.*, 1987). In man, ANF has been shown to inhibit the renin response to head-up tilt (Williams *et al.*, 1988). ANF has also been shown to inhibit the renin response to several other secretagogues including furosemide, isoproterenol (McMurray & Struthers, 1989; Fig. 6.1), prostaglandin E_2 (McMurray *et al.*, 1989) and captopril (Lang *et al.*, 1989).

Taking all these findings together, it would appear that ANF inhibits the renin response to a large number of different secretagogues so that in pharmacological terms, the renin inhibitory effect of ANF can be said to be non-specific.

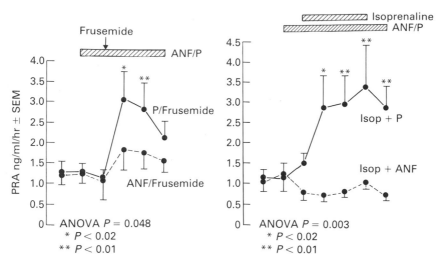

Fig. 6.1 Effects of ANF on plasma renin activity (PRA) stimulated by isoproterenol (isop) (left panel) and furosemide (right panel) in healthy salt-replete volunteers ($n = 7$). Isoproterenol (0.02 μg/kg/min) and furosemide (5-mg i.v. bolus) were given against a background infusion of 5% D-glucose (placebo) or ANF (0.025 μg/kg/min). Horizontal bars at top of figures show timing of infusions. Reproduced from McMurray & Struthers (1989a), (with permission).

Mechanism of inhibitory action of ANF on renin secretion

The mechanisms by which ANF inhibits the secretion of renin are unknown. Several theories have been postulated. In the first instance, an enhanced delivery of sodium chloride to the macula densa generated by ANF would be expected to decrease renin release rate according to the 'macula densa hypothesis'. Secondly, ANF causes afferent arteriolar dilatation which might conceivably increase the hydrostatic pressure along the afferent arteriole where 'renal baroreceptors' control renin release by the juxtaglomerular cells. Finally, ANF might cause direct inhibitory effects on juxtaglomerular cells themselves.

The macula densa theory has received support from several studies employing the 'non-filtering kidney' model, i.e. animals who had undergone ureteral ligation to prevent any changes in luminal solute. Employing this model in dogs, ANF no longer inhibited basal, norepinephrine- or prostacyclin-stimulated renin response (Opgenorth *et al.*, 1986; Deray *et al.*, 1987). Similarly in humans with end-stage renal failure (i.e. 'non-filtering kidneys') ANF failed to suppress plasma renin activity and also failed to increase urinary sodium excretion (Richards *et al.*, 1988b). This finding was not however universal as ANF has also been reported to inhibit renin release in non-filtering as well as filtering kidneys (Villareal *et al.*, 1986).

By causing changes in renal perfusion pressure, ANF might conceivably influence the 'renal baroreceptor', an event which could decrease renin secretion by the juxtaglomerular cells. The importance of this mechanism to ANF-induced inhibition of renin secretion was initially suggested by the failure of ANF to acutely reduce PRA in chronic two-kidney, one-clip hypertensive rats, and in fact caused a slight but significant increase in PRA (Volpe *et al.*, 1984b). Similar findings were also demonstrated in the early renal clamp model in anaesthetized dogs in which the ANF-induced increase in GFR and other renal haemodynamic effects were prevented (Sosa *et al.*, 1985).

The effects of ANF on renin release in juxtaglomerular cells have also been studied in *in vitro* preparations in which indirect mechanisms are not operating and here results have been conflicting. For instance, ANF has been shown to inhibit (Obana *et al.*, 1985; Antonipillai, Vogelsang & Horton, 1986; Kurtz *et al.*, 1986a), stimulate (Hackenthal, Lang & Buhrle, 1985; Hiruma, Ikemoto & Yamamoto, 1986; Itoh *et al.*, 1987) or not affect basal renin release (Rodriguez-Puyol *et al.*, 1986; Takagi *et al.*, 1988). ANF was able to directly inhibit renin release in a dose-dependent fashion in dispersed juxtaglomerular cells (Kurtz *et al.*, 1986a), but in a preparation of isolated rat glomeruli, ANF did not inhibit basal or prostaglandin-stimulated renin release (Rodriguez-Puyol *et al.*, 1986). Suggested explanations for this discrepancy are that the effective concentration of nutrients or stimuli bathing the cells may vary in kidney slices because of variable access. Alternatively, studies employing dispersed juxtaglomerular cells may be complicated by the fact that these juxtaglomerular cells may still retain their structural relationship with macula densa cells which in turn might affect the observed response. In a recent study, which attempted to avoid the above technical difficulties, a dispersed dynamic superfusion system in addition to dispersed juxta-glomerular cells was used (Takagi *et al.*, 1988a). These workers found that ANF failed to alter the renin response in both preparations suggesting that ANF has no direct effect on renin release. This has since been supported by another study employing a different preparation: the isolated rabbit afferent arteriole which contains only juxtaglomerular cells and is devoid of glomeruli, tubules or macula densa. In this study ANF pretreatment failed to inhibit the renin response to isoprenaline and frusemide (Itoh *et al.*, 1987).

In view of all these existing discrepancies, no firm conclusion can be drawn presently regarding the mechanism of the inhibitory effect on ANF on renin release. The available evidence from intact animal studies however suggests that either a 'macula densa' and/or an afferent arteriolar baroreflex mechanism are crucial and that, if direct inhibitory effects on the juxtaglomerular cells are involved, they are of only minor importance.

Cellular mechanisms involved in the inhibitory action of ANF on renin release

There is increasing evidence that cyclic guanyl monophosphate (cGMP) is the second messenger involved in this inhibition (Obana et al., 1985; Kurtz et al., 1986b) and these findings are consistent with many other reports which have clearly established the ability of ANF to activate cGMP in a variety of tissues (Winquist et al., 1984; Murad, 1986; Fiscus et al., 1987; Zeidell et al., 1987). In a recent study employing rat superficial cortical slices, the renin response to isoprenaline was blocked by atriopeptin III, nitroprusside (NP) and 8-bromoguanosine 3′,5′ cyclic monophosphate (8-BrcGMP) (Henrich et al., 1988). Both ANF and NP were shown to cause an increase in tissue cGMP. ANF is known to stimulate particulate guanylate cyclase whereas NP activates soluble guanylate cyclase; the observation that both these agents are able to inhibit renin release is evidence that activation of either form of guanylate cyclase will produce this response. Furthermore, the finding that 8-BrcGMP, an analogue for cGMP, was able to inhibit the renin response to isoprenaline whilst methylene blue, the guanylate cyclase inhibitor, effectively blocked the cGMP increase and attenuated the inhibitory effect of ANF, firmly establishes cGMP as the principal intracellular mediator.

The decline in cAMP seems to play only a minor role (Kurtz et al., 1986a). Henrich et al. (1988) confirmed this when they showed that both ANF and NP did not influence the ability of isoprenaline to induce an increase in cAMP. Kurtz et al. (1986b) had previously investigated the role of intracellular calcium and showed that ANF at 10^{-10} mmol/l had no influence on the transmembrane calcium flux, nor did it alter the intracellular calcium concentration of the juxtaglomerular cells. In contrast, they did find that the inhibitory effect of ANF on renin release could be attenuated by the calcium channel blocker verapamil suggesting that the inhibitory action of ANF might require a normal level of intracellular calcium.

Effects on ANGII actions

ANF has been shown to antagonize most of the known effects of ANGII ANF is a potent antagonist of ANGII-induced aldosterone production (Atarashi et al., 1984; Chartier et al., 1984; De Lean et al., 1984a). The mechanism of ANF-induced natriuresis, although complex, could partly be explained by its antagonistic effects on intrarenal ANGII (Siragy et al., 1988) with particular regard to its effects on glomerular permeability (De Arriba et al., 1988) and on tubular sodium reabsorption (Harris, Thomas & Morgan, 1987). There is also both animal in vitro and in vivo, evidence to show that these antagonistic actions also extend to ANGII-induced vasoconstriction (Kleinert et al., 1984) and pressor responses (Procter &

Bealer, 1987). Finally, these actions are not just confined to the periphery as the central administration of ANF has also been shown to inhibit ANGII-mediated effects on thirst, salt appetite (Nakamura *et al.*, 1985; Antunes-Rodrigues, McCann & Samson, 1986), blood pressure and renal responses (Yoshida *et al.*, 1989), as well as the release of vasopressin (Yamada *et al.*, 1986) and ACTH (Itoh *et al.*, 1986). All these actions will be discussed later in the appropriate sections.

Effects on aldosterone release

As indicated earlier, ANF inhibits aldosterone production by adrenal cortical cells *in vitro* and lowers plasma aldosterone levels in animals including man. The inhibition of aldosterone may result partly from the decrease in plasma renin activity and hence ANGII (Maack *et al.*, 1984; Freeman *et al.*, 1985) and/or by a direct action on the aldosterone response to its secretagogues (Atarashi *et al.*, 1984; Chartier *et al.*, 1984; De Lean *et al.*, 1984a; Schiffrin *et al.*, 1985a).

In vitro studies

ANF has been shown to inhibit aldosterone synthesis in adrenal glomerulosa cells isolated from the rat (Chartier *et al.*, 1984; Kudo & Baird, 1984; Atarashi, Mulrow & Franco-Saenz, 1985; Campbell, Currie & Needleman, 1985), cow (De Lean *et al.*, 1984a; Goodfriend *et al.*, 1984) and in a human adrenal tumour (Hirata *et al.*, 1985; Olansky & Kem, 1985). In these studies, ANF was shown to inhibit basal aldosterone release as well as its response to a variety of agonists including ANGII, K^+, ACTH, dibutyryl cAMP, forskolin and prostaglandin E_2. Although ANF generally antagonizes the effect of all these agonists *in vitro*, the precise effects appear to vary with each agonist. ANF shifts the ACTH dose–response curve to the right with no change in the maximal response, whereas it decreases the maximal response to ANGII and K^+ with no change in the EC_{50} (Schriffrin, Thibault & Chartier, 1985b). These workers went on to postulate that ANF could conceivably, by acting on specific receptors, produce simultaneously an apparent competitive antagonism of the action of ACTH and non-competitive antagonism of the action of ANGII and K^+.

Cellular mechanism involved in the inhibitory action of ANF on aldosterone biosynthesis

ANF appears to bind to two distinct cell-surface receptors on the zona glomerulosa (DeLean *et al.*, 1984b; Takayanagi *et al.*, 1987). Furthermore, specific receptors for ANF and for ANGII are both present and overlap each other in the adrenal zona glomerulosa (Mendelsohn *et al.*, 1987).

ANF receptors are coupled to at least two transducing enzymes, adenylate cyclase and guanylate cyclase (Anand-Srivastava *et al.*, 1984; Anand-Srivastava, Genest & Cantin, 1985; Cantin & Genest, 1985; Tremblay *et al.*, 1985). In adrenal cortical cells and cell homogenates, ANF is a potent stimulator of particulate guanylate cyclase (Waldman, Rapoport & Murad, 1984; Matsuoko *et al.*, 1985). On the other hand, neither the elevation of cGMP levels by sodium nitroprusside nor the addition of cGMP analogues produces any inhibition of aldosterone production (Matsuoko *et al.*, 1987; Ganguly *et al.*, 1989). Thus, unlike smooth muscle where cGMP is likely to be the only mediator of ANF action (Winquist *et al.*, 1984), adrenal cGMP may only be a partial mediator functioning in conjunction with other messenger(s) to bring about the inhibition of aldosterone release.

ACTH-induced aldosterone synthesis is associated with cAMP accumulation and ANF has been reported to inhibit adenylate cyclase in the adrenal cortex (Anand-Srivastava *et al.*, 1985). ANF also inhibits the aldosterone response to ACTH and to forskolin, an adenylate cyclase activator (DeLean *et al.*, 1984a), and to the pharmacological agent dbcAMP (Goodfriend *et al.*, 1984). In a recent study a rise in cGMP as well as a reduction in cellular cAMP may be required for the inhibition of steroidogenesis by ANF (Barrett & Isales, 1988). In other words, neither messenger alone could fully reproduce the inhibitory action of ANF.

The three major regulators of aldosterone (i.e. ANGII, K^+ and ACTH) act on zona glomerulosa cells through the intracellular messenger systems (Fig. 6.2). In the case of ANGII stimulation, activation of the membrane-bound enzyme phospholipase C leads to the breakdown of the membrane phospholipid phosphatidylinositol-4,5-bisphosphate (PIP_2) into 1,2-diacylglycerol (DAG) and myoinositol-1,4,5-triphosphate (IP_3). DAG activates protein kinase C. IP_3 leads to the release of calcium ions (Ca^{2+}) from the endoplasmic reticulum and to an elevation of cytosolic Ca^{2+} concentration. The liberated Ca^{2+} ions are bound to calmodulin and lead to the activation of calmodulin-dependent protein kinases. The zona glomerulosa cell is particularly sensitive to changes in extracellular K^+ concentration and is depolarized by relatively small increases of this parameter. Potassium-induced decreases in membrane potential lead to the opening of potential-dependent calcium channels and thus raise the cytosolic calcium concentration by facilitating the entry of this ion into the cell. Increases in the extracellular K^+ concentration also stimulate the production of cAMP by an unknown mechanism dependent on the influx of Ca^+ ions. ACTH interacts with a specific membrane receptor which activates adenylate cyclase and this leads to the formation of cAMP. cAMP acts as a second messenger and in turn activates a protein kinase. The activated protein kinase triggers protein phosphorylation. The specific labile protein or phosphoprotein (Protein-P) may lead to increased side-chain cleavage of cholesterol within the mitochondria (the 'early pathway'

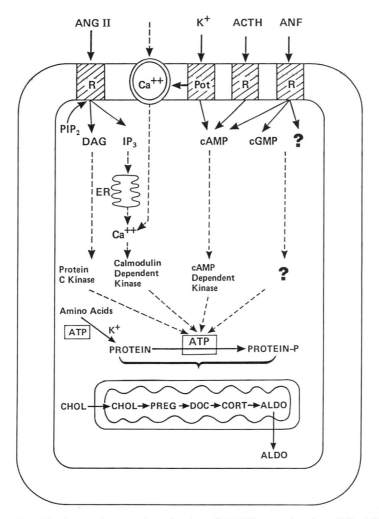

Fig. 6.2 Proposed mechanism of action of ANGII, potassium ions (K⁺), ACTH and ANF on corticosteroid biosynthesis in adrenocortical zona glomerulosa cells. R, receptor; Pot, membrane potential; DAG, 1,2-diacylglycerol; IP_3, myoinositol 1,4,5-triphosphate; ER, endoplasmic reticulum, PROTEIN-P, phosphoprotein; CHOL, cholesterol; PREG, pregnenolone; DOC, deoxycorticosterone; CORT, corticosterone; ALDO, aldosterone.

of steroidogenesis). Pregnenolone is converted to aldosterone through a series of steps referred to as the 'late pathway'.

Initial studies using rat adrenal capsular cell showed that ANF was reported to decrease the Ca^{2+} influx stimulated by ANGII, ACTH, K⁺ or the dihydropyridine Bay K 8644 (Chartier & Schiffrin, 1987). In contrast, in studies performed on bovine cells in which intracellular free calcium was monitored using the fluorescent dye Quin 2, no inhibitory effect of ANF was observed on the changes in intracellular calcium induced by either ANGII or K⁺ (Capponi et al., 1986). This work has since received support from recent studies in both rat and bovine adrenal glomerulosa cells indicating that the inhibitory effect of ANF on aldosterone production is not caused by interference with the calcium messenger system (Apfeldorf, Isales & Barrett, 1988; Takagi et al., 1988b). These findings in conjunction with a recent study in which ANF was shown not to influence the angiotensin-induced hydrolysis of phosphatidylinositol 4-5-biphosphate (Ganguly et al., 1989) suggest that the inhibitory effects of ANF would appear to occur distal to the generation of calcium.

A few studies on the intracellular mechanism of action at a site beyond calcium generation have been reported. In a recent study, it was reported that both ANGII and dbcAMP stimulated phosphorylation of a 17.6 K protein in bovine adrenal glomerulosa cells and that ANF inhibited the phosphorylation of this protein both tonically and after stimulation by ANGII and dbcAMP (Elliott & Goodfriend, 1986b, 1987; Pandey et al., 1987). However, in two recent studies this effect of ANF on protein phosphorylation was not seen in bovine (Ganguly et al., 1989) or rat glomerulosa cells (Takagi et al., 1988b).

There is conflicting data on which step in the biosynthetic pathway is inhibited by ANF. Several workers have suggested that ANF acts at a late stage in aldosterone synthesis, i.e. inhibition of the activation of corticosterone methyloxidate (Campbell et al., 1985; Nakajima et al., 1987; Schiebinger, Kem & Brown, 1988). Others have suggested a proximal effect on the 'early pathway', i.e. the step prior to the mitochondrial metabolism of cholesterol (Goodfriend et al., 1984; Racz et al., 1985; Elliott & Goodfriend, 1986a). In one study ANF was able to inhibit pregnenolone synthesis but yet was unable to inhibit the aldosterone response to exogenous progesterone (Goodfriend et al., 1984). The same study also showed that ANF had no effect on the rise in aldosterone production caused by a polar derivative of cholesterol, which suggests that ANF does not impede cholesterol side chain cleavage per se. Various possible site(s) of actions were considered which included hydrolysis of cholesterol esters, movement of cholesterol to the mitochondria and transport of cholesterol from outer to inner mitochondria. The recent discovery that adrenal cell mitochondria can directly bind ANF raises the distinct possibility that the inhibitory effects of ANF may occur directly at mitochondrial level where it might block cholesterol transport into the mitochondria (Heisler, 1989). This could account for the ability of ANF to inhibit both aldosterone biosynthesis and formation in response to a variety of agonists with dissimilar mechanisms of action.

In summary, the mechanism(s) of ANF action within the adrenal cortex remains far from clear. Although an attempt has been made to summarize the current evidence, we await further investigations to fully characterize these actions.

In vivo studies

These *in vitro* findings have since been extended to animal *in vivo* studies. Initial studies employing pharmacological doses of ANF have shown prompt suppression of basal-, ANGII-, ACTH- and K^+-stimulated aldosterone secretion (Maack *et al.*, 1984; Garcia *et al.* 1986; Takagi, Franco-Saenz & Mulrow, 1986). Recent studies with lower infusion rates of ANF designed to increase the plasma ANF levels within a physiological range have reported similar findings (Zimmerman *et al.*, 1987; Brands & Freeman, 1988). The reduction in plasma aldosterone concentration generally occurs in assocation with a fall in PRA in most studies (Maack *et al.*, 1984; Vari *et al.*, 1986; Atlas *et al.*, 1987). Recent animal studies have suggested that this action is independent of renin. In one study rats were pretreated with dexamethasone and captopril to suppress the hypothalamo–hypophyseal–adrenal axis and the renin–angiotensin system. Thereafter, a prolonged infusion of ANF still caused a lowering of basal plasma concentration of aldosterone, which indicates that the inhibitory effect is independent of both ANGII or ACTH secretion (Rebuffatt *et al.*, 1988). In another experiment in sodium-deplete rats receiving stepwise increments of ANF infusion, a high dose of ANF 45 ng/kg/min resulted in a further reduction in aldosterone without any further suppression of PRA (Brands & Freeman, 1988). This lends further support to a direct non-renin-dependent physiological action of ANF on the zona glomerulosa.

Human studies

Experimental findings in humans concur with the above intact animal studies. However, as with the effects of ANF on renin, initial studies using intravenous boluses or brief infusions did not result in inhibition of aldosterone secretion (Richards *et al.*, 1985; Tikkanen *et al.*, 1985). However, when steady-state conditions are achieved, a fall in plasma aldosterone has been unequivocally demonstrated (Cuneo *et al.*, 1986). It has also been demonstrated that the baseline sodium status of an individual influences the aldosterone response to ANF and there are several reasons for this. First, the effects of a given infusion of ANF is liable to be disproportionately greater in individuals with low endogenous levels of ANF such as sodium depletion (Sagnella *et al.*, 1985; Espiner *et al.*, 1986). Secondly, the aldosterone response to ANGII (Hollenberg *et al.*, 1974; Oelkers *et al.*, 1974) and ACTH (Tuck *et al.*, 1981) is well known to be augmented by sodium depletion. Thus, any inhibitory effect of ANF should appear greater in the salt-deplete state where aldosterone turnover is greater.

Various investigators, have investigated the effect of ANF on the

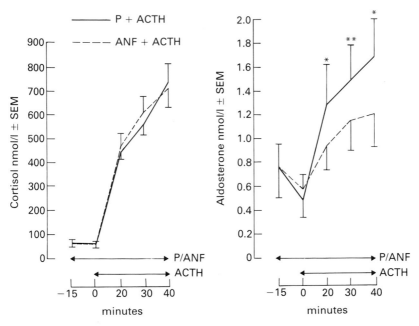

Fig. 6.3 Effects of ANF on the plasma cortisol (left panel) and aldosterone (right panel) responses to synthetic ACTH infusion in healthy salt-replete volunteers ($n = 8$). Infusion of ACTH (0.1 mi.u./kg/min) was commenced 15 min after starting infusion of either 5% D-glucose (Placebo, P) or ANF (15 pmol/kg/min). Arrows indicate nature and timing of infusions. *, $P < 0.01$; **, $P < 0.001$ for individual time point by paired t-test after MANOVA. P+ACTH (–), ANF 15 pmol/kg/min + ACTH (----). Reproduced from McMurray *et al.* (1988), (with permission).

aldosterone secretion to different secretagogues. ANF at both physiological and pharmacological doses attenuated the aldosterone response to ANGII (Anderson *et al.*, 1986; Vierhapper, Nowotny & Waldhausl, 1986; Cuneo *et al.*, 1987). Recently these inhibitory findings have been extended to ACTH-stimulated aldosterone secretion. In one study (Cuneo *et al.*, 1987), the aldosterone and cortisol responses were observed during four consecutive infusions of ACTH (6.25, 12.5, 25 and 50 mm i.v./30 min) in the presence and absence of ANF (2–3 pmol/kg/min). ANF only inhibited the aldosterone, though not the cortisol, response to the lowest dose of ACTH (6.25 m i.u./30 min). In contrast ANF inhibited the aldosterone response to all incremental doses of ANGII (0.5–4.0 ng/kg/min). This accords with the earlier hypothesis that ANF inhibited the ACTH response in a competitive manner but the ANGII response in a non-competitive manner (Schiffrin *et al.*, 1985b). McMurray *et al.* (1988) used a pharmacological dose of ANF (15 pmol/kg/min) and a high dose of ACTH to show that ANF selectively inhibited the aldosterone but not the cortisol response in healthy volunteers (Fig. 6.3). This differential effect between aldosterone and cortisol will be dealt with later on in the chapter.

Lang *et al.* (1990) have also recently demonstrated that both physiological and pharmacological doses of ANF inhibit the aldosterone response to metoclopramide, a dopamine antagonist. Taking all these findings together, it would appear that ANF inhibits aldosterone secretion in man in a non-specific manner, a finding in keeping with the animal *in vitro* studies as discussed earlier.

Effects on glucocorticoids

As regards glucocorticoids, the effects of ANF appear to be species-dependent. In most laboratories, ANF did not suppress glucocorticoid formation by rat fasciculata cells (Atarashi *et al.*, 1984; Kudo & Baird 1984; Campbell *et al.*, 1985; Hashimoto *et al.*, 1987) and this is in keeping with the lack of ANF receptors in the zona fasciculata in this species (Bianchi *et al.*, 1986). On the other hand, ANF has been shown to decrease cortisol production in bovine adrenal cells (DeLean *et al.*, 1984a). In *in vitro* studies using isolated human adrenal tissues, ANF has also been shown to depress basal as well as ACTH-stimulated cortisol secretion (Naruse *et al.*, 1987). Data from human studies have, however, been conflicting. Cody *et al.* (1986) and Weidmann *et al.* (1986) both demonstrated a modest inhibition of plasma cortisol by ANF. However, several investigators have demonstrated otherwise (McMurray *et al.*, 1988; Jungmann *et al.*, 1989; Muller-Esch *et al.*, 1990).

Inhibition of ACTH release could also contribute to glucocorticoid suppression. It has been reported that ANF can inhibit ACTH release using primary cultures of rat anterior pituitary cells (Shibasaki *et al.*, 1986; Shilo *et al.*, 1988; King & Baertschi, 1989). Furthermore, ANF has been shown to inhibit the stimulation of ACTH release caused by haemorrhage in the intact rat (Sugawara *et al.*, 1987) and sheep (Cameron *et al.*, 1988).

Renal interactions with the renin–angiotensin–aldosterone system

ANF and the renin–angiotensin system seem to interact with each other at several possible sites within the kidney. With regard to the glomerulus, specific ANF receptors have been identified in the isolated rat glomerulus (Bianchi *et al.*, 1986). Recent studies have also shown that ANF was able to inhibit the ANGII-induced glomerular mesangial cell contraction (De Arriba *et al.*, 1988). Such an effect is liable to alter the glomerular filtration surface area and hence the glomerular ultrafiltration coefficient (K_f). With regard to the proximal tubule, Harris *et al.* (1987) used the shrinking split droplet technique and found that ANF had no intrinsic effect on basal transport in the late proximal tubule but that ANF did antagonize the stimulation of proximal tubular absorption evoked by ANGII. However, other workers have disputed this finding (Cogan, 1986; Liu & Cogan, 1988).

With regard to natriuresis and diuresis, ANGII has been shown to inhibit ANF-induced natriuresis and conversely ANF has been shown to inhibit ANGII-induced antinatriuresis (Siragy et al., 1988). Similar findings have been reported in normal man using doses of ANGII and ANF which by themselves did not alter systemic blood pressure (McMurray & Struthers, 1988).

In recent years, a number of workers have investigated the effect of ACE inhibition (ACEI) on the renal actions of ANF. In vivo animal experiments showed either enhancement or no change in ANF-induced natriuresis after ACEI (Wang & Gilmore, 1985; Spinelli, Kamber & Schnell, 1986; Di Nicolantonio & Morgan, 1987; Hansell & Ulfendahl, 1987; Woods & Anderson, 1987). Similar studies in humans are divided as to whether ACEI increase (Wilkins et al., 1987) or decrease (Mann et al., 1986) endogenous plasma ANF levels, but a fall in ANF-induced natriuresis has been a consistent finding after ACEI pretreatment (Wilkins et al., 1987; Gaillard, Koomans & DorhoutMees, 1988; Wambach et al., 1989). There may be several possible reasons for this blunting of the renal actions of ANF. In the first instance, most of these initial studies have been associated with changes in blood pressure and hence presumably also reduction in renal perfusion pressure. Secondly, after ACE inhibition, endogenous ANGII levels are often reduced and it may be that some ANGII is required to maintain the glomerular pressure gradient necessary for ANF action. In a recent study in which posture and diet were carefully controlled, ACE inhibition had little effect on ANF metabolism or on its natriuretic effect at doses which had only a minor effect on blood pressure. They did however, find rather surprisingly that ACE inhibition super-imposed on a background of low-dose infusion of ANF causes an increase in the activity of the hypothalamo-pituitary-adrenal axis and sympathetic nervous system by mechanisms which remain unexplained (Richards et al., 1989).

Vascular interactions with the renin–angiotensin–aldosterone system

Full discussion on the vascular effects of ANF will be dealt with in another chapter. Suffice to say that there is still considerable disagreement concerning the mechanism by which ANF lowers arterial pressure.

Of relevance to this particular chapter, there is much evidence to suggest that ANF interacts with the renin–angiotensin–aldosterone at the vascular level. Kleinert and coworkers (1984), demonstrated that ANF exerts especially pronounced antagonism towards ANGII-induced vas-constriction in the isolated aorta. This preferential effect on angiotensin-mediated vasoconstriction would be consistent with the demonstrable action of ANF on cultured smooth muscle cells where it inhibits intracellular calcium mobilization which is the mediator by which ANGII acts in vascular smooth muscle cells (Knorr et al., 1986). In recent years, interest has spread to the study of ANF action on smaller peripheral arteries where different effects have been seen. Osol et al. (1986) examined in vitro small (210 μm diameter) cerebral and mesenteric arteries of the rat and showed that ANGII-induced vasoconstriction was insensitive to ANF. Similarly Edwards & Weidley (1987) observed that constriction of rabbit glomerular arterioles in vitro with noradrenaline or ANGII was insensitive to ANF at concentrations as high as 10^{-7} M.

Recently Procter & Bealer (1987) examined the responses of small, third-order arterioles (20–40 μm diameter) in the rat spinotrapezium muscle microcirculation. They observed that whilst ANF had no effect on the intrinsic tone, the receptor-mediated constriction of arterioles with ANGII (but not vasopressin and noradrenaline) was inhibited by ANF. In addition, constriction of intestinal arterioles with ANGII and vasopressin was inhibited by pharmacological concentrations of ANF while noradrenaline responses were unaffected (Edwards & Weidley, 1987).

As mentioned, many studies have demonstrated a depressor response to ANF (Biollaz et al., 1986). Consistent with this being due to antagonism of angiotensin ANGII-induced vasoconstriction is that ANF has a greater depressor effect in renin-dependent, two-kidney, one-clip renovacular hypertensive rats than in non-renin-dependent, one-kidney, one-clip rats (Volpe et al., 1984b). Yasujima et al. (1986) also observed that a non-hypotensive dose of ANF could modulate the vasopressor effect of a 3-day infusion of ANGII in the rat, a finding which has since been confirmed by others (Lappe, Todt & Wendt, 1987). In man, Uehlinger et al. (1986) compared the depressor effect of ANF during infusions of both noradrenaline and ANGII. In contrast to the above-mentioned studies, a preferential interaction was noted with noradrenergic as compared to angiotensinergic pressor responses. This initial finding has since received support from a recent study by Faber et al. (1988) who investigated ANF action on the rat cremaster microcirculation. Their data indicated that ANF exhibits a high potency and selectivity for reversal of α_1-adrenoceptor-mediated constriction of large arterioles and venules. Furthermore constriction produced by α_2-adrenoceptor stimulation or noradrenergic 'intrinsic' mechanisms appeared to be insensitive to ANF.

Investigators have also been interested in the effect of various vasoactive hormones including ANGII on release of ANF from the atria. All available experimental data suggest that the rise in plasma ANF during ANGII infusion is due to increased venous return caused by ANGII with subsequent atrial distension (Dietz, 1988; Shenker et al., 1988). Nevertheless, in a recent study it was reported that in ACEI-treated dogs, a low non-pressor dose of ANGII was able to induce ANF release independent of any haemodynamic changes, which suggests that angiotensin might facilitate ANF release at a cellular level (Volpe et al., 1988).

Central interactions with the renin–angiotensin–aldosterone system

There is now a growing body of evidence that ANF antagonizes the renin–angiotensin–aldosterone system centrally as well as peripherally. ANF and its binding sites have now been identified in some periventricular structures including the subfornical organ (SFO) and the organum vasculosum laminae terminals (OVLT), both of which are also rich in ANGII binding sites.

The SFO sends projections to the hypothalamus specifically to the OVLT, an area critical to fluid and electrolyte balance and to the development of experimental hypertension. Thus the SFO and its hypothalamic projection may represent the site of interaction between circulating as well as local brain neuropeptides such as ANF and ANGII. Animal in vitro studies have supported this speculation. An increased activity as well as number of binding sites for ANGII have been observed in SHR when compared with WKY rats. These animals have also been shown to have a decreased number of ANF binding sites in the SFO (Saavedra et al., 1986a,b). Furthermore, it has recently been demonstrated in rat brain slices that ANF depresses the ANGII-induced excitation of neurons in the SFO (Hattori et al., 1988).

The effects of brain ANGII receptor stimulation in various species have been a matter of intensive investigation (Phillips, 1987; Unger et al., 1988). Most of the central action of ANGII, such as elevation of blood pressure (Fitzsimons, 1980), drinking (Reid, 1984) salt preference (Avrith & Fitzsimons, 1980) release of vasopressin and ACTH release (Scholkens et al., 1982) and suppression of renin release from the kidney (Malayan et al., 1979) conform with those exerted by peripheral ANGII with one notable exception, namely the effect on renal sodium handling. While circulating ANGII tends to retain sodium, central ANGII has been shown to induce natriuresis (Brooks & Malvin, 1982; Unger et al., 1989).

With regard to the central effects of ANF on body fluid regulation, conflicting data have been reported. On the one hand, centrally administered ANF has been shown to result in natriuresis and diuresis in conscious hydrated rats (Lee et al., 1987; Israel, Torres & Barbella, 1988; Imura & Nakao, 1990). On the other hand, there is evidence to suggest that central ANF although diuretic in its action, may be antinatriuretic (Rohmeiss et al., 1990).

The central interactions between ANGII and ANF have been extensively studied. Briefly, central ANF has been shown both in vitro and *in vivo* to antagonize all of the central effects of ANGII. The blunting of ANGII-induced pressor responses by central ANF could be due to many different mechanisms such as changes in blood volume, sympathetic activity or vasopressin release (Shimizu *et al.*, 1986; Casto *et al.*, 1987; McKitrick & Calaresu, 1988; Imam *et al.*, 1989; Yoshida *et al.*, 1989). Intracerebroventricular ANF has also been shown to inhibit the natriuresis and antidiuresis induced by either central ANG II or hypertonic NaCl (Yoshida *et al.*, 1989; Rohmeiss *et al.*, 1990). ICV ANF also inhibits water intake induced by central ANGII or by dehydration (Antunes-Rodrigues *et al.*, 1985; Nakamura *et al.*, 1985). The importance of this has been underlined by the observation that the infusion of specific ANF antibodies potentiates the water intake induced by either water deprivation or ANGII. Similarly, salt-deplete rats have an exaggerated urge to consume salt water and this appetite is inhibited by ANF (Antunes-Rodrigues *et al.*, 1986).

Both ANGII and ANF play a significant role in the secretion of vasopressin (AVP). Many studies have shown that although ANF has variable effects on basal AVP, it does consistently inhibit the AVP response to osmolality, ANGII, KCL and haemorrhage (Samson, 1985; Yamada *et al.*, 1986). A number of studies have been designed to examine the mechanism and site of ANF action on AVP secretion and there are several possibilities. First, ANF could alter baroreceptor-mediated alterations in cerebral blood flow resulting in changes in AVP release. Secondly, ANF could act directly at the posterior pituitary, a site within the blood–brain barrier and also where low-density binding sites are present (Quirion *et al.*, 1984). In this regard, ANF has been shown to inhibit adenylate cyclase activity in cultured posterior pituitary cells (Anand-Srivastava *et al.*, 1985). The final possibility is that ANF could act more centrally to inhibit AVP release. Dense innervation of the paraventricular nucleus by ANF-positive axon terminals suggests a direct action on the AVP-producing cell bodies. Furthermore, Samson *et al.* (1987) demonstrated in an isolated hypothalamoneurohypophyseal explant that ANF was capable of inhibiting AVP release without affecting oxytocin release. In man, most studies have also shown a lack of effect of ANF on basal AVP but ANF does attenuate AVP release as stimulated by osmolality or posture (Allen *et al.*, 1988; Williams *et al.*, 1988). In addition to inhibiting vasopressin release, there is evidence from *in vitro* studies that ANF also antagonizes its peripheral actions. Notably it has been shown to antagonize vasopressin-induced renal vasoconstriction (Camargo *et al.*, 1984) and also to inhibit vasopressin-stimulated epithelial water transport (Dillingham & Anderson, 1986).

The presence of ANF-positive axon terminals in the external layer of the median eminence as well as the presence of ANF binding in the anterior pituitary gland itself suggest that the peptide might modulate pituitary function, especially ACTH release. We have previously discussed the ability of ANF to inhibit ACTH release in primary cultures of rat anterior pituitary cells (Shibaski *et al.*, 1986; Shilo *et al.*, 1988; King & Baertschi, 1989). Furthermore, peripherally administered ANF has been shown to inhibit the stimulation of ACTH-release caused by haemorrhage (Sugawara *et al.*, 1987; Cameron *et al.*, 1988). Itoh *et al.* (1986) have also demonstrated that an i.c.v infusion of ANF in conscious unrestrained rats inhibits corticosterone release as stimulated by central ANGII.

These findings may have important implications because critically ill patients may be dependent on these stress-related hormones which might be adversely affected if ANF levels were increased by some novel therapeutic approach. However, recent studies have produced more reassuring results. In *in vitro* studies using cultures of both normal pituitary cells as well as mouse pituitary tumour cells, ANF has had no effect on ACTH release (Heisler *et al.*, 1986; Hashimoto *et al.*, 1987). Recent human studies also support this. ANF had no effect on the CRF- and GHRH-induced release of ACTH, growth hormone or plasma cortisol in healthy volunteers (Muller-Esch *et al.*, 1990). Jungmann *et al.* (1989) also demonstrated a similar lack of effect in the stimulation of pituitary or adrenal tissues during insulin-induced hypoglycaemia.

A number of workers have also been interested in the converse process by which the brain renin–angiotensin–aldosterone system regulates ANF secretion. Itoh *et al.* (1988) demonstrated that an i.c.v. infusion of ANGII, although having no effect on basal ANF level, significantly enhanced ANF secretion in conscious rats when stimulated by volume loading. Furthermore, they demonstrated that this enhancing effect is attenuated by the i.v. administration of a V_1-receptor antagonist or by i.c.v administration of phentolamine. They concluded that the brain renin–angiotensin–aldosterone system regulates ANF secretion by the stimulation of AVP secretion and/or the activation of a central α-adrenergic pathway.

At present, little is known about the molecular mechanism of the ANGII/ANF interaction in the brain. ANGII has been shown to excite neuronal cells in a number of brain regions, including those involved in central salt and water regulation. ANF, on the other hand has recently been demonstrated to induce a short-lasting hyperpolarization followed by depolarization in cultured rat glioma cells (Reiser, Hopp & Hamprecht, 1987). In addition, ANF was reported to inhibit putative vasopressin neurons in the paraventricular nucleus (Standaert *et al.*, 1987). In view of the close anatomical relationship between ANGII- and ANF-containing cell bodies, fibres and binding sites, one could speculate that both peptides may directly interact by altering neuronal excitability within common pathways. Another possibility for the central interaction of the two peptides could be their influence on the release of a $(Na^+ + K^+)$-ATPase inhibitor from the brain. Central ANGII has been shown to release a $(Na^+ + K^+)$-ATPase inhibitor into circulation (Buckley *et al.*, 1986) and more recently, ANF had been shown to have an inhibitory effect on the release of the inhibitor from brain tissue (Crabos *et al.*, 1988).

Conclusions

In conclusion, ANF exhibits remarkable peripheral and central effects at key sites of the renin–angiotensin–aldosterone system, thus establishing its broad involvement in the regulation of blood pressure, blood volume and sodium balance. It is tempting to speculate that ANF acts as a physiologic counterpart to the renin–angiotensin–aldosterone system. Whilst the renin–angiotensin–aldosterone system plays a major role in promoting sodium and fluid balance and in supporting arterial pressure, ANF may act to oppose this system in situations involving salt/fluid overload and elevated blood pressure. Thus the two systems could operate in tandem to regulate cardiac output, arterial pressure, tissue perfusion and salt/water balance.

Acknowledgements

We are most grateful to Mrs Joy Thomson for typing the manuscript and to Miss Maureen Sneddon of the Department of Medical Illustration, Ninewells Hospital, for help with the illustrations.

References

Allen, M. J., Ang, V. T. Y., Bennett, E. D. & Jenkins, J. S. (1988). Atrial natriuretic peptide inhibits osmolality-induced arginine vasopressin release in man. *Clin. Sci.* **75**: 35–9.

Anand-Srivastava, M. B., Franks, D. J., Cantin, M. & Genest, J. (1984). Atrial natriuretic factor inhibits adenylate cyclase. *Biochem. Biophys. Res. Commun.* **121**: 855–62.

Anand-Srivastava, M. B., Genest, J. & Cantin, M. (1985). Inhibitory effect of atrial natriuretic factor on adenylate cyclase activity in adrenal cortical membranes. *FEBS Lett* **181**: 199–202.

Anderson, J. V., Donckier, J., Payne, N. N., Beecham, J., Slater, J. D. H. & Bloom, S. R. (1987). Atrial natriuretic peptide: evidence of action as a natriuretic hormone at physiological plasma concentrations in man. *Clin. Sci.* **72**: 305–512.

Anderson, J. V., Struthers, A. D., Payne, N. N., Slater, J. D. H. & Bloom, S. R. (1986). Atrial natriuretic peptide inhibit the aldosterone response to angiotensin II in man. *Clin. Sci.* **70**: 507–12.

Andersson, B., Eriksson, L., Fernandez, O., Kolmodin, C. G. & Oltner, R. (1972). Centrally mediated effects of sodium and angiotensin II on arterial blood pressure and fluid balance. *Acta Physiol. Scand.* **85**: 398–407.

Antonipillai, I., Vogelsang, J. & Horton, R. (1986). Role of atrial natriuretic factor in renin release. *Endocrinology* **119**: 318–22.

Antunes-Rodrigues, J., McCann, S. M., Rogers, L. C. & Samson, W. K. (1985). Atrial natriuretic factor inhibits dehydration and angiotensin II induced water intake in the conscious unrestrained rat. *Proc. Nat. Acad. Sci. USA* **82**: 8720–3.

Antunes-Rodrigues, J., McCann, S. M. & Samson, W. K. (1986). Central administration of atrial natriuretic factor inhibits saline preference in the rat. *Endocrinology* **118**: 1726–8.

Apfeldorf, W. J., Isales, C. M. & Barrett, P. (1988). Atrial natriuretic peptide inhibits the stimulation of aldosterone secretion but not the transient increase in intracellular free calcium induced by angiotensin II addition. *Endocrinology* **122**: 1460–5.

Atarashi, K., Mulrow, P. J. & Franco-Saenz, R. (1985). Effect of atrial peptides on aldosterone production. *J. Clin. Invest.* **76**: 1807–11.

Atarashi, K., Mulrow, P. J., Franco-Saenz, R., Snajdar, R. & Rapp, J. (1984). Inhibition of aldosterone production by an atrial extract. *Science* **224**: 992–4.

Atlas, S. A., Pecker, M. S., Cody, R. J. & Laragh, J. H. (1987). Endocrine and renal responses to physiological levels of ANF. *Abstracts of 2nd World Congress on Biologically Active Atrial Peptides*, New York, p. 181.

Avrith, D. B. & Fitzsimmons, J. T. (1980). Increased sodium appetite in the rat induced by intracranial administration of components of the renin–angiotensin system. *J. Physiol.* **301**: 349–64.

Barrett, P. Q. & Isales, C. M. (1988). The role of cyclic nucleotides in atrial natriuretic peptide-mediated inhibition of aldosterone secretion. *Endocrinology* **122**: 799–808.

Bianchi, G., Gutkowska, G., Thibault, G., Garcia, R., Genest, J. & Cantin, M. (1985). Radioautiographic localization of ^{125}I-atrial natriuretic factor (ANF) in rat tissues. *Histochemistry* **82**: 441–52.

Bianchi, C., Gutkowska, J., Thibault, G., Garcia, R., Genest, J. & Cantin, M. (1986). Distinct localization of atrial natriuretic factor and angiotensin II binding sites in the glomeruli. *Am. J. Physiol.* **251**: F594–602.

Biollaz, J., Nussberger, J., Porchet, M., Brunner-Ferber, F., Otterbein, E. S., Gomez, H. J., Waeber, B., & Brunner, H. R. (1986). Four hour infusion of synthetic atrial natriuretic peptide in normal volunteers. *Hypertension* **8** (Suppl. II): II96–105.

Brands, M. W. & Freeman, R. H. (1988). Aldosterone and renin inhibition by physiological levels of atrial natriuretic factor. *Am. J. Physiol.* **254**: R1011–16.

Brooks, V. L. & Malvin, R. L. (1982). Intracerebroventricular infusion of angiotensin II increases sodium excretion. *Proc. Soc. Exp. Biol. Med.* **169**: 532–7.

Buckley, J. P., Doursout, M. F., Liang, Y. Y. & Chelly, J. E. (1986). Central angiotensin II mechanisms and the sodium pump. *J. Hypertension* **4** (Suppl. 6): S465–7.

Burnett, J. C. Jr., Granger, J. P. & Opgenorth, T. S. (1984). Effects of synthetic atrial natriuretic factor on renal function and renin release. *Am. J. Physiol.* **247**: F863–6.

Camargo, M. J. F., Kleinert, H. D., Atlas, S. A., Sealey, J. E., Laragh, J. H. & Maack, T. (1984). Ca-dependent haemodynamic and natriuretic effects of atrial extract in isolated rat kidney. *Am. J. Physiol.* **246**: F447–56.

Cameron, V. A., Espiner, E. A., Nicholls, N. G. & Skidmore, D. S. (1988). Hormone and haemodynamic responses to atrial natriuretic peptide in conscious sheep and effect of haemorrhage. *Endocrinology* **122**: 407–14.

Campbell, W. B., Currie, M. G. & Needleman, P. (1985). Inhibition of aldosterone biosynthesis by atriopeptins in rat adrenal cells. *Circulation Res.* **57**: 113–18.

Cantin, M. & Genest, J. (1985). The heart and the atrial natriuretic factor. *Endocrine Rev.* **6**: 107–27.

Capponi, A. M., Lew, P. D., Wuthrich, R. & Vallotton, M. B. (1986). Effects of atrial natriuretic peptide on the stimulation of angiotensin II of various target cells. *J. Hypertension* **4** (Suppl. 2): S61–5.

Casto, R., Gilbig, J., Schroeder, G. & Stock, G. (1987). Atrial natriuretic factor inhibits central angiotensin II pressor responses. *Hypertension* **9**: 473–7.

Chartier, L. & Schiffrin, E. C. (1987). Role of calcium in effects of atrial natriuretic peptide on aldosterone production in adrenal glomerulosa cells. *Am. J. Physiol.* **252**: E485–91.

Chartier, L., Schiffrin, E. L., Thibault, G. & Garcia, R. (1984). Atrial natriuretic factor inhibits the stimulation of aldosterone secretion by angiotensin II, ACTH and potassium *in vitro* and angiotensin II-induced steroidogenesis *in vivo*. *Endocrinology* **115**: 2026–8.

Cody, R. J., Atlas, S. A., Laragh, J. H., Kubo, S. H., Kovit, A. B., Ryman, K. S., Shaknovich, A. *et al.* (1986). Atrial natriuretic factor in normal subjects and heart failure. *J. Clin. Invest.* **78**: 1362–74.

Cogan, M. G. (1986). Atrial natriuretic factor can increase renal solute excretion primarily by raising glomerular filtration. *Am. J. Physiol.* **250**: F710–14.

Crabos, M., Ausiello, D. A., Haupert, G. T. & Cantiello, H. F. (1988). Atrial natriuretic peptide regulates release of Na$^+$ K$^+$ ATPase inhibitor from rat brain. *Am. J. Physiol.* **254**: F912–17.

Cuneo, R. C., Espiner, E. A., Nicholls, M. G., Yandle, T. G., Joyce, J. L. & Gilchrist, N. L. (1986). Renal, haemodynamic and hormonal responses to atrial natriuretic peptide infusion in normal man, and effect of sodium intake. *J. Clin. Endocrinol. Metab.* **63**: 946–53.

Cuneo, R. C., Espiner, E. A., Nicholls, M. G., Yandle, T. G. & Livesey, J. H. (1987). Effects of physiological levels of atrial natriuretic peptide on hormone secretion: Inhibition of angiotensin-induced aldosterone secretion and renin release in normal man. *J. Clin. Endocrinol. Metab.* **65**: 765–72.

De Arriba, G., Barrio, V., Olivera, A., Rodriguez-Puyol, D. & Lopez-Novoa, J. M. (1988). Atrial natriuretic peptide inhibits angiotensin II-induced contraction of isolated glomeruli and cultured glomerular mesangial cells of rats: the role of calcium. *J. Lab. Clin, Med.* **III**: 466–74.

DeLean, A., Gutkowska, J., McNicoll, N,, Schiller, P. W., Cantin, M. & Genest, J. (1984b). Characterisation of specific receptors for atrial natriuretic factor in bovine adrenal zona glomerulosa. *Life Sci.* **35**: 2311–18.

DeLean, A., Racz, K., Gutkowska, J., Nguyen, T.-T., Cantin, M. & Genest, J. (1984a). Specific receptor mediated inhibition by synthetic atrial natriuretic factor of bovine-stimulated steroidogenesis in cultured bovine adrenal cells. *Endocrinology* **115**: 1636–8.

Deray, G., Branch, R. A., Herzer, W. A., Ohnishi, A. & Jackson, E. K. (1987). Effects of atrial natriuretic factor on hormone induced renin release. *Hypertension* **9**: 513–17.

Dietz, J. R. (1988). The effect of angiotensin II and ADH on the secretion of atrial natriuretic factor. *Proc. Soc. Exp. Biol. Med.* **187**: 366–9.

Dillingham, M. A. & Anderson, R. J. (1986). Inhibition of vasopressin action by atrial natriuretic factor. *Science* **231**: 1572–3.

Di Nicolantonio, R. & Morgan, T. O. (1987). Captopril attenuates diuretic and natriuretic actions of furosemide but not natriuretic peptide. *Clin. Exp. Hypertension* **A9**: 19–32.

Edwards, R. M. & Weidley, E. F. (1987). Lack of effect of atriopeptin II on rabbit glomerular arterioles *in vitro*. *Am. J. Physiol.* **252**: F317–21.

Elliot, M. E. & Goodfriend, T. L. (1986a). Inhibition of aldosterone synthesis by atrial natriuretic factor. *Fed. Proc.* **45**: 2376–81.

Elliot, M. E. & Goodfriend, T. L. (1986b). Atrial natriuretic peptide inhibits protein phosphorylation stimulated by angiotensin II in bovine adrenal glomerulosa cells. *Biochem. Biophys. Res. Commun.* **140**: 814–20.

Elliot, M. E. & Goodfriend, T. L. (1987). Effects of atrial natriuretic peptide, angiotensin, cyclic AMP and potassium on protein phosphorylation in adrenal glomerulosa cells. *Life Sci.* **41**, 2517–24.

Espiner, E. A., Nicholls, M. G., Yandle, T. G., Crozier, K., Cuneo, R. C., McCormick, D. & Ikram, H. (1986). Studies on the secretion, metabolism and action of atrial natriuretic peptide in man. *J. Hypertension* **4** (Suppl. 2): S85–91.

Faber, J. E., Gettes, D. R. & Gianturc, D. P. (1988). Microvascular effects of atrial natriuretic factor: interaction with α_1 and α_2 adrenoceptors. *Circulation Res.* **63**: 415–28.

Fiscus, R. R., Robles, B. J., Waldman, S. A. & Murad, F. (1987). Atrial natriuretic factors stimulate cyclic GMP accumulation and efflux in C6-2B rat glioma and PC-12 rat phaeochromocytoma cell culture. *J. Neurochem.* **48**: 522–8.

Fitzsimons, J. T. (1980). Angiotensin stimulation of the central venous system. *Rev. Physiol. Biochem. Pharmacol.* **87**: 117–67.

Freeman, R. H., Davis, J. O. & Vari, R. C. (1985). Renal response to atrial natriuretic factor in conscious dogs with caval constriction. *Am. J. Physiol.* **248**: R495–500.

Gaillard, C. A., Koomans, H. A. & DorhoutMees, E. J. (1988). Enalapril attenuates natriuresis of atrial natriuretic factor in humans. *Hypertension* **11**: 160–5.

Ganguly, A., Chiou, S., West, L. A. & Davis, J. S. (1989). Atrial natriuretic factor inhibits angiotensin induced aldosterone secretion not through cGMP or interference with phospholipase C. *Biochem. Biophys. Res. Commun.* **159**: 148–54.

Garcia, R., Thibault, G., Gutkowska, J. & Cantin, M. (1986). Effect of chronic infusion of atrial natriuretic factor on plasma and urinary aldosterone, plasma renin activity, blood pressure and sodium excretion in 2K-1C hypertensive rats. *Clin. Exp. Hypertension* **8**: 1127–34.

Goodfriend, T. L., Elliot, M. & Atlas, S. A. (1984). Actions of synthetic atrial natriuretic factor on bovine adrenal glomerulosa. *Life Sci.* **35**: 1675–82.

Hackenthal, E., Lang, R. E. & Buhrle, C. P. (1985). Atrial natriuretic factor stimulates renin release from the isolated rat kidney. *J. Hypertension* **3** (Suppl. 3): S323–5.

Hansell, P. & Ulfendahl, H. R. (1987). Effects of atrial natriuretic peptide (ANP) during converting enzyme inhibition. *Acta Physiol. Scand.* **130**: 393–9.

Harris, P. J., Thomas, D. & Morgan, T. O. (1987). Atrial natriuretic peptide inhibits angiotensin-stimulated proximal tubular sodium and water transport. *Nature* **326**: 697–8.

Hashimoto, K., Hattori, T., Suemaru, S., Sugawara, M., Takao, T., Kageyama, J. & Ota, Z. (1987). Atrial natriuretic peptide does not affect corticotropin-releasing factor, arginine vasopressin—and angiotensin II-induced adrenocorticotrophic hormone release *in vivo* or *in vitro*. *Regul. Peptides* **17**: 53–60.

Hattori, Y., Kasai, M., Vesugi, S., Kawata, M. & Yamashita, H. (1988). Atrial natriuretic polypeptide depresses angiotensin II induced excitation of neurons in the rat subfornical organ *in vitro. Brain Res.* **443**: 355–9.

Heisler, S. (1989). Direct binding of atrial natriuretic factor to adrenocorticortical mitochondria. *Eur. J. Pharmacol.* **162**: 281–8.

Heisler, S., Simard, J., Assayag, E., Mehri, Y. & Labrie, F. (1986). Atrial natriuretic factor does not affect basal forskolin and CRF stimulated adenylate cyclase activity, cAMP formation or ACTH secretion, but does stimulate cGMP synthesis in anterior pituitary. *Molec. Cell. Endocrinol.* **44**: 125–31.

Henrich, W. L., McAlister, E. A., Smith, P. B. & Campbell, W. B. (1988). Guarosine 3′,5′-cyclic monophosphate as a mediator of inhibition of renin release. *Am. J. Physiol.* **255**: F474–8.

Henrich, W. L., Needleman, P. & Campbell, W. B. (1986). Effect of atriopeptin III on renin release *in vitro. Life Sci.* **39**: 993–1001.

Hirata, Y., Tomita, M., Yoshimi, H., Kuramochi, M., Ito, K. & Ikeda, M. (1985). Effect of synthetic human atrial natriuretic peptide on aldosterone secretion by dispersed aldosterone producing adenoma cells *in vitro. J. Clin. Endocrinol. Metab.* **61**: 677–80.

Hiruma, M., Ikemoto, F. & Yamamoto, K. (1986). Rat atrial natriuretic factor stimulates renin release from renal cortical slices. *Eur. J. Pharmacol.* **125**: 151–3.

Hollenberg, N. K., Chenitz, W. R., Adams, D. F. & Williams, G. H. (1974). Reciprocal influence of salt intake on adrenal glomerulosa and renal vascular responses to angiotensin II in normal man. *J. Clin. Invest.* **54**: 34–2.

Imam, K., Maddens, M., Mohanty, P. K., Felicetta, J. V. & Sowers, J. R. (1989). Atrial natriuretic peptide attenuates the reflex sympathetic responses to lower body negative pressure. *Am. J. Med. Sci.* **298**: 1–7.

Imura, H. & Nakao, K. Atrial natriuretic peptide in the central nervous system and its possible function. In: *UCLA Symposium Series. Biological and Molecular Aspects of Atrial Factors* (Needleman, P. ed.). New York: Liss, in press.

Israel, A., Torres, M. & Barbella, Y. (1988). Natriuretic and diuretic action of centrally administered rat atrial natriuretic peptide (99–126): possible involvement of aldosterone and sympathoadrenal system. *Can. J. Physiol. Pharmacol.* **66**: 295–300.

Itoh, H., Nakao, K., Katsuura, G., Morii, N., Yamada, T., Shiono, S., Sakamoto, M. *et al.* (1986). Possible involvement of central atrial natriuretic polypeptide in regulation of hypothalamo–pituitary–adrenal axis in conscious rats. *Neurosci. Lett.* **69**: 254–8.

Itoh, H., Nakao, K., Yamada, T., Morii, N., Shiono, S., Sugawara, A., Saito, Y., Mukoyama, M., Arai, H. & Imura, H. (1988). Brain renin angiotensin. Central control of secretion of atrial natriuretic factor from the heart. *Hypertension* **11** (Suppl. I): 157–61.

Itoh, S., Abe, K., Nushiro, N., Omata, K., Yasajima, M. & Yoshinaga, K. (1987). Effect of atrial natriuretic factor on renin release in isolated afferent arterioles. *Kidney Int.* **32**: 493–7.

Jungmann, E., Konzok, C., Holl, E., Fassbinder, W. & Schoffling, K. (1989). Effect of human atrial natriuretic peptide on blood glucose concentrations and hormone stimulation during insulin induced hypoglycaemia in healthy man. *Eur. J. Clin. Pharmacol.* **36**: 593–7.

King, M. S. & Baertschi, A. J. (1989). Physiological concentrations of atrial natriuretic factors with intact N-terminal sequences inhibit corticotrophin releasing factor-stimulated adrenocorticotropin secretion from cultured anterior pituitary cells. *Endocrinology* **124**: 286–92.

Kleinert, H. D., Maack, T., Atlas, S. A., Januszewicz, A., Sealey, J. E. & Laragh, J. H. (1984). Atrial natriuretic factor inhibits angiotensin-, norepinephrine- and potassium-induced vascular contractility. *Hypertension* **6** (Suppl. I): II43–7.

Knorr, M., Locher, R., Stimpel, M., Edwards, D. & Vetter, W. (1986). Effect of atrial natriuretic polypeptide on angiotensin II induced increase of cytosolic free calcium in cultured smooth muscle cells. *J. Hypertension* **4** (Suppl. 2): S67–9.

Kudo, T. & Baird, A. (1984). Inhibition of aldosterone production in the adrenal glomerulosa by atrial natriuretic factor. *Nature* **312**: 756–7.

Kurtz, A., Della Bruna, R., Pfeilschifter, J. & Bauer, C. (1986a). Effect of synthetic atrial natriuretic peptide on rat renal juxtaglomerular cells. *J. Hypertension* **4** (Suppl. 2): 557–60.

Kurtz, A., Della Bruna, R., Pfeilschifter, J., Taugner, R. & Bauer, C. (1986b). Atrial natriuretic peptide inhibits renin release from juxtaglomerular cells by a cGMP-mediated process. *Proc. Nat. Acad. Sci. USA* **83**: 4769–73.

Lang, C. C., McMurray, J. J., Balfour, D. J. K. & Struthers, A. D. (1989). Atrial natriuretic factor and atriopeptin III both inhibit ACE inhibitor induced renin release in man. *Br. J. Clin. Pharmacol.* **28**: 219P (abstract).

Lang, C. C., Rahman, A. R., Coutie, W. J., Balfour, D. J. K. & Struthers, A. D. (1990). Atrial natriuretic factor inhibits the aldosterone response to metoclopramide in man. *Br. J. Clin. Pharmacol.* (abstract) **29**: 606P

Lappe, R. W., Todt, J. A. & Wendt, R. L. (1987). Effects of atrial natriuretic factor on the vasoconstrictor actions of the renin angiotensin system in conscious rats. *Circulation Res.* **61**: 134–40.

Lee, J., Feng, J. Q., Malvin, R. L., Huang, B. S. H. & Grekin, R. J. (1987). Centrally administered atrial natriuretic factor increases renal water excretion. *Am. J. Physiol.* **252**: F1011–15.

Liu, F. Y. & Cogan, M. R. (1988). Atrial natriuretic factor does not inhibit basal or angiotensin II stimulated proximal transport. *Am. J. Physiol.* **225**: F434–7.

McKitrick, D. J. & Calaresu, F. R. (1988). Cardiovascular responses to microinjection of ANF into dorsal medulla of rats. *Am. J. Physiol.* **255**: R182–7.

McMurray, J., Coutie, W. J., McFarlane, L. & Struthers, A. D. (1988). Atrial natriuretic factor inhibits ACTH stimulated aldosterone, but not cortisol secretion in man. *Eur. J. Clin. Pharmacol.* **35**: 409–12.

McMurray, J. J., McFarlane, L., Coutie, W. J., Balfour, D. & Struthers, A. D. (1989). Atrial natriuretic factor attenuates prostaglandin E_2 stimulated plasma renin activity in man. *J. Cardiovasc. Pharmacol.* **14**: 326–30.

McMurray, J. & Struthers, A. D. (1988). Effects of angiotensin II and atrial natriuretic peptide alone and in combination on urinary water and electrolyte excretion in man. *Clin. Sci.* **74**: 419–25.

McMurray, J. J. & Struthers, A. D. (1989). Atrial natriuretic factor inhibits isoproterenol- and furosemide-stimulated renin release in humans. *Hypertension* **13**: 9–14.

Maack, T., Marion, D. N., Camargo, M. J. F., Kleinert, H. D., Laragh, J. H., Vaughan, E. D. Jr. & Atlas, S. A. (1984). Effects of auriculin (atrial natriuretic factor) on blood pressure, renal function, and the renin aldosterone system in dogs. *Am. J. Med.* **77**: 1069–75.

Malayan, S. A., Keil, L. C., Ramsay, D. J. & Reid, A. I. (1979). Mechanism of suppression of plasma renin activity by centrally administered angiotensin II. *Endocrinology* **104**: 672–5.

Mann, F. E., Lang, R. E., Leidig, M. & Ritz, E. (1986). Effect of angiotensin I-converting enzyme inhibition on circulating atrial natriuretic peptide in humans. *Klin. Wochenschr.* **64** (Suppl. VI): 13–15.

Matsuoko, H., Ishii, M., Hirata, Y., Atarashi, K., Sugimoto, T., Kangawa, K. & Matsuo, H. (1987). Evidence for lack of a role of cGMP in effect of alpha-hANP on aldosterone inhibition. *Am. J. Physiol.* **252**: 643–7.

Matsuoko, H., Ishii, M., Sugimoto, T., Hirata, Y., Sugimoto, T., Kangawa, K. & Matsuo, H. (1985). Inhibition of aldosterone production by α-human atrial natriuretic polypeptide is associated with an increase in cGMP production. *Biochem. Biophys. Res. Commun.* **127**: 1052–6.

Mendelsohn, F. A., Allen, A. M., Chai, S. Y., Sexton, P. M. & Figdor, R. (1987). Overlapping distributions of receptors for atrial natriuretic peptide and angiotensin II visualized by *in vitro* autoradiography: morphological basis of physiological antagonism. *Can. J. Physiol. Pharmacol.* **65**: 1517–21.

Muller-Esch, G., Klingler, W., Alt, J., Gerzer, R., Lawrenz, R. & Scriba, P. C. Interaction between atrial natriuretic peptide (αhANP) and hypothalamic pituitary function in normal man. *Am. J. Hypertension* (in press).

Murad, F. (1986). Cyclic guanosine monophosphate as a mediator of vasodilation. *J. Clin. Invest.* **78**: 1–5.

Nakajima, S., Suzuki, H., Saito, I. & Saruta, T. (1987) Effects of atrial natriuretic peptide dopamine and ouabain on aldosterone synthesis. *Acta Endocrinol.* **115**: 57–62.

Nakamura, M., Katsuura, G., Nakao, K. & Imura, H. (1985). Antidipsogenic action of α-human atrial natriuretic polypeptide administered intracerebroventricularly in rats. *Neurosci. Lett.* **58**: 1–6.

Naruse, M., Obana, K., Naruse, K., Yamaguchi, H., Demura, H., Inagami, T. & Shizume, K. (1987). Atrial natriuretic polypeptide inhibits cortisol secretion as well as aldosterone secretion *in vitro* from human adrenal tissue. *J. Clin. Endocrinol. Metab.* **64**: 10–16.

Obana, K., Naruse, M., Naruse, K., Sakurai, H., Demura, H., Inagami, T. & Shizume, K. (1985). Synthetic rat atrial natriuretic factor inhibits *in vitro* and *in vivo* renin secretion in rats. *Endocrinology* **117**: 1282–4.

Oelkers, W., Brown, J. J., Fraser, R., Lever, A. F., Morton, J. J. & Robertson, J. I. S. (1974). Sensitization of the adrenal cortex to angiotensin II in sodium deplete man. *Circulation Res.* **34**: 69–77.

Olansky, L. & Kem, D. C. (1985). Human aldosterone-producing adenoma cells respond to ACTH and atrial natriuretic factor. *Endocrinol. Suppl.* **116**: 173.

Opgenorth, T. J., Burnett, J. C. Jr., Granger, J. P. & Scriven, T. A. (1986). Effects of atrial natriuretic peptide on renin secretion in non-filtering kidney. *Am. J. Physiol.* **250**: F798–801.

Osol, G., Halpern, W. & Tesfamariam, B., Nakayama, K. & Weinberg, D. (1986). Synthetic atrial natriuretic factor does not dilate resistance-sized arteries. *Hypertension* **8**: 606–10.

Pandey, K. N., Inagami, T., Girard, P. R., Kuo, J. F. & Misono, K. S. (1987). New signal transduction mechanisms of phosphorylation of protein kinase C and A 240 kDa protein in adrenal cortical plasma membrane by cGMP dependent and independent mechanisms. *Biochem. Biophys. Res. Commun.* **148**: 589–95.

Phillips, M. I. (1987). Functions of angiotensin in the central nervous system. *Ann. Rev. Physiol.* **49**: 413–35.

Procter, K. G. & Bealer, S. L. (1987). Selective antagonism of hormone induced vasoconstriction by synthetic atrial natriuretic factor (ANF) in rat microcirculation. *Circulation Res.* **61**: 42–9.

Quirion, R., Dalpe, M., DeLean, A., Gutkowska, J., Cantin, M. & Genest, J. (1984). Atrial natriuretic factor (ANF) binding sites in brain and related structures. *Peptide* **5**: 1167–72.

Racz, K., Kuchel, O., Cantin, M. & DeLean, A. (1985). Atrial natriuretic factor inhibits the early pathway of steroid biosynthesis in bovine adrenal cortex. *FEBS Lett.* **192**: 19–22.

Rebuffatt, P., Mazzocchi, G., Gottardi, G., Meneghelli, V. & Nussdorfer, G. G. (1988). Further investigation of the atrial natriuretic factor induced inhibition of the growth and steroidogenic capacity of rat adrenal zona glomerulosa *in vivo*. *J. Ster. Biochem.* **29**: 605–9.

Reid, I. A. (1984). Actions of angiotensin II on the brain: mechanisms and physiologic role. *Am. J. Physiol.* **246**: F533–43.

Reiser, G., Hopp, H. P. & Hamprecht, B. (1987). Atrial natriuretic polypeptide hormones induce membrane potential responses in cultured rat glioma cells. *Brain Res.* **402**: 164–7.

Richards, A. M., Ikram, H., Yandle, T. G., Nicholls, M. G., Webster, M. W. I. & Espiner, E. A. (1985). Renal, haemodynamic and hormonal effects of human alpha atrial natriuretic peptide in healthy volunteers. *Lancet* **i**: 545–9.

Richards, A. M., McDonald, D., Fitzpatrick, M. A., Nicholls, M. G., Espiner, E. A., Ikram, H., Jans Siegried, J. *et al.* (1988a). Atrial natriuretic hormone has biological effects in man at physiological plasma concentrations. *J. Clin. Endocrinol. Metab.* **67**: 1134–9.

Richards, A. M., Rao, G., Espiner, E. A. & Yandle, T. (1989). Interaction of angiotensin converting enzyme inhibition and atrial natriuretic factor. *Hypertension* **13**: 193–9.

Richards, A. M., Tonolo, G., Tree, M., Robertson, J. I., Montorsi, P., Leckie, B. J. & Polonia, J. (1988b). Atrial natriuretic peptides and renin release. *Am. J. Med.* **84**(3A): 112–18.

Rodriuguez-Puyol, D., Arriba, G., Blanchart, A., Santos, J. C., Caramelo, C., Fernandez-Cruz, A., Hernando, L. *et al.* (1986). Lack of a direct regulatory effect of atrial natriuretic factor on prostaglandins and renin release by isolated rat glomeruli. *Biochem. Biophys. Res. Commun.* **138**: 496–501.

Rohmeiss, P., Demmert, G.. Rettig, R. & Unger, T. (1989). Centrally administered atrial natriuretic factor inhibits central angiotensin-induced natriuresis. *Brain Res.* **502**; 198–203.

Saavedra, J., Correa, F. M. A., Kurihara, M. & Shigematsu, K. (1986a). Increased number of angiotensin II receptors in the subfornical organ of spontaneously hypertensive rats. *J. Hypertension* **4** (Suppl. 5): S27–30.

Saavedra, J. M., Correa, F. M. A., Plunkett, L. M., Israel, A., Kurihara, M. & Shigematsu, K. (1986b). Binding of angiotensin and atrial natriuretic peptide in brain of hypertensive rats. *Nature* **320**: 758–60.

Sagnella, G. A., Markandu, N. D., Shore, A. C. & MacGregor, G. A. (1985). Effects of changes in dietary sodium intake and saline infusion on immunoreactive atrial natriuretic peptide in human plasma. *Lancet* **ii**: 1208–10.

Samson, K. W. (1985). Atrial natriuretic factor inhibits dehydration and haemorrhage induced vasopressin release. *Neuroendocrinology* **40**: 277–9.

Samson, W. K., Aguila, M. C., Martinovic, J., Antunes-Rodrigues, J. & Norris, M. (1987). Hypothalamic action of atrial natriuretic factor to inhibit vasopressin secretion. *Peptides* **8**: 449–54.

Schiebinger, R. J., Kem, D. C. & Brown, R. D. (1988). Effect of atrial natriuretic peptide on ACTH, dibutyryl cAMP, angiotensin II and potassium-stimulated aldosterone secretion by rat adrenal glomerulosa cells. *Life Sci.* **42**: 919–26.

Schriffin, E., Chartier, L., Thibault, G., St Louis, J., Cantin, M. & Genest, J. (1985a). Vascular and adrenal receptors for atrial natriuretic factor in the rat. *Circulation Res.* **56**: 801–7.

Schiffrin, E., Thibault, G. & Chartier, L. (1985b). Regulation of aldosterone secretion by atrial natriuretic factor. *Endocrinology* **116**: 15 (abstract).

Scholkens, B. A., Jung, W., Rascher, W., Dietz, R. & Ganten, D. (1982). Intracerebroventricular angiotensin increases arterial blood pressure in rhesus monkeys by stimulation of pituitary hormones and the sympathetic nervous system. *Experimentia* **38**: 469–70.

Shenker, Y., Bates, E. R., Egon, B. H., Hammond, J. & Grekin, R. J. (1988). Effect of vasopressin on atrial natriuretic factor and haemodynamic function in humans. *Hypertension* **12**: 20–5.

Sheuer, D. A., Trasher, T. N., Quillen, E. W. Jr., Metzler, C. H. & Ramsay, D. J. (1987). Atrial natriuretic peptide blocks renin response to hypotension. *Am. J. Physiol.* **252**: R423–7.

Shibasaki, T., Naruse, M., Yamauchi, N., Masuda, A., Imaki, T., Naruse, K., Demura, H. *et al.* (1986). Rat atrial natriuretic factor suppresses pro-opio melano cortico-derived peptides secretion from both anterior and intermediate lobe cells and growth hormone release from anterior lobe cells of rat pituitary *in vitro. Biochem. Biophys. Res. Commun.* **135**: 1035–41.

Shilo, L., Pomeranz, A., Rathaus, M., Weiss, E., Bernheim, J. & Shenkman, L. (1988). Atrial natriuretic peptide administration to normal and salt depleted rats … effects on digoxin-like immunoreactive factor, aldosterone, ACTH and renal function. *Life Sci.* **42**: 1855–9.

Shimizu, T., Katsuura, G., Nakamura, M., Nakao, K., Morii, N., Itoh, Y., Shiono, S. *et al.* (1986). Effect of intracerebroventricular atrial natriuretic polypeptide on blood pressure and urine production in rats. *Life Sci.* **39**: 1263–70.

Siragy, H. M., Lamb, N. E., Rose, C. E. Jr., Peach, M. J. & Carey, R. M. (1988). Angiotensin II modulates the intrarenal effects of atrial natriuretic peptide. *Am. J. Physiol.* **255**: F545–51.

Sosa, R. E., Volpe, M., Marion, D. N., Glorioso, N., Laragh, J. H., Vaughan, E. D. Jr., Maack, T. *et al.* (1985). Effect of atrial natriuretic factor on renin secretion, plasma renin and aldosterone in dogs with acute unilateral renal artery constriction. *J. Hypertension* **3** (Suppl. 3): S299–302.

Spinelli, F., Kamber, B. & Schnell, C. (1986). Observations on the natriuretic response to intravenous infusions of atrial natriuretic factor in water-loaded anaesthetized rats. *J. Hypertension* **4** (Suppl. 2): S25–9.

Standaert, D. G., Cechetto, D. F., Needleman, P. & Saper, C. B. (1987). Inhibition of the firing of vasopressin neurons by atrio peptin. *Nature* **329**: 151–3.

Struthers, A. D., Anderson, J. V., Payne, N. N., Causon, R. C., Slater, J. D. H. & Bloom, S. R. (1986). The effect of atrial natriuretic peptide on plasma renin activity, plasma aldosterone and urinary dopamine in man. *Eur. J. Clin. Pharmacol.* **31**: 223–6.

Sugawara, M., Hattori, T., Hashimoto, K., Inoue, H., Suemaru, S., Takao, T., Kageyana, J. *et al.* (1987). Atrial natriuretic peptide inhibited a haemorrhage induced ACTH secretion. In: *Biologically Active Atrial Peptides* (Brenner, B. M. & Laragh, J. H., eds). New York: Raven Press, pp. 309–10.

Takagi, M., Franco-Saenz, R. & Mulrow, P. J. (1986). Effect of atrial natriuretic factor on the plasma aldosterone response to potassium infusion in rats … *in vivo* study. *Life Sci.* **39**: 359–64.

Takagi, M., Takagi, M., Franco-Saenz, R. & Mulrow, P. G. (1988a). Effect of atrial natriuretic peptide on renin release in a super fusion system of kidney slices and dispersed juxtaglomerular cells. *Endocrinology* **122**: 1437–42.

Takagi, M., Takagi, M., Franco-Saenz, R., Mulrow, P. J. & Reimann, E. M. (1988b). Effects of dibutyryl adenosine 3′5′ monophosphate, angiotensin II and atrial natriuretic factor on phosphorylation of a 17,600-dalton protein in adrenal glomerulosa cells. *Endocrinology* **123**: 2419–23.

Takayanagi, R., Inagami, T., Snajdar, R. M., Imada, T., Tamura, M. & Misono, K. (1987). Two distinct forms of receptors for atrial natriuretic factor in bovine adrenocortical cells. Purification, ligand binding, and peptide mapping. *J. Biol. Chem.* **262**: 12104–13.

Tikkanen, I., Fyhrquist, R., Metsarinne, K. & Leidenius, R. (1985). Plasma atrial natriuretic peptide in cardiac disease and during infusion in healthy volunteers. *Lancet* **ii**: 66–9.

Tremblay, J., Gerzer, R., Vinay, P., Pang, S. C., Beliveau, R. & Hamet, P. (1985). The increase of cGMP by atrial natriuretic factor correlates with the distribution of particulate guanylate cyclase. *FEBS Lett.* **181**: 17–22.

Tuck, M. L., Sowers, J. R., Asp, N. D., Viosca, S. P., Berg, G. & Mayes, D. M. (1981). Mineralocorticoid response to low dose adrenocorticotropin infusion. *J. Clin. Endocrinol. Metab.* **52**: 440–6.

Uehlinger, D. E., Weidmann, P., Gnadinger, M. P., Shaw, S. & Lang, R. E. (1986). Depressor effects and release of atrial natriuretic peptide during norepinephrine or angiotensin II infusion in man. *J. Clin. Endocrinol. Metab.* **63**: 669–74.

Unger, T, Badoer, E., Ganten, D., Lang, R. E. & Rettig, R. (1988). Brain angiotensin: pathways and pharmacology. *Circulation* **77**: 140–54.

Unger, T., Horst, P. J., Bauer, M., Demmert, G., Rettig, R. & Rohmeiss, P. (1989). Natriuretic action of central angiotensin II in conscious rats. *Brain Res.* **486**: 33–8.

Vari, R. C., Freeman, R. H., Davis, J. O., Villareal, D. & Verburg, K. M. (1986). Effect of synthetic atrial natriuretic factor on aldosterone secretion in the rat. *Am. J. Physiol.* **251**: R48–52.

Vierhapper, H., Nowotny, P. & Waldhausl, W. (1986). Prolonged administration of human atrial natriuretic factor in healthy man: reduced aldosteronotropic effect of angiotensin II. *Hypertension* **8**: 1040–3.

Villareal, D., Freeman, R. H., Davis, J. O., Verburg, K. M. & Vari, R. C. (1986). Renal mechanisms for suppression of renin secretion by atrial natriuretic factor. *Hypertension* **8** (Suppl. 2): II28–35.

Volpe, M., Odell, G. & Kleinert, H. D. (1984a). Effect of atrial natriuretic factor on blood pressure, renin and aldosterone in Goldblatt hypertension. *Hypertension* **7** (Suppl. I): I43–8.

Volpe, M., Odell, G. & Kleinert, H. D. (1984b). Antihypertensive and aldosterone lowering effects of synthetic atrial natriuretic factor in renin-dependent renovascular hypertension. *J. Hypertension* **2** (Suppl. 3): S313–15.

Volpe, M., Sosa, E. R., Atlas, S., Sealey, J. & Laragh, J. H. (1988). Angiotensin II stimulates atrial peptide (ANF) secretion which modulates aldosterone and renal responses to AII. *Hypertension* **12**: 346 (abstract).

Waldman, S. A., Rapoport, R. M. & Murad, F. (1984). Atrial natriuretic factor selectively activates particulate guanylate cyclase and elevates cGMP in rat tissues. *J. Biol. Chem.* **259**: 14332–4.

Wambach, G., Schittenhelm, U., Stimpel, M., Bonner, G. & Kaufman, W. (1989). Natriuretic action of ANP is blunted by ACE inhibition in humans. *J. Cardiovasc. Pharmacol.* **13**: 748–53.

Wang, S. L. & Gilmore, J. P. (1985). Renal responses to atrial natriuretic factor during converting enzyme inhibition. *Can. J. Physiol. Pharmacol.* **63**: 220–3.

Weidmann, P., Hasler, L., Gnadinger, M. P., Lang, R. E., Uehlinger, D. E., Shaw, S., Rascher, W. *et al.* (1986). Blood levels and renal effects of atrial natriuretic peptide in normal man. *J. Clin. Invest.* **77**: 734–42.

Wilkins, M. R., Lewis, H. M., West, M. J., Kendall, M. J. & Lote, C. J. (1987). Captopril reduces the renal response to intravenous natriuretic peptide in normotensives. *J. Human Hypertension* **1**: 47–51.

Williams, T. D. M., Walsh, K. P., Lightman, S. L. & Sutton, R. (1988). Atrial natriuretic peptide inhibits postural release of renin and vasopressin in humans. *Am. J. Physiol.* **255**: R368–72.

Winquist, R. J., Faison, E. P., Waldman, S. A., Schwartz, K., Murad, F. & Rapoport, R. M. (1984). Atrial natriuretic factor elicits an endothelium-independent relaxation and activates particulate guanylate cyclase in vascular smooth muscle. *Proc. Nat. Acad. Sci. USA* **81**: 7661–4.

Woods, R. C. & Anderson, W. P. (1987). Natriuretic and diuretic effects of atrial natriuretic peptide (ANP) are not dependent on the renin angiotensin system in conscious dogs. *Austral. NZ J. Med.* **17**: 155 (abstract).

Yamada, T., Nakao, K., Morii, N., Itoh, H., Shiono, S., Sakamoto, M., Sugawara, A. *et al.* (1986). Central effect of atrial natriuretic polypeptide on angiotensin II-stimulated vasopressin secretion in conscious rats. *Eur. J. Pharmacol.* **125**: 453–6.

Yasujima, M., Abe, K., Kohzuki, M., Tanno, M., Kasai, Y., Sato, M., Omata, K. *et al.* (1986). Effect of atrial natriuretic factor on angiotensin II-induced hypertension in rats. *Hypertension* **8**: 748–53.

Yoshida, K., Kawano, Y., Kawamura, M., Kuramochi, M. & Omae, T. (1989). Effects of intracerebroventricular atrial natriuretic factor on angiotensin or sodium-induced blood pressure elevation and natriuresis. *J. Hypertension* **7**: 639–43.

Zeidell, M. L., Silva, P., Brenner, B. M. & Seifler, J. L. (1987). cGMP mediates effects of atrial peptides on medullary collecting duct cells. *Am. J. Physiol.* **252**: F551–9.

Zimmerman, R. S., Schirger, J. S., Edwards, B. S., Schwab, T. R., Heublein, D. M. & Burnett, J. C., Jr. (1987). Cardiorenal endocrine dynamics during stepwise infusion of physiologic and pharmacologic concentrations of atrial natriuretic factor in the dog. *Circulation Res.* **60**: 63–9.

Chapter 7
Atrial natriuretic factor in hypertension

A. M. Richards

Introduction

Atrial natriuretic factor (ANF) has a wide variety of actions all of which
may be pertinent to pressure and volume homeostasis. These include
enhanced natriuresis, changes in renal haemodynamics with a rise in renal
filtration fraction, inhibition of renin–angiotensin–aldosterone activity, a
direct vasodilator action and possible inhibitory effects on arginine
vasopressin and sympathetic nervous system activity. ANF also induces
contraction of plasma volume by inducing a shift of fluid from the
intravascular to the extravascular space. Clearly, deficiencies of one or
more of these actions of ANF have the potential to be prohypertensive.
Conversely, enhanced ANF activity could conceivably compensate for
other hypertensive stimuli. These possibilities have led to an intensive
international effort to document the behaviour of the endogenous ANF
system in hypertension. Tissue and plasma concentrations of ANF have
been measured in a variety of animal models of hypertension and in
hypertensive man. In addition, tissue ANF receptor density and affinity
have been studied in renal, endocrine, vascular and central nervous
systems. The effects of administration of ANF initially in pharmacologic
and more recently in physiologic doses and for periods of up to 13 days
have been reported in various animal models of hypertension. Exciting
data have recently been published indicating important biological effects of
physiological doses of ANF infused for periods of between 3 h and 5 days
in hypertensive man.

Animal studies

Investigation of the behaviour of the ANF system in animal models of
hypertension has been directed to the following questions:
1 Are tissue and/or plasma concentrations of ANF abnormal in
hypertension?
2 Are end-organ responses to ANF abnormal in hypertension?

141

Prior to publication of the amino-acid sequence of atrial natriuretic factor, studies were confined to assessment of the activity of atrial extracts. Sonnenberg and colleagues (Sonnenberg et al., 1983) tested the effect of atrial extracts from spontaneously hypertensive rats (SHR) as opposed to Wistar–Kyoto rats (WKY), as judged by their ability to induce natriuresis in anaesthetized Sprague–Dawley rats. SHR atrial extract exhibited diminished natriuretic effect. This led to the early suggestion that tissue levels of ANF are diminished in this model of hypertension and the speculation that this may have some importance in the generation and maintenance of hypertension. With publication of the amino-acid sequence of ANF and the development of radioimmunoassays for this peptide in many centres around the globe, investigators were able to directly measure concentrations of ANF in both tissue and plasma. Morii and colleagues (Morii et al., 1986) documented increased plasma concentrations and decreased atrial (particularly of the left atrial appendage) content of ANF in SHR when compared to WKY rats. Other rat models have demonstrated similar abnormalities of plasma and tissue ANF levels. Gutkowska and colleagues (Gutkowska et al., 1986) observed that plasma concentrations of ANF rise in parallel with blood pressure in SHR. These workers support what now appears to be a consensus view that increased plasma levels of ANF reflect an increased turnover and secretion of ANF from the atria with secondary depletion of tissue levels of the peptide. The same group (Garcia et al., 1987b) have reported similar changes in tissue and plasma ANF in the one-kidney, one-clip model of hypertension in the rat.

However in Dahl salt-sensitive rats, atrial content of ANF appears to be higher than in salt-resistant animals (Snajdar & Rapp, 1985). These workers went on to compare ANF release from isolated heart–lung preparations from Dahl salt-sensitive and resistant animals (Onwochei & Rapp, 1989). Prehypertensive salt-sensitive animals exhibited hypo-secretion of ANF for any given atrial load but once hypertension was established, salt-sensitive rats became hypersecretors of ANF. These observations lead to the hypothesis that deficient ANF release from atria may be a primary lesion contributing to the hypertension of salt-sensitive animals. The concept that hypertension may be associated with deficient release of plasma ANF has received some support from other workers. Although resting levels of plasma ANF tend to be elevated in SHR, further increases in response to stimuli such as volume expansion appear to be attenuated in this model of hypertension (Petterson et al., 1985).

As already mentioned it has been frequently proposed that decreased atrial tissue content of ANF and increased plasma concentrations of ANF reflect increased secretion of the peptide in rat models of hypertension with enhanced turnover of ANF and subsequent tissue depletion. Atrial stretch is accepted as the primary stimulus for ANF release and it seems likely that increased left atrial work secondary to left ventricular hypertrophy (and diminution in left ventricular compliance) because of hypertension may well constitute the stimulus for the changes in tissue and plasma ANF observed in hypertension. In support of this, correlations were found between cardiac hypertrophy and plasma concentrations of ANF in assorted models of hypertension in the rat (Garcia, Thibault & Gantin, 1987d). In this work, two-kidney one-clip, one-kidney one-clip, DOC-salt and adrenal regeneration models of hypertension in the rat all showed increased plasma concentrations of the peptide which correlated with concomitant blood pressure and with cardiac weight in each of these models ($r = 0.69$–0.83; $P < 0.01$ all models). An alternative or additional explanation for this relationship between plasma ANF and left ventricular hypertrophy is the possibility that the hypertrophied ventricle may be recruited to make a significant contribution to secretion of ANF. Certainly evidence suggests that in cardiac failure, the ventricles of the heart make a significant contribution to circulating ANF.

A number of reports have appeared concerning ANF receptor number and affinity in models of hypertension. Schiffrin and colleagues (Schiffrin et al., 1986) demonstrated specific ANF binding in the vasculature and adrenal glomerulosa of the rat. They were unable to detect any change in receptor density in response to sodium depletion or modest sodium loading. However, in a hypertensive rat model consisting of reduced renal mass combined with sodium loading, they did observe down-regulation, i.e. a fall in receptor density in both tissues. Concomitant with this, the vasorelaxant response to ANF of precontracted aortic rings from renal hypertensive rats was attenuated. The authors suggested that decreased vascular relaxation secondary to reduced responsiveness to ANF may play a role in elevation of blood pressure or maintenance of raised blood pressure in some models of experimental hypertension with expansion of circulating volume. Other workers have studied the vascular receptor for ANF with manipulations of sodium balance and with DOC-salt hypertension in the rat (Morton, Lyall & Wallace, 1987). They found that high or low salt ingestion in normal rats did not result in any detectable change in plasma concentrations of ANF but that in the hypertensive DOC-salt rat, plasma ANF concentrations were enhanced and this was associated with an apparent down-regulation of vascular ANF receptors.

Some data are available concerning the binding and content of ANF in the central nervous system of rat hypertensive models. Binding sites of ANF have been found in the subfornical region of the brain in SHR in a similar distribution to angiotensin II (ANG II) receptors (Saavedra et al., 1986). The density of such ANF binding sites appears to be reduced in both young and mature SHR compared with age-matched Wistar–Kyoto rats. This has led to speculation concerning a potential role for both ANF and ANG II in the central nervous system in the pathogenesis of genetic hypertension. It seems likely these peptides fulfil neurotransmitter roles and act as mutual antagonists in brain areas involved in the control of blood pressure and fluid regulation. Kuchel *et al.*, 1988) have found immunoreactivity to antisera raised against both carboxy and amino terminals of pro-ANF in the brain, peripheral sympathetic nervous system, parasympathetic ganglia and spinal cord of the rat. This suggests local generation of ANF in these neural structures. The overall content of ANF in SHR has been reported as enhanced by this group but receptor density in the brain and peripheral ganglia appeared to be diminished in this hypertensive model. Whether these variations in ANF tissue content and receptor characteristics in SHR reflect a primary state or a compensatory response to high blood pressure remains uncertain.

Several groups have studied isolated vascular smooth muscle cells derived from SHR and their normotensive Wistar–Kyoto controls in an attempt to discern whether receptor characteristics differ in the tissue of hypertensive origin and whether cyclic guanosine monophosphate (cGMP, the putative intracellular second messenger mediating the effects of ANF) responses are altered in hypertensive models. The data are conflicting. While one group suggests decreased affinity and increased number of ANF receptors with decreased production of cyclic GMP in cells from SHR (Nakamura *et al.*, 1988), another has previously published exactly contrary observations (Takayanagi *et al.*, 1986)! Recently Garcia and coworkers (Garcia *et al.*, 1989) described an age-related increase in glomerular ANF receptor density in WKY but not SHR. Receptor density was higher in WKY than SHR at 8, 12 and 16 weeks of age but binding affinity was greater in SHR (8 and 12 weeks). cGMP production from isolated glomeruli was reduced in SHR.

Work has begun concerning the effect of other hormones and of pharmacological agents on ANF receptors. Vascular smooth muscle cells incubated with ANGII for a period of 18 h exhibited a fall in ANF receptor numbers and this effect was inhibited by the ANGII antagonist, saralasin. However ANF was unable to alter ANGII receptors (Chabrier *et al.*, 1988). The ANGII-induced down-regulation of ANF receptors was paradoxically associated with an enhanced cGMP response to ANF and the effect on receptors appeared to be confined to the non-guanylate cyclase coupled ANF receptor subtype. The authors hypothesized that this may represent a mechanism that opposes the long-term vasopressor effects of ANGII. The vasorelaxant effect of ANF on precontracted aortic strips is potentiated by amiloride (Linz *et al.*, 1988). cGMP production is not affected by amiloride alone in this experimental situation but exhibits a dose-dependent increase in the presence of ANF. Amiloride appears to induce an increase in the total number of ANF binding sites. The blood pressure lowering effect of ANF in SHR is also potentiated by amiloride. This early work may offer some insight into the mechanism of action of amiloride as a blood pressure lowering agent and clearly the other antihypertensive modalities should be similarly investigated.

In summary, plasma concentrations of ANF are generally elevated in animal models of hypertension and atrial ANF content is reduced. Circulating concentrations of the peptide are related to blood pressure and also to left ventricular mass, perhaps reflecting the stimulus of hypertension-induced changes in central haemodynamics on ANF secretion. In some models several strands of evidence point to a deficient ANF secretory response as a prehypertensive phenomenon perhaps of pathogenetic significance in the development of hypertension. Whether ANF receptor number and affinity differ in any systematic fashion in vascular or other tissues in hypertension remains to be confirmed. Similarly, whether there is a disturbed relationship between ANF, receptor numbers and cGMP responses in hypertension remains uncertain.

Over the last 5 years a substantial body of data has accumulated concerning the effect of ANF administered in rat models of hypertension. At least two groups have reported a deficient natriuretic response to ANF in Dahl salt-sensitive rats (Hirata et al., 1984: Snajdar & Rapp, 1985). Both these studies were conducted when both salt-sensitive and salt-resistant rats were normotensive prior to the administration of high salt diet to render the sensitive rats hypertensive. Hence renal hypo-responsiveness to ANF, together with deficient ANF release (see above), may contribute to the pathogenesis of hypertension in this model.

However, once hypertension is established both in Dahl salt-sensitive animals and other models of hypertension, the natriuretic response to ANF appears to be enhanced (Snajdar & Rapp, 1985). These latter findings are consistent with the observation that ANF-induced natriuresis is dependent upon renal perfusion pressure (Sosa et al., 1986; Davis & Briggs, 1987). In renovascular models of hypertension ANF has significant hypotensive effects in association with inhibition of renin and aldosterone levels. Volpe et al. (1985) investigated two-kidney one-clip and one-kidney one-clip rats divided according to their hypotensive response to administration of saralasin. Using very high doses of ANF these authors found that both the vascular and adrenal effects of ANF appeared enhanced when renin–angiotensin–aldosterone system activity was increased. Garcia and colleagues (1987c) similarly separated two-kidney one-clip rats into saralasin-sensitive and resistant subgroups. Using far lower doses of ANF (approximately 2 pmol/kg/min) given as a chronic infusion over a period of 6 days, these workers found the most significant hypotensive effects (systolic pressures falling from 180 to < 130 mmHg) occurred only in the saralasin-sensitive group. Observations such as these have promoted the idea that the hypotensive effect of ANF is renin-dependent.

However, other models of hypertension such as the SHR, DOC-Na and one-kidney one-clip rat (none of which are dependent upon the renin–angiotensin system for maintenance of hypertension and two of which are in fact volume-expanded models of hypertension) also show significant hypotensive responses to ANF. Seymour *et al.* (1985) studied the effects of administering ANF across a very broad dose range (from 0 to 10 000 pmol/kg/min) in normotensive, DOC-Na, 2K-1C and 1K-1C rats. They found ANF to be natriuretic in all rat models but this effect was surprisingly most pronounced in 2K-1C rats. Their other major finding was that the dose eliciting maximum natriuresis was consistently lower than that dose producing the maximum blood pressure lowering effect. In fact, it appears that the greatest natriuretic response depended upon minimizing concomitant reductions in blood pressure. These findings reinforce the concept that ANF-induced natriuresis depends upon renal perfusion pressure.

Perhaps the most exciting data concerning ANF administered in animal models of hypertension have been generated by Garcia and colleagues who have documented the effects of chronic infusion of low doses of ANF. Early work with relatively high dose infusions (approximately 30 pmol/kg/min) administered to two-kidney one-clip rats resulted in a fall in systolic blood pressure from 183 ± 4 to 116 ± 5 mmHg by days 6 and 7 of infusions. In association with this salutary fall in blood pressure, plasma renin activity was also inhibited, dropping from 8.56 ng/ml/h to as low as 1.81 ng/ml/h. Natriuresis fell in parallel with blood pressure over the study period. This group went on to study the effects of chronic administration of ANF to two-kidney one-clip rats at lower and near-physiological doses (approximately 2 pmol/kg/min for 6 days) which were insufficient to induce measurable increases in plasma concentrations of the peptide (Garcia *et al.*, 1987c). These animals were divided into saralasin-sensitive and resistant subgroups. Once again, an important fall in systolic blood pressure from 181 to 128 mmHg was observed in association with falls in plasma renin activity and aldosterone concentrations. These changes were all restricted to the saralasin-sensitive group of animals. However, consistent with data from short-term studies by Seymour *et al.* (1985) chronic infusion studies in non-renin-dependent models of hypertension demonstrate that the hypotensive action of ANF does not depend upon renin–angiotensin–aldosterone system activation. Seven-day low-dose infusions of ANF in SHR (Garcia *et al.*, 1985d) reduced systolic blood pressure from 177 to 133 mmHg by day 6. In contrast, no significant change in blood pressure was seen in the ANF-infused normotensive control WKY rats. Interestingly, over the period of 7 days there was no difference in natriuresis or diuresis when SHR receiving ANF were compared with non-infused rats. These workers (Garcia *et al.*, 1987a) have also attempted to document changes in total blood volume, plasma volume, extracellular fluid and interstitial space volume during 5-day low-dose infusions of ANF (ANF 101–126) in both SHR and WKY animals. Systolic blood pressure fell from 176 to 133 mmHg in SHR but there were no measurable interstrain differences in any of these volume measurements at day 5.

De Mey et al. (1987) infused ANF 103–126 at doses of 6.7 and 67 pmol/kg/min into SHR for a period of 7 days. Both doses resulted in an important fall in systolic arterial pressure from 212 to 177 and 210 to 155 mmHg at lower and higher doses, respectively. Even the lower of these two doses is still somewhat higher than the chronic dose regimes employed by the Canadian group (approximately 2 pmol/kg/min) and in contrast to findings by Garcia and colleagues, De Mey did not notice any tendency for blood pressure to return towards basal levels beyond day 5 of chronic infusions. De Mey and colleagues were unable to define the mechanisms underlying the hypotensive effect observed in their studies but were able to essentially rule out modulation of renovascular resistance or major change in renal function, plasma renin activity or plasma aldosterone concentrations as being of importance. Hence, the mechanism by which chronic low-dose infusion of ANF lowers blood pressure in such animal models remains unclear.

Parkes et al. (1988) studied the effects of 5-day low-dose infusions of ANF in sheep (ANF 99–126 at 2–3 pmol/kg/min). Interpretation of the data is limited by the lack of a time-matched concurrent control study but is nevertheless suggestive. On day 1 ANF caused a fall in cardiac output and stroke volume and blood volume together with a small fall in arterial pressure. Heart rate and total peripheral resistance rose. However, by days 4 and 5 this haemodynamic profile had altered with the return of cardiac output towards basal values but persistent further falls in arterial pressure and hence a drop in calculated total peripheral resistance. In this animal model, little change in plasma renin activity or protein concentrations was observed. Hence it seems possible that the short-term and chronic effects of ANF on haemodynamic indices differ. Short-term effects reflect the consequences of an acute natriuresis and diuresis with additional contraction of circulating volume by shifts of fluid from the intravascular to the extravascular space, a subsequent decrease in venous return, in cardiac output and hence a fall in blood pressure. In the longer term, work by the Canadian group (Garcia et al., 1987a–d) and others (Parkes et al., 1988) suggests that the blood pressure lowering effect of ANF may at least be partly dependent upon a reduction in peripheral vascular resistance.

In summary, experience with infusion of ANF into animal models of hypertension indicates that this peptide has potent blood pressure lowering effects in both renin- and volume-dependent models of hypertension. Chronic infusion of very low doses of ANF with no obvious acute hypotensive action has a salutary blood pressure lowering effect over a period of several days. The mechanisms underlying short-term and long-term hypotensive effects of ANF appear to differ with the former being more dependent on the acute effects of natriuresis and extrarenal plasma volume contraction whilst longer term effects may well reflect a chronic reduction in peripheral vascular resistance.

Studies in hypertensive man

There is a consensus in the literature that plasma concentrations of ANF in patients with severe or complicated hypertension are elevated compared with age- and sex-matched normotensive control subjects. However, whether essential hypertensives with mild, uncomplicated hypertension have raised plasma ANF remains controversial.

Sugawara et al. (1985) reported plasma ANF concentrations in patients with essential hypertension to be twice that seen in age-matched normotensive control subjects. They also described a significant correlation between plasma ANF concentrations and both systolic and diastolic arterial pressure. These findings were essentially confirmed by Sagnella et al. (1986) in a larger group (n = 28) of essential hypertensive patients matched as closely as possible for age, sex and race to 24 normotensive control patients. Mean arterial pressure in the hypertensive group was greater than 120 mmHg compared with approximately 94 mmHg in the normotensive group. These authors suggested that the increased plasma levels of ANF observed in hypertension may reflect a compensatory reaction to a diminished renal capacity for sodium excretion. They also noticed an increase in plasma ANF with age in the normotensive group. This latter finding has been confirmed by other workers (Richards et al., 1986; Ohashi et al., 1987). Richards and colleagues (1986) and other workers (Iimura et al., 1987; Kohno et al., 1987) reported very similar findings to those published by Sagnella et al. and in addition Richards et al. documented extreme elevation of plasma ANF in three patients with malignant phase hypertension. Plasma concentrations of the peptide fell with effective treatment of accelerated hypertension.

There appears to be little dispute that essential hypertension of at least a moderate degree is associated with a rise in plasma ANF and there appears to be a correlation between arterial pressure and plasma ANF levels with progressive levels of hypertension. However there is a large body of contradictory data concerning plasma ANF concentrations in the majority of hypertensive patients who have mild and uncomplicated hypertension. Yamaji and colleagues (1986) published an early report indicating that plasma ANF concentrations were not raised in 41 patients with uncomplicated essential hypertension (class 1 or 2, WHO classification) compared with 108 normotensive control subjects. In support of this, the Canadian group (Larochelle *et al.*, 1987) found virtually identical plasma ANF concentrations in 44 patients with mild uncomplicated untreated essential hypertension as compared with 48 normotensive control subjects (13.2 ± 1.5 ng/l and 13.0 ± 1.3 ng/l in hypertensive and normotensive control subjects, respectively). By far the largest series has been published by Nilsson and colleagues (1987) who measured plasma ANF concentrations in 391 hypertensive patients and 328 normotensive control subjects. They observed no difference in concentrations irrespective of whether the hypertension was treated or untreated in comparison with normotensive subjects. However, the major drawback with this study is that plasma ANF concentrations were measured using direct radioimmunoassay of unextracted plasma. There is ample evidence to suggest that this technique may be very poor at distinguishing differences in plasma ANF concentrations at the lower part of the pathophysiological range and varying only by factors of 1 or 2 (Richards *et al.*, 1987; Poole *et al.*, 1988).

Much of the controversy concerning the presence or absence of elevated plasma ANF concentrations in mild, uncomplicated hypertension may well reflect inadequate standardization of relevant background factors. For example, plasma ANF concentrations are clearly affected by dietary sodium intake, age, posture, physical activity and possibly by race. Inadequate attention to such potentially confounding factors coupled with assay techniques which may lack the necessary sensitivity may well be sufficient to obscure a subtle but significant systematic elevation of plasma ANF in mild uncomplicated essential hypertension. With this in mind, Montorsi *et al.* (1987) undertook a study in which hypertensive and normotensive subjects were as closely paired as possible in a prospective fashion (i.e. prior to the measurement of plasma ANF concentrations) for sex, age, renal function (creatinine clearance) and sodium intake. The data were also analysed by both parametric and non-parametric paired and unpaired statistical methods. As previously reported, there was a wide overlap of plasma ANF concentration between hypertensive and normotensive groups. However, there was a subtle increase in mean plasma ANF in the hypertensive group (45 ± 3 pg/ml vs. 36 ± 3 pg/ml). Simple parametric statistical analysis revealed no statistical difference. However, careful, paired non-parametric analysis indicated a statistically significant elevation of ANF within the hypertensive group. Hence it remains possible that with appropriate matching of normotensive and hypertensive subjects for the potentially confounding factors listed above, mild hypertension is associated with a subtle elevation in plasma ANF concentrations.

These findings of course remain to be confirmed and an alternative explanation may be that in the early phase of essential hypertension an abnormal lack of compensatory rise in plasma ANF with the increase in blood pressure may play some pathogenetic role in maintaining or exacerbating the hypertension. This would be consistent with the findings of the workers in such animal models of hypertension as the Dahl salt-sensitive rat.

In support of this concept, Ferrier and colleagues (1988) have presented preliminary data suggesting that the offspring of hypertensive parents fail to raise plasma concentrations of ANF with increased dietary sodium intake when compared with the offspring of normotensive parents. It remains possible that an inadequate ANF response to dietary sodium challenge is a prehypertensive event in essential hypertension.

Deficient plasma ANF responses have also been documented in Gordon's syndrome (Tunny, Higgins & Gordon, 1986b). This hypertensive state is the mirror image of Bartter's syndrome in that hypertension is present in association with hyperkalaemia and relative volume expansion. These workers found plasma ANF to be present at near-normal concentrations in this condition, which may be interpreted as an inappropriate lack of response in plasma ANF. In addition, challenge of such patients with an intravenous saline load induced a subnormal increase in plasma ANF levels when compared with the response in patients with Bartter's syndrome, in whom increases in plasma ANF were inappropriately enhanced. Hence, although Gordon's syndrome certainly does not represent a syndrome of absolute ANF deficiency, it may well be a condition in which ANF responses are attenuated, thus contributing to the volume-expanded state and hypertension.

However, in established essential hypertension Sorenson *et al.* (1989) found a modest but significant increase in basal concentrations of plasma ANF in essential hypertension as opposed to normotensive control subjects and in response to an intravenous hypertonic saline challenge, hypertensive subjects exhibited an enhanced rise in plasma ANF concentrations in association with an exaggerated natriuresis and an exaggerated increase in fractional sodium excretion. Hence, in established essential hypertension, both resting and stimulated plasma ANF concentrations appear enhanced. Matsubara and colleagues (1987) examined the relationship between hypertonic-saline-induced natriuresis in essential hypertension and concomitant changes in plasma ANF concentrations in patients with essential hypertension who were first divided into 'renin-responsive' and 'renin-unresponsive' subgroups. The 'renin-unresponsive' group exhibited an enhanced increase in peak fractional sodium excretion. Plasma ANF concentrations were both higher at rest and showed a clear increase with hypertonic challenge as opposed to renin-responsive patients in whom plasma ANF did not increase. The authors suggested that enhanced secretion of ANF was an important determinant of the exaggerated natriuresis observed in patients with renin-unresponsive hypertension.

Plasma concentrations of ANF have also been documented in

secondary and complicated hypertension. Patients with primary aldo-steronism exhibit an appropriate elevation of plasma ANF concentrations which is corrected by excision of the adrenal adenoma or by aldosterone antagonists (Espiner *et al.*, 1985; Tunny & Gordon, 1986a; Yamaji *et al.*, 1986; Yandle *et al.*, 1986; Iimura *et al.*, 1987; Sugawara *et al.*, 1988). Renovascular hypertension and hypertension associated with chronic renal impairment are also associated with elevated ANF concentrations provided that hypertension is of at least moderate severity (Arendt *et al.*, 1986; Iimura *et al.*, 1987).

Regardless of the aetiology of hypertension, there appears to be good agreement that plasma ANF rises in parallel with increasing severity of hypertension and there is a relationship between cardiac hypertrophy presumably via effects on central haemodynamic indices and plasma ANF similar to that described in animal studies. In support of this concept, Kohno and colleagues (1987) documented marked elevation of plasma ANF in a subgroup of hypertensives with left ventricular hypertrophy. Similarly Montorsi and colleagues (1987) found markedly enhanced plasma concentrations of ANF in patients with left ventricular hyper-trophy when compared with similarly hypertensive patients without LVH. In addition these authors found a correlation between the radiographic cardiac trans-thoracic ratio and plasma ANF concen-trations. More recently published data (Wambach *et al.*, 1988) have confirmed significant correlations between a number of echocardiographic and electrocardiographic indices of increased left atrial or ventricular size and/or mass on the one hand and plasma concentrations of ANF on the other in a group of 36 patients with untreated hypertension. However, as yet there is no substantial series documenting the relationship between central haemodynamic indices as measured by invasive catheterization techniques and plasma ANF concentrations in hypertensive patients.

One apparent exception to the generally applicable rule that essential haemodynamics dictate or are at least directly related to plasma ANF concentrations is found in work reported by Visser *et al.* (1987) concerning patients with untreated pre-eclampsia. In this group, although plasma ANF concentrations are clearly elevated to at least twice those found in normotensive pregnant women, pulmonary capillary wedge pressure and right atrial pressures as measured per catheter were significantly lower than in normotensive control subjects. In addition there was no relationship between atrial pressures and plasma ANF. Hence, the cause of elevated plasma ANF in the pre-eclamptic state is unknown. It is possible that metabolic clearance of ANF is impaired in this condition.

There are few data available describing changes in plasma ANF concentrations in response to treatment of hypertension by various modalities. In general, it is found that diuretics lead to a fall in ANF levels but β-adrenergic blockade leads to an increase in plasma ANF (Nakaoka *et al.*, 1987). These workers studied 31 patients undergoing long-term treatment with β blockade. Multivariate analysis demonstrated age, pretreatment mean arterial pressure and plasma cGMP concentrations as being significant independent predictors of plasma ANF concentrations. Hence, in treated hypertension, plasma ANF and plasma cGMP concentrations are related. The rise in plasma ANF concentrations may be a part of the compensatory response to the central haemodynamic effects of β blockade and conceivably contributes to the longer term blood pressure lowering effects of β blockade.

Schiffrin and coworkers (Schiffrin, St Louis & Essiambre, 1988) have published data concerning platelet receptor numbers and their relationship to plasma concentrations of ANF in patients with essential hypertension. They found that the receptor density on platelets is reduced in hypertensive patients and exhibits an inverse relationship to plasma concentrations. With introduction and withdrawal of diuretic treatment, platelet receptor numbers altered inversely with plasma ANF concentrations.

The relationship between plasma ANF and cGMP has been investigated in hypertensive man by Bruun *et al.* (1989). These authors found that plasma ANF concentrations were less on low sodium compared with high sodium intake in normotensive subjects but plasma cGMP levels did not differ between low and medium sodium diets. In hypertensive subjects, the converse was true in that plasma ANF showed little change with change in sodium intake but plasma cGMP was elevated above levels found in normotensives at all levels of dietary sodium intake. The authors suggests that hypertensives may exhibit an enhanced cellular production of cGMP for any given level of ANF. However, these data were derived from small groups and require confirmation.

In summary, plasma ANF concentrations are progressively elevated in human hypertension in parallel with increasing severity of hypertension. This is likely to represent a compensatory response to increased central (atrial) pressures. Although there is some hint that in the prehypertensive phase, humans may show some deficiency of ANF secretion in response to assorted stimuli, this is not supported by findings in established hypertension. Whether there is some distortion of the relationship between plasma ANF and generation of cGMP in hypertension remains to be confirmed.

Administration of ANF to hypertensive man

Studies investigating the effect of ANF administered to patients with hypertension have evolved from short-term experiments in which pharmacologic doses of the peptide were given as a single bolus through to the current literature which contains a small number of key reports documenting the effect of sustained physiological dose infusions of ANF in hypertensive man. Initial studies confirmed the natriuretic and hypotensive effects of ANF in human hypertension but the doses employed induced compensatory reflex responses from both the sympathetic nervous and the renin–angiotensin systems. Such responses tended to disguise the primary inhibitory effect of ANF on the renin–angiotensin–aldosterone system and possibly also the sympathetic nervous system. These effects become apparent when ANF is given in a sustained fashion at physiological dose.

In the first published report of ANF given to hypertensive patients, Richards *et al.* (1985) documented the renal, haemodynamic and hormonal impact of injecting 100 μg of ANF 99–126 as an intravenous bolus. Six patients were studied under standardized conditions of posture and dietary electrolyte intake. Natriuresis rose to sixfold time-matched placebo values and enhanced sodium excretion persisted for some 2.5 h following the bolus injection. However the impact on blood pressure was minimal. Mean arterial pressure fell within the first 2 min following the injection but returned to basal values within 10 min. However the heart rate remained elevated above time-matched placebo values for the 3-h follow-up period of the study. These effects differed slightly from those seen in a similarly studied group of normal volunteers (Richards *et al.*, 1985). Natriuresis was clearly enhanced in the hypertensive group in spite of similar baseline rates of sodium excretion in both normotensive and hypertensive groups. Both within groups and when data from both groups were combined, pretreatment blood pressures were positively correlated with the natriuretic effect of the peptide bolus. This provided some of the first evidence in man that arterial pressure and therefore renal perfusion pressure is pivotal indicating the natriuretic response to ANF (as has been observed in animal studies). The short-lived hypotensive response seen in the hypertensive group differed from the effects seen in our normotensive subjects in that the latter group exhibited a minor but statistically significant fall in mean arterial pressures which lasted for at least 3 h after the time of the bolus injection. Heart rate responses were very similar in both groups. These data lead to speculation concerning possible relative resistance to the hypotensive effects of ANF in hypertensive man. The effect on circulating hormones was similar in both groups. Despite natriuresis and the acute hypotensive effect, plasma renin activity was not enhanced. Aldosterone concentrations tended to fall in the normotensive group and in hypertensive patients showed a clear fall to half of time-matched placebo levels. Plasma noradrenaline concentrations showed a transient rise immediately after the injection of the peptide in the hypertensive group only, presumably reflecting a baroreflex-mediated activation of the sympathetic nervous system. In contrast to this, in both normotensive and hypertensive groups, plasma adrenalin concentrations were suppressed over a similar time-span compared to placebo data.

Swiss workers (Weidmann *et al.*, 1986) have studied the impact of a 50-μg bolus of ANF 99–126 followed by a 45-min high-dose infusion (over

30 pmol/kg/min) in groups of 10 normotensive and 10 hypertensive patients. These studies were conducted without time-matched control data and intra-infusion data are hence compared with baseline values. Plasma ANF was enhanced to far above the pathophysiologic range observed in hypertensive patients. Blood pressure was reduced from severely hypertensive values of 181/127 to a nadir of 165/109 mmHg. An impressive natriuresis was observed to 665% of baseline values. There were similar increases in excretion of urine volume, chloride, phosphorous and other urinary electrolytes. In addition, these authors carefully calculated and demonstrated an increase in free water clearance. Urinary amino-acid excretion was also increased. In addition, biphasic changes in renal haemodynamic indices were observed. Initially both glomerular filtration rate and effective renal blood flow were enhanced by 40 and 30% respectively but then tended to return to baseline and in the case of renal blood flow fell below baseline levels. However renal filtration fraction was consistently enhanced throughout the study. Plasma renin activity was stimulated by this high dose of ANF in association with the abrupt hypotensive effect. During the infusion no effect on plasma aldosterone or cortisol concentrations was evident but at completion of the infusion a 'rebound' rise in plasma levels of both hormones was observed. The authors noted no change in plasma concentrations of arginine vasopressin, urine prostaglandins (E_2, $F_2\alpha$) or in urinary dopamine. Compared with similarly studied normotensive subjects, natriuresis was enhanced but the hypotensive impact of this high dose of ANF was similar in both hypertensive and normotensive groups. Taken together, these initial studies by Richards *et al.* and Weidmann *et al.* confirmed an enhanced natriuretic response to ANF in hypertension but hinted at a relative resistance to the hypotensive effects of ANF in such patients.

Janssen and coworkers (Janssen *et al.*, 1986) described the effect of administering relatively low doses of ANF over periods of 4 h in hypertensive patients receiving two different levels of dietary sodium intake (50 and 200 mmol/day). The salient observation made by this group was that of the acute onset of profound hypotension in association with bradycardia which occurred in all three subjects after 2–3 h of infusion. There was some suggestion that this was more likely to occur in patients on the lower sodium intake. The authors generated dose–response curves relating dose of ANF administered to change in blood pressure induced (prior to any acute hypotensive reaction). The number of patients in the study ($n = 3$) was markedly limited and thus the data must be interpreted with caution. However, a leftward shift in this dose relationship was observed. The authors also demonstrated a marked curtailment of the natriuretic effect of ANF with the onset of abrupt hypotensive episodes.

More recent work (Weder *et al.*, 1987) also assessed the effect of ANF administered at different doses to hypertensive patients receiving different levels of dietary sodium. ANF 99–126 was administered at doses of 9.6, 64 and 144 pmol/kg/min for 1 h at each dose with each dose administered on a separate day. An increase in heart rate and a fall in blood pressure was observed at the middle and higher doses and this was not enhanced by reduction of dietary sodium (in contrast to the data derived from a small group of subjects by Janssen *et al.* (1986)). The hypotensive effect of ANF appeared to be sustained for more than 2 h after infusions ceased. Four out of eight subjects experienced sudden episodes of bradycardia and profound hypotension. Three of these four were on the lower sodium intake at the time the adverse event occurred. This tends to reinforce the suggestion by Janssen *et al.* that sodium depletion may lower the threshold for such acute hypotensive reactions to the peptide. As previously noted, Weder and colleagues observed a dose-related increase in urinary excretion of volume, sodium chloride, calcium and phosphorous. These urinary effects were enhanced by a high sodium diet. A major strength of this study is that it offers data within the same individuals of different doses of ANF administered separately in time. The dose response of the urinary indices offers little new information. However, this study confirmed for the first time in hypertensive subjects what had hitherto been only indirectly inferred, that low doses of ANF primarily inhibit both renin and aldosterone but at higher doses at which an acute fall in blood pressure is observed compensatory responses abolish this effect of ANF. The 'low' dose of ANF (9.6 pmol/kg/min) lowered plasma renin activity and plasma aldosterone concentrations to a statistically significant degree (renin declined by 12% below placebo values and aldosterone by 45%: $P < 0.01$). These effects were not observed at the intermediate or higher doses.

Cusson and coworkers (Cusson *et al.*, 1987) also investigated the impact of serial doses of ANF administered to patients with hypertension (approximately 3.7, 7.4 and 14.8 pmol/kg/min. However, these were administered in three serial 30-min periods immediately after one another and hence 'carry over' effect from one dose to another may well confound interpretation of results. These authors documented for the first time an enhancement of plasma concentrations of cGMP in response to administration of ANF in hypertension. At the lower dose, no significant effect on blood pressure or heart rate was observed in either subject group. At the intermediate dose both ANF and plasma cGMP concentrations were similarly enhanced in both groups. Natriuresis and urinary excretion of cGMP also rose to a similar degree. At the highest dose an acute hypotensive effect was observed in three control subjects. This led to a change in protocol whereby hypertensive patients were studied in the supine posture whereas the normotensive control group had been studied seated upright. This element partially limits our ability to compare data from the two groups. At the peak dose, the increase in plasma ANF concentrations, diuresis, natriuresis and urinary cGMP excretion were similar in both groups. However, plasma cGMP rose to more than twice the level observed in the normotensive group. The authors suggest that in mild essential hypertension, patients may exhibit an enhanced cGMP response to administered ANF, but similar ANF end-organ effects compared with normotensive control subjects. This study stands in contrast to other work which has been essentially consistent in demonstrating enhanced natriuresis in hypertensive subjects. The authors did not publish the intra-infusion blood pressures in either group. Furthermore, to date, most studies comparing normotensive/hypertensive subjects with respect to their response to administered ANF are somewhat bedevilled by relatively poor matching of groups for characteristics other than their blood pressure. Generally hypertensive subjects have been older and heavier than their normotensive controls.

Administration of doses of ANF varying between 0.0017 and 0.5 pmol/min/100 ml of forearm volume given via the brachial artery have been used to examine the dose–response relationship between ANF-induced effects on forearm blood flow and forearm vascular resistance. Bolli et al. (1987) conducted such studies on 12 normotensive and 12 hypertensive patients. They found that ANF increased forearm blood flow and reduced forearm vascular resistance in a dose-dependent fashion. Compared with the normotensive group this effect appeared to be enhanced at lower doses of ANF in the hypertensive patients and showed a lower ED50 value in this patient group. However, at higher doses differences between the two groups disappeared. A fall in systemic blood pressure was noted at high dose in the hypertensive but not the normotensive group. The forearm vasodilator effect of ANF was inversely related with baseline renin activity with greater effects observed in patients with low renin levels. Theses data stand in contradistinction to suggestions from the studies by Richards et al. and by Weidmann et al. that hypertensives have a relative resistance to the vasodepressor actions of ANF. In addition, they contradict the suggestion in animal studies that the vasodepressor effects of ANF are enhanced in the presence of high basal activation of the renin–angiotensin system. These data are in need of confirmation but they do suggest there is no major qualitative abnormality in the peripheral vasodilator response to ANF in hypertensive patients.

Data are now available from at least four studies in which near-physiological (low) doses of ANF have been administered to patients with hypertension in a sustained fashion for periods of between 3 h to 5 days. Tonolo et al. (1989) administered ANF 99–126 to patients with untreated essential hypertension at doses of 1 and 2 pmol/kg/min for 2 h at each dose. The doses were given in fixed sequence. Plasma ANF rose to concentrations which were still well within the pathophysiological range observed among hypertensive patients. After 2 h, the lower dose of peptide induced a significant fall (approximately 10 mmHg) in systolic blood pressure which was further accentuated after a further 2 h at the higher dose (20 mmHg). However, no effect on diastolic arterial pressure was observed. Plasma volume contraction occurred even with the lower dose as evidenced by an increase in haematocrit above time-matched placebo values and this effect was accentuated with the higher dose. Effects on both haematocrit and on blood pressure were sustained for more than 2 h after cessation of infusions. Natriuresis exhibited a statistically insignificant trend upwards during the first dose with a clear-cut increase in sodium excretion at the higher dose. Glomerular filtration rate was not significantly altered by either dose of ANF. In these patients who were sodium replete and studied in the supine posture, no further suppression of already very low baseline levels of renin, ANG II or plasma aldosterone was observed. Similarly, sympathetic nervous system activity as assessed by measurement of plasma catecholamine concentrations was not altered. Central haemodynamics as assessed by Swan–Ganz catheter demonstrated a trend downwards in both right atrial and pulmonary capillary wedge pressures. Cardiac output fell and calculated peripheral vascular resistance was unchanged. Hence this careful placebo-controlled study employing invasive high-fidelity techniques demonstrated an acute hypotensive effect of physiological doses of ANF administered for a total of 4 h which was independent of effects on renal haemodynamics, renin–angiotensin–aldosterone system activity, global sympathetic nervous system activity, peripheral vasodilation and appeared to depend primarily on plasma volume contraction with a reduction in cardiac output. These data are consistent with the initial effects of ANF observed in short-term studies of animals (Parkes et al., 1988).

Richards and coworkers (Richards et al., 1989) have administered an even lower dose of ANF 99–126 (0.75 pmol/kg/min) for 3 h to well-matched groups of patients with essential hypertension and normotensive control subjects (similar age and weight). Infusions at this level induce a mere doubling of plasma concentrations of ANF which remain entirely confined to the normal resting range. Even these subtle perturbations of plasma ANF concentrations induced natriuresis to 50 % above time-matched placebo values. The natriuretic effect was more pronounced in the hypertensive group. Urinary excretion of cGMP rose to more that double placebo values in both groups. In both groups, plasma renin activity was consistently suppressed to less than 50 % of time-matched placebo values as were plasma aldosterone concentrations. In addition, for the first time, plasma noradrenaline levels also fell significantly below placebo values although this effect was restricted to the hypertensive group. At this very low dose level of ANF given for only 3 h, no significant impact on blood pressure was observed. In addition, urine volume, excretion of electrolytes other than sodium, haematocrit, effective renal plasma flow, glomerular filtration rate and renal filtration fraction were unaffected by ANF. These data suggest that minor shifts in plasma ANF (which might be expected to accompany day-to-day variations in stimuli such as dietary sodium intake and physical activity) are of physiological relevance in mild hypertension and probably contribute to volume homeostasis in this condition.

ANF 99–126 has been administered intravenously at the even lower dose of 0.5 pmol/kg/min over 12 h in six patients with mild to moderate essential hypertension and in a group of six normotensive volunteers (Cusson et al., 1989). This dose of ANF (which is right at the threshold at which induced changes in plasma ANF concentrations can be detected by radioimmunoassay) was sufficient to significantly enhance plasma cGMP concentrations (from 2.8 ± 0.4 to 5.1 ± 0.5 nmol/l: $P < 0.05$). Urinary output and sodium excretion were enhanced in the hypertensive group but not significantly altered in normal subjects. Haematocrit increased significantly in both groups. No hypotensive effect was observed in normotensive controls but systolic blood pressure tended to fall over the latter 8 h of the infusion by about 5 % ($P = 0.06$). The authors concluded that prolonged infusion of ANF at a physiological dose caused a modest increase in plasma cGMP, haemoconcentration, a trend towards reduction in systolic blood pressure and natriuresis (with the latter two effects being evident in patients with mild hypertension but not in normal subjects).

Janssen and coworkers (Janssen et al., 1989) have undertaken the logistically difficult task of continuously infusing low doses of ANF over a 5-day period in six patients with essential hypertension. This study represents the cutting edge of our current knowledge concerning the effects of sustained subtle increments in plasma ANF concentrations in hypertensive man. The infusion rate (approximately 1 pmol/kg/min) was sufficient to merely double basal plasma concentrations of ANF. Patients exhibited enhanced urinary sodium excretion with a regaining of sodium balance after 24 h in association with a net loss of some 70 mmol of sodium. After 12 h of infusion, both systolic and diastolic blood pressure began to gradually decrease, reaching a stable new lower level after 36 h, having fallen by 11.5 ± 1.5 and $10.3 \pm 0.8\%$ below baseline levels respectively. Heart rate and haematocrit both rose. Changes in blood pressure, heart rate and haematocrit were sustained throughout the remainder of the infusion period. The achieved mean arterial pressures were within the normotensive range. After infusions were halted, sodium balance returned to baseline values within 36 h. In contrast, blood pressures, although returning towards baseline values, were still significantly below preinfusion levels at 3 days postinfusion. Haematocrit fell to a new lower steady state value within 36 h. In the absence of haemodynamic data beyond blood pressure and heart rate measurement it is difficult to be certain of the exact effect of these prolonged infusions of ANF on cardiac output and peripheral vascular resistance. It seems reasonable to suggest that the observed negative volume balance, reduced weight and stable increase in haematocrit reflect plasma volume contraction which may well have contributed to falls in arterial pressure. However, the drop in diastolic pressure plus the rather slow return towards baseline values of blood pressure (in spite of the quick return to baseline sodium balance and haematocrit) suggests that an additional action(s) inducing peripheral vasodilation was at work.

In summary, sustained physiological doses of ANF can cause a moderate negative shift in sodium balance in association with a significant fall in arterial pressure in human hypertension without major reflex activation of compensatory mechanisms including the renin–angiotensin–aldosterone and the sympathetic nervous systems and without the catastrophic hypotensive–bradycardiac phenomena observed at higher doses. These data suggest that ANF-like analogues or agents which inhibit degradation of endogenous ANF may offer a new therapeutic avenue in hypertension. Such an inhibitor has been exhibited in normal subjects and patients with mild heart failure (Jardine *et al.*, 1989: Northridge *et al.*, 1989) with induction of enhanced plasma ANF levels, natriuresis and a fall in cardiac filling pressures. The scene is now set for acute and chronic dosing studies of such agents in human hypertension.

References

Arendt, R. M., Gerbes, A. L., Ritter, D., Stangl, E., Bach, P. & Zahringer, J. (1986). Atrial natriuretic factor in plasma of patients with arterial hypertension, heart failure or cirrhosis of the liver. *J. Hypertension* **4** (Suppl. 2): 5131–5.

Bolli, P., Muller, F. B., Linder, L., Raine, A. E. G., Resink, T. J., Erne, P., Kiowski, W. *et al.* (1987). Greater vasodilator responsiveness to atrial natriuretic peptide in low-renin essential hypertensives. *J. Hypertension* **5** (Suppl. 5): S55–8.

Bruun, N. E., Nielsen, M. D., Skott, P., Giese, J., Leth, A., Schutten, H. J. & Rasmussen, S. (1989). Changed cyclic guanosine monophosphate atrial natriuretic factor relationship in hypertensive man. *J. Hypertension* **7**: 287–91.

Cachofeiro, V., Schiffrin, E. L., Thibault, G., Cantin, M. & Garcia, R. (1989). Effect of a chronic infusion of atrial natriuretic factor on glomerular and vascular receptors in spontaneously hypertensive rats. *J. Hypertension* **7**: 335–42.

Chabrier, P., Roubert, P., Longchamps, M., Plas, P. & Braquet, P. (1988). Interaction between atrial natriuretic factor and angiotensin II receptors in the regulation of blood pressure. *J. Hypertension* **6**: S290–1.

Cusson, J. R., Hamet, P., Gutkowska, J., Kuchel, O., Genest, J., Cantin, M. & Larochell, P. (1987). Effects of atrial natriuretic factor on natriuresis and cGMP in patients with essential hypertension. *J. Hypertension* **5**: 435–43.

Cusson, J. R., Thibault, G., Cantin, M. & Larochelle, P. (1989). Cardiovascular, renal and endocrine responses to low doses of atrial natriuretic factor in mild essential hypertension. *J. Human Hypertension* **3**: 89–96.

Davis, C. L. & Briggs, J. P. (1987). Effect of reduction in renal artery pressure on atrial natriuretic peptide-induced natriuresis. *Am. J. Physiol.* **252**: F146–53.

De Mey, J. G., Defreyn, G., Lenaers, A., Calderon, P. & Roba, J. (1987). Arterial reactivity, blood pressure, and plasma levels of atrial natriuretic peptides in normotensive and hypertensive rats: Effects of acute and chronic administration of atriopeptin III. *J. Cardiovasc. Pharmacol.* **9**: 525–35.

Espiner, E. A., Crozier, I. G., Nicholls, M. G., Cuneo, R., Yandle, T. G. & Ikram, H. (1985). Cardiac secretion of atrial natriuretic peptide. *Lancet* **i**: 398–9.

Ferrier C., Weidmann, P., Hollmann, R., Dietler, R. & Shaw, S. (1988). Impaired response of atrial natriuretic factor to high salt intake in persons prone to hypertension. *New Engl. J. Med.* **319**: 1223–4.

Garcia, R., Cantin, M., Genest, J., Gutkowska, J. & Thibault, G. (1987a). Body fluids and plasma atrial peptide after its chronic infusion in hypertensive rats. *Proc. Soc. Exp. Biol. Med.* **185**: 352–8.

Garcia, R., Cantin, M., Gutkowska, J. & Thibault, G. (1987b). Atrial natriuretic factor during development and reversal of one-kidney, one clip hypertension. *Hypertension* **9**: 144–9.

Garcia, R., Gauquelin, G., Thibault, G., Cantin, M. & Schiffrin, E. L. (1989). Glomerular atrial natriuretic factor receptors in spontaneously hypertensive rats. *Hypertension* **13**: 567–74.

Garcia, R., Gutkowska, J., Cantin, M. & Thibault, G. (1987c). Renin dependency of the effect of chronically administered atrial natriuretic factor in two-kidney, one clip rats. *Hypertension* **9**: 88–95.

Garcia, R., Thibault, G. & Cantin, M. (1987d). Correlation between cardiac hypertrophy and plasma levels of atrial natriuretic factor in non-spontaneous models of hypertension in the rat. *Biochem. Biophys. Res. Commun.* **145** (1): 532–41.

Garcia, R., Thibault, G., Gutkowska, J., Hamet, P., Cantin, M. & Genest, J. (1985a). Effect of chronic infusion of synthetic atrial natriuretic factor (ANF 8–33) in conscious two-kidney, one-clip hypertensive rats. *Proc. Soc. Exp. Biol. Med.* **178**: 155–9.

Garcia, R., Thibault, G., Gutkowska, J., Horky, K., Hamet, P., Cantin, M. & Genest, J. (1985b). Chronic infusion of low doses of atrial natriuretic factor (ANF Arg 101–Tyr 126) reduces blood pressure in conscious SHR without apparent changes in sodium excretion. *Proc. Soc. Exp. Biol. Med.* **179**: 396–401.

Gutkowska, J., Horky, K., Lachance, C., Racz, K., Garcia, R., Thibault, G., Kuchel, O. *et al.* (1986). Atrial natriuretic factor in spontaneously hypertensive rats. *Hypertension* **8** (Suppl. I): I137–40.

Hirata, Y., Ganguli, M., Tobian, L. & Iwai, J. (1984). Dahl S rats have increased natriuretic factor in atria but are markedly hyporesponsive to it. *Hypertension* **6**(Suppl. I): I148–55.

Iimura, O., Shimamoto, K., Ando, T., Ura, N., Ishida, H., Nakagawa, M., Yokoyama, T. *et al.* (1987). Plasma levels of human atrial natriuretic peptide in patients with hypertensive diseases. *Can. J. Physiol. Pharmacol.* **65**: 1701–5.

Janssen, W. M. T., de Jong, P. E., van der Hem, G. K. & Zeeuw, D. (1986). Effect of human atrial natriuretic peptide on blood pressure after sodium depletion in essential hypertension. *Br. Med. J.* **293**: 351–3.

Janssen, W. M. T., de Zeeuw, D., van der Hem, G. K. & de Jong, P. E. (1989). Antihypertensive effect of a 5-day infusion of atrial natriuretic factor in humans. *Hypertension* **13**: 640–6.

Jardine, A., Connell, J. M. C., Dilly, S. G., Northridge, D., Leckie, B., Cussans, N. J. & Lever, A. F. (1989). Pharmacological elevation of endogenous atrial natriuretic factor in man using the atriopeptidase inhibitor (UK 69578). *J. Am. Coll. Cardiol.* **13** (2): 76A.

Kohno, M., Yasunari, K., Matsuura, T., Murakawa, K. & Takeda, T. (1987). Circulating atrial natriuretic polypeptide in essential hypertension. *Am. Heart J.* **113**: 1160–3.

Kuchel, O., Debinski, W., Thibault, G., Gantin, M. & Genest, J. (1988). Ganglionic, spinal cord and hypothalamic atrial natriuretic factor: its distribution, origin and possible role in spontaneously hypertensive rats. *J. Hypertension* **6** (Suppl. 4): S279–81.

Larochelle, P., Cusson, J. R., Gutkowska, J., Schiffrin, E. L., Hamet, P., Kuchel, O., Genest, J. *et al.* (1987). Plasma atrial natriuretic factor concentrations in essential and renovascular hypertension. *Br. Med. J.* **294**: 1249–51.

Linz, W., Albus, U., Wiemer, G., Breipohl, G., Knolle, J. & Scholkens, B. A. (1988). Amiloride potentiates the vascular effects of atrial natriuretic factor. *J. Hypertension* **6** (Suppl. 4): S300–2.

Matsubara, H., Umeda, Y., Yamane, Y., Nishikawa, M., Taniguchi, T. & Inada, M. (1987). Role of atrial natriuretic polypeptides for exaggerated natriuresis in essential hypertension. *Am. J. Cardiol.* **60**: 708–14.

Montorsi, P., Tonolo, G., Polonia, J., Hepburn, D. & Richards, A. M. (1987). Correlates of plasma atrial natriuretic factor in health and hypertension. *Hypertension* **10**: 570–6.

Morii, N., Nakao, K., Kihara, M., Sugawara, A., Sakamoto, M., Yamori, Y. & Imura, H. (1986). Decreased content in left atrium and increased plasma concentration of atrial natriuretic polypeptide in spontaneously hypertensive rats (SHR) and SHR stroke-prone. *Biochem. Biophys. Res. Commun.* **135**: 74–81.

Morton, J. J., Lyall, F. & Wallace, E. C. H. (1987). Rat atrial natriuretic peptide vascular receptor: effect of alterations in sodium balance and of DOC hypertension. *J. Hypertension* **5**: 475–9.

Nakamura, M., Nakamura, A., Fine, B. & Aviv, A. (1988). Blunted cGMP response to ANF in vascular smooth muscle cells of SHR. *Am. Physiol. Soc.* **24**: C573–80.

Nakaoka, H., Kitahara, Y., Amano, M., Imataka, K., Fujii, J., Ishibashi, M. & Yamaji, T. (1987). Effect of β-adrenergic receptor blockade on atrial natriuretic peptide in essential hypertension. *Hypertension* **10**: 221–5.

Nilsson, P., Lindholm, L., Schersten, B., Rudiger, H., Melander, A. & Hesch, R. D. (1987). Atrial natriuretic peptide and blood pressure in a geographically defined population. *Lancet* 883–5.

Northridge, D. B., Findlay, I. N., Jardine, A., Dilly, S. G. & Dargie, H. J. (1989). Acute effects of atriopeptidase inhibition on plasma atrial natriuretic factor in chronic heart failure. *J. Am. Coll. Cardiol.* **13**: 76A.

Ohashi, M., Fujio, N., Nawata, H., Kato, K., Ibayashi, H., Kangawa, K. & Matsuo, H. (1987). High plasma concentrations of human atrial natriuretic polypeptide in aged men. *J. Clin. Endocrinol. Metab.* **64**: 81–5.

Onwochei, M. O. & Rapp, J. P. (1989). Hyposecretion of atrial natriuretic factor by pre-hypertensive Dahl salt-sensitive rat. *Hypertension* **13**: 440–8.

Parkes, D. G., Coghlan, J. P., McDougall, J. G. & Scoggins, B. A. (1988). Long-term hemodynamic actions of atrial natriuretic factor (99–126) in conscious sheep. *Heart Circ. Physiol.* **23**: H811–15.

Petterson, A., Ricksten, S., Towle, A., Hedner, J. & Hedner, T. (1985). Plasma atrial natriuretic peptide and haemodynamics in conscious normotensive and spontaneously hypertensive rats after acute blood volume expansion. *J. Hypertension* **3**: S311–13.

Poole, S., Gaines Das, R. E., Dzau, V. J., Richards, A. M. & Robertson, J. I. S. (1988). The international standard for atrial natriuretic factor calibration by an international collaborative study. *Hypertension* **12**: 629–34.

Richards, A. M., Espiner, E. A., Ikram, H. & Yandle, T. G. (1989). Atrial natriuretic factor in hypertension: bioactivity at normal plasma levels. *Hypertension* **14**: 261–8.

Richards, A. M., Nicholls, M. G., Espiner, E. A., Ikram, H., Yandle, T. G., Joyce, S. L. & Cullens, M. M. (1985). Effects of α-human atrial natriuretic peptide in essential hypertension. *Hypertension* **7**: 812–17.

Richards, A. M., Tonolo, G., McIntyre, G. D., Leckie, B. J. & Robertson, J. I. S. (1987). Radioimmunoassay for plasma alpha human atrial natriuretic peptide: A comparison of direct and pre-extracted methods. *J. Hypertension* **5**: 227–36.

Richards, A. M., Tonolo, G., Tillman, D., Connell, J. M., Hepburn, D. & Robertson, J. I. S. (1986). Plasma atrial natriuretic peptide in stable and accelerated essential hypertension. *J. Hypertension* **4**: 790–1.

Saavedra, J. M., Correa, M. A., Plunkett, L. M., Israel, A., Kurihara, M. & Shigematsu, K. (1986). Binding of angiotensin and atrial natriuretic peptide in brain of hypertensive rats. *Nature* **320**: 758–60.

Sagnella, G. A., Markandu, N. D., Shore, A. C. & MacGregor, G. A. (1986). Raised circulating levels of atrial natriuretic peptides in essential hypertension. *Lancet* i: 179–81.

Schiffrin, E. L., St-Louis, J. & Essiambre, R. (1988). Platelet binding sites and plasma concentration of atrial natriuretic peptide in patients with essential hypertension. *J. Hypertension* **6**: 565–72.

Schiffrin, E. L., St-Louis, J., Garcia, R., Thibault, G., Cantin, M. & Genest, J. (1986). Vascular and adrenal binding sites for atrial natriuretic factor effects of sodium and hypertension. *Hypertension* **8** (Suppl. I): I141–5.

Seymour, A. A., Marsh, E. A., Mazack, E. K., Stabilito, I. I. & Blaine, E. H. (1985). Synthetic atrial natriuretic factor in conscious normotensive and hypertensive rats. *Hypertension* **7** (Suppl. I): I35–42.

Snajdar, R. M. & Rapp, J. P. (1985). Atrial natriuretic factor in Dahl-sensitive rats—atrial content and renal and aortic responses. *Hypertension* **7**: 775–82.

Sonnenberg, H., Milojevic, S., Chong, C. K. & Veress, A. T. (1983). Atrial natriuretic factor: reduced cardiac content in spontaneously hypertensive rats. *Hypertension* **5**: 672–5.

Sorensen, S. S., Danielsen, H., Amdisen, A. & Pedersen, E. B. (1989). Atrial natriuretic peptide and exaggerated natriuresis during acute hypertonic volume expansion in essential hypertension. *J. Hypertension* **7**: 21–9.

Sosa, R. E., Volpe, M., Marion, D. N., Atlas, S. A., Laragh, J. H., Vaughan, E. D. & Maack, T. (1986). Relationship between renal hemodynamic and natriuretic effects of atrial natriuretic factor. *Am. J. Physiol.* **250**: F520–4.

Sugawara, A., Nakao, K., Kono, T., Morii, N., Yamada, T., Itoh, H., Shiono, S. *et al.* (1988). Atrial natriuretic factor in essential hypertension and adrenal disorders. *Hypertension* **11** (Suppl. I): I212–16.

Sugawara, A., Nakao, K., Sakamoto, M., Morii, N., Yamada, T., Itoh, H., Shiono, S. *et al.* (1985). Plasma concentration of atrial natriuretic polypeptide in essential hypertension. *Lancet* **ii**: 1426–7.

Takayanagi, R., Imada, T., Grammer, R. T., Misono, K. S., Naruse, M. & Inagami, T. (1986). Atrial natriuretic factor in spontaneously hypertensive rats: concentration changes with the progression of hypertension and elevated formation of cyclic GMP. *J. Hypertension* **4**: S303–7.

Tonolo, G., Richards, A. M., Manunta, P., Pazzola, A., Pala, F. & Glorioso, N. (1989). Low dose infusion of atrial natriuretic factor in mild essential hypertension. *Circulation* **80**: 893–902.

Tunny, T. J. & Gordon, R. D. (1986). Plasma atrial natriuretic peptide in primary aldosteronism (before and after treatment) and in Bartter's and Gordon's syndromes. *Lancet* **i**: 272–3.

Tunny, T. J., Higgins, B. A. & Gordon, R. D. (1986). Plasma levels of atrial natriuretic peptide in man in primary aldosteronism, in Gordon's syndrome and in Bartter's syndrome. *Clin. Exp. Pharmacol. Physiol.* **13**: 341–5.

Visser, W., van den Dorpel, M. A., Derkx, F. H. M., Wallenburg, H. C. S. & Schalekamp, M. A. D. H. (1987). Atrial natriuretic peptide and haemodynamics in untreated pre-eclampsia. *J. Hypertension* **5** (Suppl. 5): S33–5.

Volpe, M., Odell, G., Kleinert, H. D., Muller, F., Camargo, M. J., Laragh, J. H. & Maack, T. (1985). Effect of atrial natriuretic factor on blood pressure, renin, and aldosterone in Goldblatt hypertension. *Hypertension* **7** (Suppl. I): I43–8.

Wambach, G., Bonner, G., Stimpel, M. & Kaufmann, W. (1988). Relationship between plasma atrial natriuretic peptide and left atrial and left ventricular involvement in essential hypertension. *J. Hypertension* **6**: 573–7.

Weder, A. B., Sekkarie, M. A., Takiyyuddin, M., Schork, N. J. & Julius, S. (1987). Anti-hypertensive and hypotensive effects of atrial natriuretic factor in men. *Hypertension* **10**: 582–9.

Weidmann, P., Gnadinger, M. P., Ziswiler, H. R., Shaw, S., Bachmann, C., Rascher, W., Uehlinger, D. E. *et al.* (1986). Cardiovascular, endocrine and renal effects of atrial natriuretic peptide in essential hypertension. *J. Hypertension* **4** (Suppl. 2): S71–83.

Yamaji, T., Ishibashi, M., Sekihara, H., Takaku, F., Nakaoka, H. & Fujii, J. (1986). Plasma levels of atrial natriuretic peptide in primary aldosteronism and essential hypertension. *J. Clin. Endocrinol. Metab.* **63**: 815–18.

Yandle, T. G., Espiner, E. A., Nicholls, M. G. & Duff, H. (1986). Radioimmunoassay and characterization of atrial natriuretic peptide in human plasma. *J. Clin. Endocrinol. Metab.* **61**: 72–8.

Chapter 8
The pathophysiology of atrial natriuretic factor in congestive heart failure
Robert J. Cody

Introduction

Atrial natriuretic factor (ANF) is an important modulator of sodium excretion. From the time of its identification in 1981 (deBold *et al.*, 1981), to the current time, ANF has been the focus of an explosive volume of research activity (Fig. 8.1). One of the most important areas where abnormal ANF secretion suggested potential therapeutic application was in those patients with chronic congestive heart failure. High circulating levels of ANF, the less than impressive response to pharmacologic infusions of ANF and the need for parenteral administration of ANF, led to a degree of frustration regarding the potential for ANF modulation in heart failure patients.

In view of the temporal distance since these initial studies, it is reasonable to reassess the importance of ANF in congestive heart failure and to determine what role, if any, may exist for modulating ANF levels in patients with chronic congestive heart failure. Therefore, this chapter provides an overview of the background development and current thinking regarding ANF in congestive heart failure.

Background

Under normal conditions, the majority of sodium ingested in the diet is excreted in the urine, allowing for small losses in sweat and other bodily secretions. Sodium excretion is functional dependent on the glomerular filtration rate (GFR) and sodium reabsorption. GFR represents the first factor controlling sodium excretion, and the hormonal control of sodium

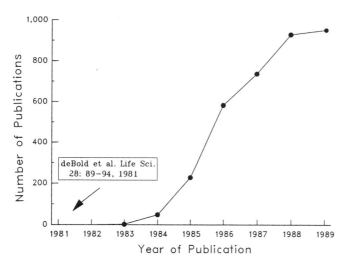

Fig. 8.1 ANF publications since the reference publication by deBold *et al.* (1981). Citations were generated using the major descriptor 'natriuretic–peptides–atrial', from the MedLine database.

reabsorption, or second factor, is primarily the effects of aldosterone at the distal tubule of the kidney. A 'third factor' had been suspected for several decades. Hypotheses included physical and mechanical factors within the kidney, tubular effects of well-described hormonal pathways, or a putative substance that remained to be described (deWardener, Mills & Clapham, 1961).

Evidence that changes in atrial tension were somehow closely related to sodium excretion had been suspected for many years, in that the atria of the mammalian heart appeared to participate in the regulation of intravascular volume. Very early studies had demonstrated that mechanical stretch of the atria produced a rapid diuresis (Henry & Pearce, 1956; Wood, 1963; Epstein, 1978; Linden, 1979), and this was initially felt to be related to the degree to which parasympathetic nervous system activity was stimulated (Henry & Pearce, 1956; Ledsome & Linden, 1968; Sealey Kirschman & Laragh, 1969). It was postulated that changes in vagal nerve traffic would, in addition, release vasopressin (Henry & Pearce, 1956), with changes in efferent sympathetic traffic to the kidney (Linden, 1979). These observations led to a growing belief that secretion of a natriuretic-factor-promoted diuresis during volume expansion (deWardener *et al.* 1961; Bourgoignie, Klarh & Bricker, 1971; Sonneberg, Veress & Pearce, 1972; Buckalew & Nelson, 1974; deWardener, 1977) and coincided with the identification of membrane-bound secretory granules in atrial myocytes (Kisch, 1956; Jamieson, 1964), that responded to alterations of intravascular volume (Marie, Guillemot & Hatt, 1976; deBold, 1979).

Such studies set the stage for the landmark study by deBold and colleagues (deBold *et al.* 1981). These investigators demonstrated that a crude atrial extract could induce rapid reversible increases of sodium and water excretion thereby producing a direct demonstration of a natriuretic hormone, and firmly establishing a tie between the heart and the kidney in the control of sodium and water excretion. This was also the first unequivocal demonstration of a tissue source for this natriuretic hormone. The evidence summarized elsewhere in this text, and previously published (Cantin & Genest, 1985; deBold, 1985; Needleman *et al.*, 1985; Atlas, 1986; Atlas & Laragh, 1986; Ballermann & Brenner, 1986; Laragh *et al.*, 1986; Schwartz, Katsube & Needleman, 1986; Cody, Atlas & Laragh, 1987b; Genest & Cantin, 1987; Lang, Unger & Ganten, 1987; Nicholls *et al.*, 1987; Sonnenberg, 1987; Trippodo, 1987; Genest *et al.*, 1988), provide a summary of a now large database which demonstrates that ANF fulfils the criteria of the putative 'third factor'.

The potential role of ANF secretion in heart failure is readily apparent, as this disorder is characterized by sodium and water retention and vasoconstriction. Both factors are readily attributable to the abnormal neurohormonal milieu of the heart failure state. Excessive sodium and water retention is readily explained by the abnormal activation of the renin system and the influence of angiotensin II (ANGII), and aldosterone, but is also influenced by increased sympathetic nervous system activity, and vasopressin release. None the less, these and other factors (abnormal prostaglandin activity in the kidney, etc.) may not provide a full picture of abnormalities of sodium and water regulation. The location of ANF in secretory granules in the myocardium provided a logical focus of ANF as a regulator of sodium and water excretion in that abnormalities of atrial tension could explain abnormalities of ANF secretion. This will be discussed in greater detail below. Since ANF is a potent vasodilator, it would seem reasonable that either decreased secretion of ANF, or a decreased vascular responsiveness to circulating levels of ANF, could contribute to the overall vasoconstrictor environment within the heart failure circulation.

ANF concentration within the circulation

The precursor peptide of ANF (proANF) is a 126-amino-acid residue peptide and is stored in atrial myocytes of mammalian tissue (Seidman *et al.*, 1985). Structurally related ANF segments have been isolated by numerous investigators (Flynn, deBold & deBold, 1983; Atlas *et al.*, 1984, 1985; Currie *et al.*, 1984; Inagami *et al.*, 1984, 1987; Kangawa & Matsuo, 1984; Kangawa *et al.*, 1984; Matsuo & Kangawa, 1984; Misono *et al.*, 1984; Needleman *et al.*, 1985; Richards *et al.*, 1987). These biologically active peptides are derived from the C-terminus of proANF and their biological activity is due to a core sequence of amino acids that comprise

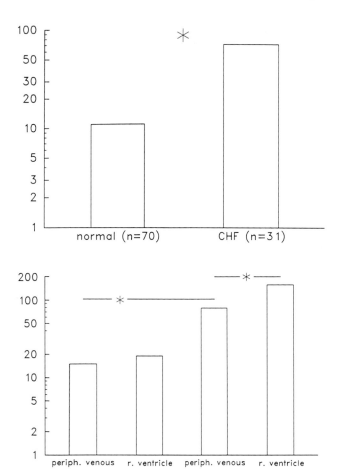

Fig. 8.2 (a) Immunoreactive ANF, comparing normal subjects and patients with congestive heart failure. ANF is expressed in fmol/ml. Conversion to pg/ml is achieved by multiplying these values by approximately 3.1. Note that the values are expressed on a logarithmic scale. The patients with congestive heart failure display ANF levels which span a wide range, from high-normal, through markedly elevated levels. (b) Incremental values of ANF at the level of the right ventricle in normal subjects and heart failure, consistent with active secretion of the peptide into the circulation, from the coronary sinus. Fig. 8.2(a) and (b) are derived from Cody et al. (1986).

a 17-residue ring, which is formed by an intrachain disulphide bridge. There are some species differences in the composition of this peptide chain. For instance, at position number 110 of the precursor, there is an isoleucine residue in the rat species, whereas this position is occupied by methionine in man. These aspects of ANF production and release are discussed elsewhere in this text. Specific ANF receptors have been identified in various target organs (Hirata et al., 1984; McKenzie et al., 1985; Osol et al., 1986; Kurihara et al., 1987; Maack et al., 1987; Morton,

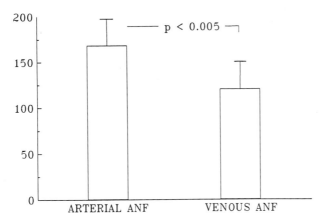

Fig. 8.3 Clearance of ANF across the vascular bed is indicated by the fall of ANF values, comparing simultaneous brachial artery and basilic vein blood samples in heart failure patients. Derived from Cody *et al.* (1987a).

Lyall & Wallace, 1987; Suzuki *et al.*, 1987; Swithers, Stewart & McCarty, 1987; Garcia *et al.*, 1988; Gauquelin *et al.*, 1988).

Circulating levels of ANF in patients with congestive heart failure, compared to levels from normal subjects, are shown in Fig. 8.2a. In normal subjects, the range of plasma ANF was from 2 to approximately 30 fmol/ml, with a mean value of approximately 12 fmol/ml. While the mean value for congestive heart failure (73 fmol/ml) was approximately sixfold greater than the mean value in normal subjects, there was, none the less, some overlap of values.

Plasma ANF levels demonstrate a dynamic response to a number of physiologic stimuli. The wide range of ANF values suggests active secretion, and this is readily identified by simultaneous measurements of peripheral venous and central circulation ANF (Cody *et al.*, 1986; Cody, Atlas & Laragh, 1988a). Since ANF is secreted by atrial (and under certain conditions, ventricular) myocytes, it has been demonstrated that the highest concentration of ANF in the circulation is in the coronary sinus (Crozier *et al.*, 1986; Lindop *et al.*, 1987). Coronary sinus sampling is difficult, however, particularly during physiological testing. The coronary sinus effluent mixes completely with peripheral venous return at the level of the right ventricle.

In normal subjects, and heart failure patients, there is an approximate twofold step up of plasma ANF concentration at the level of the right ventricle (Fig. 8.2b), consistent with active secretion of the peptide by myocytes. It has been demonstrated that ANF is cleared across several vascular beds, which would be consistent with utilization of ANF at receptor sites, or metabolism by peripheral tissues. This is demonstrated in the skeletomuscular bed by evaluating simultaneous ANF concentration across the forearm (Fig. 8.3; Cody *et al.*, 1987a), where an approximate 50% reduction of ANF across the forearm is consistent with binding of ANF to a specific receptor in vascular myocytes, linked to activation of particulate guanylate cyclase (Hirata *et al.*, 1984; Waldman, Rapoport & Murad, 1984; Winquist *et al.*, 1985; Hamet *et al.*, 1986; Shirasaki *et al.*, 1986; Leitman & Murad, 1987; Otsuka *et al.*, 1988), the rate-limiting enzyme governing the formation of cyclic guanyl mono-phosphate (cGMP). cGMP is a potent cellular mediator of vasodilatation and provides a plausible cellular mechanism for the vasodilator effect of ANF.

ANF secretion during physiological manoeuvres

Since ANF is readily measured in the plasma, and its secretion and clearance are consistent with active production and target organ effects, the response of ANF to stimuli that potentially increase or decrease its secretion can be readily assessed (Rankin, 1987). An early hypothesis was that ANF release was directly related to changes in intravascular volume; with increased atrial volume, and increased atrial distension, ANF would be secreted as a means to augment sodium and water secretion by the kidney to reduce intravascular volume. This hypothesis is readily tested by several manoeuvres that increase or decrease atrial tension. For instance, total body submersion to the level of the neck redistributes intravascular volume to the central circulation, thereby increasing atrial volume (Epstein, 1978). In normal subjects this manoeuvre results in a rapid and marked increase of ANF concentrations in the circulation, and aug-mentation of sodium and water excretion (Epstein *et al.*, 1986, 1987).

Alteration of atrial tension and volume can also be achieved by performing tilt studies (Hodsman *et al.*, 1986). Head-up tilt will decrease atrial volume and tension, thereby decreasing ANF secretion, whereas head-down tilt will increase atrial volume and tension, similar to water immersion, producing an increase of ANF concentration.

Lower body negative pressure, by inducing a redistribution of blood from the central circulation to the periphery, results in a reduction of atrial pressure and tension. In response to this manoeuvre, there is a reduction of circulating levels of atrial natriuretic peptide.

A more intensive physiological stress to increase atrial volume and tension, is maximal exercise (Cody *et al.*, 1987b). Despite the high basal level of ANF secretion in congestive heart failure, the left ventricular dysfunction and increased atrial tension of exercise produces a doubling of circulating ANF (Fig. 8.4). Teleologically, it is unlikely that exercise-induced ANF secretion is meant to increase sodium and water excretion but rather, to augment vasodilatation (Winquist *et al.*, 1984; Cody *et al.*, 1986; Bolli *et al.*, 1987; Mulvany, 1987) and promote haemoconcentration

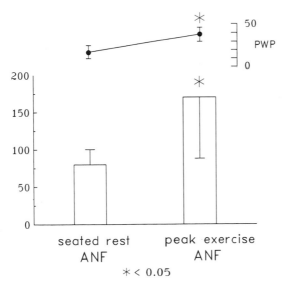

Fig. 8.4 Circulating ANF and pulmonary wedge pressure before and after exercise in congestive heart failure (derived from Cody *et al.* 1987b).

(deBold, 1985; Maack *et al.*, 1986; Cody *et al.*, 1987). The latter effect appears to be achieved by sequestration of fluid outside of the vascular space. Volume expansion or depletion also produces the anticipated response.

Infusion of saline or other colloids tends to increase ANF secretion (Sonneberg *et al.*, 1972; Espiner *et al.*, 1986; Hollister *et al.*, 1986; Khraibi *et al.*, 1987; Morris, Cain & Chalmers, 1987). However, this is not a uniform response, and may depend to a certain degree on the myocardial response to volume challenge. These studies therefore provide direct evidence for a link between atrial haemodynamic status, blood volume, and the extent to which ANF is secreted. At the same time the studies firmly establish the fact that ANF is truly a hormone: there is a site of active production and secretion (the heart), with blood-borne transport, and physiological effects at distant target organ sites (kidney, adrenal glands, vascular smooth muscle).

ANF secretion and myocardial morphological adaptation in congestive heart failure

Ventricular remodelling and hypertrophy, secondary to congestive heart failure or long-standing hypertension, may be a stimulus for ANF secretion. The messenger RNA encoding for ANF synthesis has been identified within ventricular myocytes (Day *et al.*, 1987). Furthermore, immunohistological staining of ventricular myocytes has identified secretory granules within these cells, clearly demonstrating the ability to recruit ventricular production in hypertension and congestive heart failure (Edwards *et al.*, 1988). In view of ventricular synthesis and storage, ANF secretion may be increased in the presence of concentric or regional hypertrophy. It is difficult, however, to differentiate whether the stimulus for ANF release is primary morphological hypertrophy or the secondary increase of atrial distention which hypertrophy produces. None the less, one cannot diminish the significant impact of ventricular myocytes recruitment for the production of ANF.

ANF and renal function in congestive heart failure

Abnormalities of renal function in congestive heart failure have been previously summarized. (Cody, 1988; Cody *et al.*, 1988a,b,c, 1989) The pivotal role of the kidney in heart failure is based on three major influences. First, the role of the kidney as the ultimate regulator of sodium excretion. Secondly, the importance of the kidney as the major source of renin secretion in the circulation and thus its importance as the regulator of renin endocrine function. Thirdly, the fact that the kidney is the target for a number of hormonal pathways which interact in a complex way to influence renal haemodynamics, tubular function, sodium excretion, and renin release. Since these factors are influenced by the failing heart, the ischaemic kidney and the neurohormonal environment, it is difficult to isolate the influence of ANF in clinical studies.

Exogenous administration of ANF

ANF has been given to both normal subjects and patients with congestive heart failure (Winquist *et al.*, 1984; Richards *et al.*, 1985; Cody *et al.*, 1986; Ishii *et al.*, 1986; Janssen *et al.*, 1986; MacGregor & Sagnella, 1987; Mantero *et al.*, 1987a,b; Nicholls *et al.* 1987; Nicholls *et al.*, 1987; Volpe *et al.*, 1987; Weder *et al.*, 1987). The rationale is twofold: first, to gain additional information regarding the physiological effects of ANF; secondly, to determine the potential therapeutic efficacy of ANF administration. Since ANF is a peptide that can be degraded by the gastrointestinal tract, it requires an intravenous route of administration. ANF has been administered as a synthetic peptide based on the 25-amino-acid rat sequence, or the 28-amino-acid human sequence. Thus far, no major difference in response has been detected between the two different forms of peptide. The first peptide infusions consisted of relatively large or pharmacological doses of ANF. These were administered either as a bolus, or as a steady-state infusion at one or more doses.

In normal subjects, ANF administration has diverse effects (Cody *et al.*, 1986, 1987b). The haemodynamic response to administration consists of vasodilatation, reduction of blood pressure, and variable effects on heart rate and cardiac output. In some normal subjects, heart rate is unchanged, and cardiac output tends to increase in response to vasodilatation. In other subjects, there is a marked reduction of heart rate and significant drop in blood pressure. This latter response is not necessarily dose-dependent, may not be associated with a particular characteristic haemodynamic prodrome and has many of the characteristics of a vagal response, including changes in skin colour, sweating, and nausea. The response is not immediately reversible with discontinuation of peptide infusion, and gradually resolves with or without intravenous volume expansion. Cardiac output changes range from a slight decrease, to a slight increase.

The renal effects of ANF administration are perhaps the most striking. In normal subjects, there is a prompt and marked increase in sodium and water excretion. There is a tendency for GFR to increase and renal blood flow to decrease, so that there is a net significant increase of filtration fraction. While this may represent a direct glomerular effect as well as a vascular mediated effect there is also evidence that this may be influenced by changes in tubular sodium reabsorption.

The net diuresis consists of an increase of both free water and osmolar clearance. The hormonal response to ANF infusion includes a reduction of plasma renin activity, and aldosterone, with no major effect on cortisone. As previously mentioned, the reduction of plasma renin activity may reflect the primary change in renin secretory rate, but its greatest effect is most likely due to enhanced delivery of sodium to the distal nephron, thereby suppressing the macula densa signal for renin release.

An additional effect of ANF is its potent haemoconcentrating effect. During administration, there is a significant and prompt increase in haematocrit that far exceeds the losses that can be attributed to sodium and water excretion. Furthermore, this response is reversible following discontinuation of peptide administration. The haemoconcentration appears to be related to an increase of vascular hydraulic permeability.

For the most part, these effects appear blunted in the congestive heart failure patient. The renal response to the peptide is markedly diminished, perhaps related to the abnormal baseline conditions of renal function in this clinical population. There is virtually no increase of sodium and water secretion when the peptide is administered. Likewise, renin secretion is unchanged, and does not demonstrate the suppression that one sees in normal subjects. Furthermore, haemoconcentration does not occur.

A vasodilatory effect can be demonstrated in both systemic infusions, and isolated perfusion of the forearm vascular bed. Under the latter conditions, where compensatory and reflex changes can be excluded, the magnitude of vasodilatation was less than that of normal subjects. However, when corrected for the maximal vasodilatory capacity (in response to ischaemic flow), the proportionate increase of vasodilator response was similar to normal subjects. These findings, together with the findings of the renal response to ANF are consistent with the fact that ANF exerts a counter-regulatory influence on the vasoconstrictory influence of the renin–angiotensin system. To more accurately identify the physiological response to ANF infusion, it is necessary to administer the peptide at a low rate in order to maintain a circulating concentration of ANF that is consistent with ambient resting values of ANF. In such studies, MacGregor and coworkers have stressed that ANF produces a small but significant natriuresis (MacGregor & Sagnella, 1987). A similar observation has been made in a group of four congestive heart failure patients (Burnett, Edwards & Zimmerman, 1986). These patients had clinically evident heart failure, although to a lesser degree than heart failure patients in other reports. Infusion of peptide at a rate of 8 mg/kg/min produced a significant increase of sodium excretion during the infusion. The clinical experience of ANF infusion in heart failure is notable for a lack of a large clinical trial, controlling for severity of heart failure, concomitant medications and volume status, and the conditions surrounding ANF infusion.

Thus, parenteral administration of ANF to normal subjects and congestive heart failure patients has helped to identify the physiological activity of ANF in man, complementing studies of endogenous ANF secretion. While there is potential applicability for a therapeutic role of ANF as a diuretic and a vasodilator, widespread use of the peptide is unlikely. In terms of natriuresis and diuresis, the magnitude of the effect of ANF does not approach that of loop diuretics. Likewise, its vasodilatory potential does not appear to be comparable to that of currently existing vasodilators, and the sometimes sudden and uncontrolled reduction of blood pressure which it produces is not appealing.

Of interest are preliminary observations with the administration of an orally active endopeptidase inhibitor (Jardine *et al.*, 1989; Northridge *et al.*, 1989). This compound appears to inhibit, in a fairly specific manner, the endopeptidase that normally degrades ANF to inactive metabolites. The endopeptidase inhibitor produces a significant increase in the circulatory level of ANF. Thus, this orally active compound permits an increase of endogenous ANF on a chronic basis. Although exciting, the long-term persistence and clinical significance of this response is not certain and requires considerably more research. However, one can imagine that this increase of ANF, particularly in combination with other therapeutic interventions, may provide clinical benefit to at least some heart failure patients within somewhat specific clinical conditions. While some investigators have argued that such a favourable effect can be readily mimicked by an oral diuretic, there may be specific advantages to an endogenously produced hormone. It is important to carefully delineate

Table 8.1 Clinical conditions in congestive heart failure that are favourably affected by endogenous ANF secretion.

1. **Acute pulmonary oedema**
    —diuresis
    —vasodilatation
    —fluid sequestration
2. Maintenance of chronic net sodium excretion
3. Prevention of the transition from asymptomatic
    to symptomatic left ventricular dysfunction

the pharmacological effects of ANF from the likely beneficial effect of endogenous secretion of ANF in congestive heart failure under stimulated conditions. That is, ANF is already secreted to a circulating level that can exceed a five- or 10-fold increase compared to normal subjects, and further increases in ANF with either low-dose or high-dose infusions could be questioned.

There are, however, several conditions with high endogenous ANF secretion that could exert beneficial clinical effects (Table 8.1). First, a rapid marked increase of ANF may occur during acute and rapid atrial distension, such as clinical conditions associated with pulmonary oedema. Under these conditions, the physiological effects of ANF may contribute to natriuresis, vasodilatation, and fluid sequestration. Secondly, in chronic congestive heart failure, ANF probably accounts for a small but important fraction of total daily sodium excretion. If this portion of sodium excretion is as little as 5–10%, it is none the less important.

Sodium retention in heart failure is a chronic cumulative phenomenon, and 'the absence of effective ANF activity could contribute to fluid retention roughly equivalent to 2 l of isotonic saline in the course of a month. The blunting of effective ANF activity could help explain the cyclic nature of fluid retention in those subjects whose renal response to ANF is impaired, producing the oedematous clinical characteristics of heart failure. This loss of ANF effectiveness may explain the transition from asymptomatic left ventricular dysfunction, to symptomatic failure. Thirdly, it is likely that ANF constantly exerts a counterbalancing effect against both ANGII and aldosterone that is operative in all stages of heart failure.

Summary

ANF is a hormone, secreted by cardiac myocytes, with several target sites of action, confirming the fact that the heart is an endocrine organ. In congestive heart failure, ANF secretion and circulating peptide levels are increased, but can predictably respond under most conditions to perturbations of atrial tension. Exogenous administration of ANF as a pharmacological intervention reveals blunted responsiveness, compared to normal subjects, and the short-term nature of such infusions does not provide sufficient inferential data for long-term clinical efficacy. In this regard, inhibition of endogenous ANF degradation by oral administration of endopeptidase inhibitors offers some promise; however, broader clinical and experimental experience with these agents is required.

References

Atlas, S. A. (1986). Atrial natriuretic factor: a new hormone of cardiac origin. *Rec. Prog. Hormone Res.* **42**: 207–49.

Atlas, S. A., Cody, R. J., Camargo, M. J. F., Pecker, M. S., Volpe, M. & Laragh, J. H. (1989). Atrial natriuretic factor and its role in circulatory physiology. In: *Recent Advances in Endocrinology and Metabolism*, Vol. 3 (Edwards, C. R. W. & Lincoln, D. W., eds)., pp. 281–313.

Atlas, S. A., Kleinert, H. D., Camargo, M. J., Januszewicz, A., Sealey, J. E., Laragh, J. H., Schilling, J. W. *et al.* (1984). Purification, sequencing and synthesis of natriuretic and vasoactive rat atrial peptide. *Nature* **309**: 717–19.

Atlas, S. A., Kleinert, H. D., Camargo, M. J., Volpe, M., Laragh, J. H., Lewicki, J. A. & Maack, T. (1985). Atrial natriuretic factor (auriculin): structure and biological effects. *J. Clin. Hypertension* **1**(2): 187–98.

Atlas, S. A. & Laragh, J. H. (1986). Atrial natriuretic peptide: a new factor in hormonal control of blood pressure and electrolyte homeostasis. *Annu. Rev. Med.* **37**: 397–414 (review).

Atlas, S. A. & Maack, T. (1987). Effects of atrial natriuretic factor on the kidney and the renin–angiotensin–aldosterone system. *Endocrinol. Metab. Clin. N. Am.* **16**: 107–43.

Atlas, S. A., Volpe, M., Sosa, R. E., Laragh, J. H., Camargo, M. J. & Maack, T. (1986). Effects of atrial natriuretic factor on blood pressure and the renin–angiotensin–aldosterone system. *Fed. Proc.* **45**: 2115–21 (review).

Ballermann, B. J. & Brenner, B. M. (1986). George E. Brown Memorial lecture. Role of atrial peptides in body fluid homeostasis. *Circulation Res.* **58**: 619–30.

Biollaz, J., Nussberger, J., Porchet, M. & Brunner-Ferber, F. (1986). Four-hour infusions of synthetic atrial natriuretic peptide in normal volunteers. *Hypertension* **8**: II96–105.

Blaine, E. H., Heinel, L. A., Schorn, T. W., Marsh, E. A. & Whinnery, M. A. (1986). The character of the atrial natriuretic response: pressure and volume effects. *J. Hypertension* (Suppl.) **4**: S17–24.

Bolli, P., Muller, F. B., Linder, L. *et al.* (1987). The vasodilator potency of atrial natriuretic peptide in man. *Circulation* **75**: 221–8.

Bourgoignie, J., Klarh, S. & Bricker, N. S. (1971). Inhibition of transepithelial sodium transport in the frog skin by a low molecular weight fraction of uremic serum. *J. Clin. Invest.* **50**: 303–11.

Buckalew, V. M. & Nelson, D. B. (1974). Natriuretic and sodium transport inhibitory activity in plasma of volume-expanded dogs. *Kidney Int.* **5**: 12–22.

Burnett, J. C. Jr., Edwards, B. S. & Zimmerman, R. S. (1986a). Renal–cardiovascular–endocrine response to atrial natriuretic factor in humans with congestive heart failure. *Clin. Res.* **34**: 970A (abstract).

Burnett, J. C. Jr., Opgenorth, T. J. & Granger, J. P. (1986b). The renal action of atrial natriuretic peptide during control of glomerular filtration. *Kidney Int.* **30**: 16–19.

Bussien, J. P., Biollaz, J., Waeber, B., Nussberger, J., Turini, G. A., Brunner, H. R., Brunner-Ferber, F. *et al.* (1986). Dose-dependent effect of atrial natriuretic peptide on blood pressure, heart rate, and skin blood flow of normal volunteers. *J. Cardiovasc. Pharmacol.* **8**: 216–20.

Cantin, M. & Genest, J. (1985). The heart and the atrial natriuretic factor. *Endocrine Rev.* **6**: 107–27 (review).

Cantin, M. & Genest, J. (1986). The heart as an endocrine gland. *Sci. Am.* **254**: 76–81.

Cody, R. J. (1988). Sodium and water retention in congestive heart failure: the pivotal role of the kidney. *Am. J. Hypertension* **1**: 395S–401S.

Cody, R. J., Atlas, S. A. & Laragh, J. H. (1987a). Physiological and pharmacological studies of atrial natriuretic factor, a natriuretic and vasoactive peptide. *J. Clin. Pharmacol.* **27**: 927–36.

Cody, R. J., Atlas, S. A. & Laragh, J. H. (1988a). Renal responses to atrial natriuretic factor in patients with congestive heart failure. *Eur. Heart J.* (Suppl. H) **9**: 29–33.

Cody, R. J., Atlas, S. A. & Laragh, J. H. (1988b). ANF as a regulator of sodium and water in congestive heart failure. In: *Advances in Atrial Peptide Research* (Brenner, B. M. & Laragh, J. H., eds). New York: Raven Press, pp. 133–40.

Cody, R. J., Atlas, S. A., Laragh, J. H., Kubo, S. H., Covit, A. B., Ryman, K. S., Shaknovich, A. *et al.* (1986). Atrial natriuretic factor in normal subjects and heart failure patients: plasma levels and renal, hormonal, and hemodynamic responses to peptide infusion. *J. Clin. Invest.* **78**: 1362–74.

Cody, R. J., Atlas, S. A., Kubo, S. H., Shaknovich, A. & Laragh, J. H. (1987b). Identification of enhanced secretion of atrial natriuretic factor during exercise in chronic congestive heart failure. *Circulation* **76** (Suppl. IV): IV-135.

Cody, R. J., Ljungman, S., Covit, A. B., Kubo, S. H., Sealey, J. E., Pondolfino, K., Clark, M. *et al.* (1988c). Regulation of glomerular filtration rate in chronic congestive heart failure patients. *Kidney Int.* **34**: 361–7.

Cody, R. J., Torre, S., Clark, M. & Pondolfino, K. (1989). Age-related hemodynamic, renal, and hormonal differences in patients with congestive heart failure. *Arch. Int. Med.* **149**: 1023–8.

Cogan, M. G. (1986). Atrial natriuretic factor can increase renal solute excretion primarily by raising glomerular filtration. *Am. J. Physiol.* **250**: F710–14.

Cole, B. R., Kuhnline, M. A. & Needleman, P. (1985). Atriopeptin III. A potent natriuretic, diuretic, and hypotensive agent in rats with chronic renal failure. *J. Clin. Invest.* **76**: 2413–5.

Crozier, I. G., Nicholls, M. G., Ikram, H., Espiner, E. A., Yandle, T. G. & Jans, S. (1986). Atrial natriuretic peptide in humans. Production and clearance by various tissues. *Hypertension* **8**: III1–15.

Currie, M. G. *et al.* (1984). Purification and sequence analysis of bioactive atrial peptides (atriopeptins). *Science* **223**: 67–9.

Day, M. L., Schwartz, D., Weigand, R. C., Stockman, P. T., Brunnert, S. R., Tolunay, H. E., Currie, M. G. *et al.* (1987). Ventricular atriopeptin. Unmasking of messenger RNA and peptide synthesis by hypertrophy or dexamethasone. *Hypertension* **9**: 485–91.

deBold, A. J. (1979). Heart atria granularity effects of changes in water-electrolyte balance. *Proc. Soc. Exp. Biol. Med.* **161**: 508–11.

deBold, A. J. (1985). Atrial natriuretic factor: a hormone produced by the heart. *Science* **230**: 767–70.

deBold, A. J., Borenstein, H. B., Yeress, A. T. & Sonnenberg, H. (1981). A rapid and potent natriuretic response to intravenous injection of atrial myocardial extract in rats. *Life Sci.* **28**: 89–94.

deWardener, H. E. (1977). Natriuretic hormone. *Clin. Sci. Molec. Med.* **53**: 1–8.

deWardener, H. E., Mills, I. H. & Clapham, W. F. (1961). Studies on the efferent mechanisms of the sodium diuresis which follows the administration of intravenous saline in the dog. *Clin. Sci.* **21**: 249–58.

Dzau, V. J., Baxter, J. A., Cantin, M., de Bold, A., Ganten, D., Gross, K., Husain, A. *et al.* (1987). Report of the Joint Nomenclature and Standardization Committee of the International Society of Hypertension, American Heart Association and the World Health Organization. *J. Hypertension* **5**: 507–11.

Edwards, B. S., Ackermann, D. M., Lee, M. E., Reeder, G. S., Wold, L. E. & Burnett, J. C. Jr. (1988). Identification of atrial natriuretic factor within ventricular tissue in hamsters and humans with congestive heart failure. *J. Clin. Invest.* **81**: 82–6.

Epstein, M. (1978). Renal effects of head out water immersion in man: implications for an understanding of volume homeostasis. *Physiol. Rev.* **58**: 529–81.

Epstein, M., Loutzenhiser, R. D., Friedland, E., Aceto, R. M., Camargo, M. J. & Atlas, S. A. (1986). Increases in circulating atrial natriuretic factor during immersion-induced central hypervolaemia in normal humans. *J. Hypertension* (Suppl.) **4**: S93–9.

Epstein, M., Loutzenhiser, R., Friedland, E., Aceto, R. N., Camargo, M. J. & Atlas, S. A. (1987). Relationship of increased plasma atrial natriuretic factor and renal sodium handling during immmersion-induced central hypervolemia in normal humans. *J. Clin. Invest.* **79**: 738–45.

Espiner, E. A., Nicholls, M. G., Yandle, T. G., Crozier, I. G., Cuneo, R. C., McCormick, D., Ikram, K. (1986). Studies on the secretion, metabolism and action of atrial natriuretic peptide in man. *J. Hypertens.* **4** (Suppl 1): 85–91.

Flynn, T. G., deBold, M. L. & deBold, A. J. (1983). The amino acid sequence of an atrial peptide with potent diuretic and natriuretic properties. *Biochem. Biophys. Res. Commun.* **117**: 859–65.

Frohlich, E. D. (1988). The heart in hypertension: unresolved conceptual challenges. Special lecture. *Hypertension* **11**: I19–24 (review).

Gaillard, C. A., Koomans, H. A. & Mees, E. J. (1988). Enalapril attenuates natriuresis of atrial natriuretic factor in humans. *Hypertension* **11**: 160–5.

Gaillard, C. A., Koomans, H. A., Rabelink, A. J. & Mees, E. J. (1987). Effects of indomethacin on renal response to atrial natriuretic peptide. *Am. J. Physiol.* **253**: F868–73.

Ganau, A., Devereux, R. B., Atlas, S. A., Pecker, M., Roman, M. J., Vargiu, P., Cody, R. J. *et al.* (1989). Plasma atrial natriuretic factor in essential hypertension: relationship to cardiac size, function and systemic hemodynamics. *J. Am. Coll. Cardiol.* **14**: 715–24.

Gauquelin, G., Garcia, R., Carrier, F., Cantin, M., Gutkowska, J., Thibault, G. & Schiffrin, E. L. (1988). Glomerular ANF receptor regulation during changes in sodium and water metabolism. *Am. J. Physiol.* **254**: F51–5.

Genest J. & Cantin, M. (1987). Atrial natriuretic factor. *Circulation* **75**: I118–24 (review).

Genest, J., Larochelle, P., Cusson, J. R., Gutowska, J. & Cantin, M. (1988). The atrial natriuretic factor in hypertension. State of the art lecture. *Hypertension* **11**: I3–7 (review).

Goodfriend, T. L., Elliott, T. L. & Atlas, S. A. (1984). Action of synthetic atrial natriuretic factor on bovine adrenal golerulosa. *Life Sci.* **35**: 1675–82.

Granger, J. P., Opgenorth, T. J., Salazar, J., Romero, J. C. & Burnett, J. C. Jr. (1986). Long-term hypotensive and renal effects of atrial natriuretic peptide. *Hypertension* **8**: II112–16.

Haller, B. G., Zust, H., Shaw, S., Gnadinger, M. P., Uehlinger, D. E. & Weidmann, P. (1987). Effects of posture and ageing on circulating atrial natriuretic peptide levels in man. *J. Hypertension* **5**: 551–6.

Hamet, P., Tremblay, J., Pang, S. C., Skuherska, R., Schiffrin, E. L., Garcia, R., Cantin, M. *et al.* (1986). Cyclic GMP as mediator and biological marker of atrial natriuretic factor. *J. Hypertension* (Suppl.) **4**: S49–56.

Henry, J. P. & Pearce, J. W. (1956). The possible role of cardiac atrial stretch receptors in the induction of changes in urine flow. *J. Physiol.* **131**: 572–85.

Hirata, Y., Tomita, M., Yoshimi, H. & Ikeda, M. (1984). Specific receptors for atrial natriuretic factor (ANF) in cultured vascular smooth muscle cells of rat aorta. *Biochem. Biophys. Res. Commun.* **125**: 562–8.

Hodsman, G. P., Phillips, P. A., Ogawa, K. Z. & Johnston, C. I. (1986). Atrial natriuretic factor in normal man: effects of tilt, posture, exercise and haemorrhage. *J. Hypertension* (Suppl.) **4**: S503–5.

Hollister, A. S., Tanaka, I., Imada, T., Onrot, J., Biaggioni, I., Robertson, D. & Inagami, T. (1986). Sodium loading and posture modulate human atrial natriuretic factor plasma levels. *Hypertension* **8**: II106–11.

Inagami, T., Misono, K. S., Fukumi, H., Maki, M., Tanaka, I., Takayanagi, R., Imada, T. *et al.* (1987). Structure and physiological actions of rat atrial natriuretic factor. *Hypertension* **10**: I113–17 (review).

Inagami, T., Misono, K. S., Maki, M., Fukumi, H., Takyanagi, R., Grammer, R. T., Tibbetts, C. *et al.* (1984). Atrial natriuretic factor; purification of active peptides, cloning of cDNA and determination of structures of active peptides and precursors. *J. Hypertension* (Suppl.) Andersson *et al.* (1986) S317–19.

Ishii, M., Sugimoto, T., Matsuoka, H., Hirata, Y., Ishimitsu, T., Fukui, K., Sugimoto, T. *et al.* (1986). A comparative study on the hemodynamic, renal and endocrine effects of alpha-human atrial natriuretic polypeptide in normotensive persons and patients with essential hypertension. *Jap. Circulation J.* **50**: 1181–4.

Jamieson, J. D. (1964). Specific granules in atrial muscle cells. *J. Cell Biol.* **23**: 151–72.

Janssen, W. M., de Jong, P. E., van der Hem, G. K. & de Zeeuw, D. (1986). Effect of human atrial natriuretic peptide on blood pressure after sodium depletion in essential hypertension. *Br. Med. J.* **293**: 351–3.

Jardine, A., Connel, J. M. C., Dilly, S. G., Northridge, D. B., Leckie, B., Cussano, N. J. & Lever, A. F. (1989). Pharmacologic elevation of endogenous atrial natriuretic factor in man using the atriopeptidase inhibitor (UK69578). *J. Am. Coll. Cardiol.* **13**: 76A (abstract).

Kangawa, K., Fukuda, A., Kubota, I., Hayashi, Y., Minamitake, Y. & Matsuo, H. (1984). Human atrial natriuretic polypeptides (hANP): purification, structure synthesis and biological activity. *J. Hypertension* (Suppl.) **2** (Suppl 3): 321–3.

Kangawa, K. & Matsuo, H. (1984). Purification and complete amino acid sequence of alpha-human atrial natriuretic polypeptide (alpha-hANP). *Biochem. Biophys. Res. Commun.* **118**: 131–9.

Kato, J., Kida, O., Nakamura, S., Sasaki, A., Kodama, K. & Tanaka, K. (1987). Atrial natriuretic polypeptide (ANP) in the development of spontaneously hypertensive rats (SHR) and stroke-prone SHR (SHRSP). *Biochem. Biophys. Res. Commun.* **143**: 316–22.

Khraibi, A. A., Granger, J. P., Burnett, J. C. Jr., Walker, K. R. & Knox, F. G. (1987). Role of atrial natriuretic factor in the natriuresis of acute volume expansion. *Am. J. Physiol.* **252**: R921–4.

Kisch, B. (1956). Electron microscopy of atrium of the heart: I. Guinea pig. *Exp. Med. Sur.* **114**: 99–112.

Kohno, M., Yasunari, K., Matsuura, T., Murakawa, K. & Takeda, T. (1987). Circulating atrial natriuretic polypeptide in essential hypertension. *Am. Heart J.* **113**: 1160–3.

Kohno, M., Yasunari, K., Takaori, K. & Takeda, T. (1986). Increased plasma atrial natriuretic polypeptide in patients with severe essential hypertension and its decline with antihypertensive therapy with nifedipine (letter). *Arch. Intern. Med.* **1**: 1226–7.

Kramer, H. J. & Lichardus, B. (1986). Atrial natriuretic hormones—thirty years after the discovery of atrial volume receptors. *Klin. Wochenschr.* **64**: 719–31.

Kudo, T. & Baird, A. (1984). Inhibition of aldosterone production in the adrenal glomerulosa by atrial natriuretic factor. *Nature* **312**: 756–7.

Kurihara, M., Castren, E., Gutkind, J. S. & Saavedra, J. M. (1987). Lower number of atrial natriuretic peptide receptors in thymocytes and spleen cells of spontaneously hypertensive rats. *Biochem. Biophys. Res. Commun.* **149**: 1132–40.

Lang, R. E., Unger, T. & Ganten, D. (1987). Atrial natriuretic peptide: a new factor in blood pressure control. *J. Hypertension* **5**: 255–71 (review).

Lappe, R. W., Todt, J. A. & Wendt, R. L. (1986). Hemodynamic effects of infusion versus bolus administration of atrial natriuretic factor. *Hypertension* **8**: 866–73.

Laragh, J. H., Cody, R. J., Covit, A. B. & Atlas, S. A. (1986). The renin system and atrial natriuretic hormone in congestive heart failure. *Acta Med. Scand.* (Suppl.) **707**: 45–53.

Ledsome, J. R. & Linden, R. J. (1968). The role of left atrial receptors in the diuretic response to left atrial distension. *J. Physiol.* **198**: 487–503.

Leitman, D. C. & Murad, F. (1987). Atrial natriuretic factor receptor heterogeneity and stimulation of particulate guanylate cyclase and cyclic GMP accumulation. *Endocrinol. Metab. Clin. N. Am.* **16**: 79–105 (review).

Linden, R. J. (1979). Atrial reflexes and renal function. *Am. J. Cardiol.* **44**: 879–83.

Lindop, G. B., Mallon, E. A., Hair, J., Downie, T. T. & MacIntyre, G. (1987). ANF (99–126) and its propetide, ANF (1–16) are secreted simultaneously from the human atrial myocyte. *J. Hypertension* **5**: 533–6.

McKenzie, J. C., Tanaka, I., Misono, K. S. & Inagami, T. (1985). Immunocytochemical localization of atrial natriuretic factor in the kidney, adrenal medulla, pituitary, and atrium of rat. *J. Histochem. Cytochem.* **33**: 828–32.

MacGregor, G. A. & Sagnella, G. A. (1987). Are the atrial peptides a natriuretic hormone? *Eur. Heart J.* (Suppl. B): 111–16 (review).

Maack, T., Atlas, S. A., Camargo, M. D. & Cogan, M. D. (1986). Renal hemodynamic and natriuretic effects of atrial natriuretic factor. *Fed. Proc.* **45**: 2128–32.

Maack, T., Suzuki, M., Almeida, F. A., Nussenzveig, D., Scarborough, R. M., McEnroe, G. A. & Lewicki, J. A. (1987). Physiological role of silent receptors of atrial natriuretic factor. *Science* **238**: 675–8.

Mantero, F., Rocco, S., Pertile, F., Carpene, G., Fallo, F. & Menegus, A. (1987b). Alpha-h-ANP injection in normals, low renin hypertension and primary aldosteronism. *J. Ster. Biochem.* **27**: 935–40.

Mantero, F., Rocco, S., Pertile, F., Carpene, G., Fallo, F., Leone, L. & Boscaro, M. (1987a). Effect of alpha-human atrial natriuretic peptide in low renin essential hypertension and primary aldosteronism. *Clin. Exp. Hypertension: Part A. Theory Pract.* **9**: 1505–13.

Marie, J. P., Guillemot, H. & Hatt, P. Y. (1976). Le degré de granulation des cardicytes auriculaires: etude planimé trique au cours de différents apports d'eau et du sodium chez le rat. *Pathol. Biol.* **24**: 549–54.

Mark, A. L. (1987). Sensitization of cardiac vagal afferent reflexes at the sensory receptor level: an overview. *Fed. Proc.* 36–40 (review).

Matsubara, H., Umeda, Y., Yamane, Y., Nishikawa, M., Taniguchi, T. & Inada, M. (1987). Role of atrial natriuretic polypeptides for exaggerated natriuresis in essential hypertension. *Am. J. Cardiol.* **60**: 708–14.

Matsuo, H. & Kangawa, K. (1984). Human and rat atrial natriuretic polypeptides (hANP & rANP) purification, structure and biological activity. *Clin. Exp. Hypertension: Part A. Theory Pract.* **6**: 1717–2.

Mendez, R. E., Dunn, B. R., Troy, J. L. & Brenner, B. M. (1986). Modulation of the natriuretic response to atrial natriuretic peptide by alterations in peritubular Starling forces in the rat. *Circulation Res.* **59**: 605–11.

Misono, K. S., Grammer, R. T., Fukumi, H. & Inagami, T. (1984). Rat atrial natriuretic factor: isolation, structure and biological activities of four major peptides. *Biochem. Biophys. Res. Commun.* **123**: 444–51.

Morris, M., Cain, M. & Chalmers, J. (1987). Complementary changes in plasma atrial natriuretic peptide and antidiuretic hormone concentrations in response to volume expansion and haemorrhage: studies in conscious normotensive and spontaneously hypertensive rats. *Clin. Exp. Pharmacol. Physiol.* **14**: 283–9.

Morton, J. J., Lyall, F. & Wallace, E. C. (1987). Rat atrial natriuretic peptide vascular receptor: effect of alterations in sodium balance and of DOC hypertension. *J. Hypertension* **5**: 475–9.

Mulvany, M. J. (1987). Enhanced dilatation by atrial natriuretic peptide of renal arcuate arteries from young, but not adult, spontaneously hypertensive rats. *Clin. Exp. Hypertension: Part A. Theory Pract.* **9**: 1789–1801.

Murray, R. D., Itoh, S., Inagami, T., Misono, K., Seto, S., Scicli, A. G. & Carretero, O. A. (1985). Effects of synthetic atrial natriuretic factor in the isolated perfused rat kidney. *Am. J. Physiol.* **249**: F603–9.

Nakagawa, M., Shimamoto, K., Yamaguchi, Y., Masuda, A., Saito, S., Ando, T., Watarai, I. *et al.* (1987). The radioimmunoassay for human plasma atrial natriuretic peptide—its application to uremic patients. *Jap. J. Med.* **26**: 46–9.

Needleman, P., Adams, S. P., Cole, B. R., Currie, M. G., Geller, D. M., Michener, M. L., Saper, C. B. *et al.* (1985). Atriopeptins as cardiac hormones. *Hypertension* **7**: 469–82 (review).

Nicholls, M. G., Ikram, H., Crozier, I. G., Espiner, E. A. & Yandle, T. G. (1987). Atrial natriuretic peptides in man. *Can. J. Physiol. Pharmacol.* **65**: 1697–1700 (review).

Northridge, D. B., Findlay, I. N., Jardine, A., Dilly, S. G. & Dargie, H. J. (1989). Acute effects of atriopeptidase inhibition on plasma atrial natriuretic factor in chronic heart failure. *J. Am. Coll. Cardiol.* **13**: 76A (abstract).

Osol, G., Halpern, W., Tesfamariam, B., Nakayama, K. & Weinberg, D. (1986). Synthetic atrial natriuretic factor does not dilate resistance-sized arteries. *Hypertension* **8**: 606–10.

Otsuka, Y., DiPiero, A., Hirt, E., Brennaman, B. & Lockette, W. (1988). Vascular relaxation and cGMP in hypertension. *Am. J. Physiol.* **254**: H163–9.

Rankin, A. J. (1987). Mechanisms for the release of atrial natriuretic peptide. *Can. J. Physiol. Pharmacol.* **65**: 1673–9 (review).

Rappelli, A., Dessi-Fulgheri, P., Madeddu, P. & Glorioso, N. (1987). Studies on the natriuretic effect of nifedipine in hypertensive patients: increase in levels of plasma atrial natriuretic factor without participation of the renal kallikrein-kinin system. *J. Hypertension* (Suppl.) **5**: S61–5.

Richards, A. M., Tonolo, G., Cleland, J. G., Leckie, B. J., McIntyre, G. D., Ingram, M., Dargie, H. J. *et al.* (1986). Plasma atrial natriuretic peptide: responses to modest and severe sodium restriction. *J. Hypertension* (Suppl.) **4**: S559–63.

Richards, A. M., Tonola, G., McIntyre, G. D., Leckie, B. J. & Robertson, J. I. (1987). Radio-immunoassay for plasma alpha human atrial natriuretic peptide: a comparison of direct and pre-extracted methods. *J. Hypertension* **5**: 227–36.

Schwartz, D., Katsube, N. C. & Needleman, P. (1986). Atriopeptins in fluid and electrolyte homeostasis. *Fed. Proc.* **75**: 2361–5 (review).

Sealey, J. E., Kirschman, J. D. & Laragh, J. H. (1969). Natriuretic activity in plasma and urine of salt-loaded man and sheep. *J. Clin. Invest.* **48**: 2210.

Seidman, C. E., Bloch, K. D., Zisfein, J., Smith, J. A., Haber, E., Homcy, C., Duby, A. D. *et al.* (1985). Molecular studies of the atrial natriuretic factor gene. *Hypertension* **7**: 131–4.

Seino, M., Abe, K., Nushiro, N. & Yoshinaga, K. (1988). Nifedipine enhances the vasodepressor and natriuretic effects of atrial natriuretic peptide. *Hypertension* **11**: 34–40.

Showalter, C. J., Zimmerman, R. S., Schwab, T. R., Edwards, B. S., Opgenorth, T. J. & Burnett, J. C. Jr. (1988). Renal response to atrial natriuretic factor is modulated by intrarenal angiotension II. *Am. J. Physiol.* **254**: R453–6.

Smith, S., Anderson, S., Ballermann, B. J. & Brenner, B. M. (1986). Role of atrial natriuretic peptide in adapatation of sodium excretion with reduced renal mass. *J. Clin. Invest.* **77**: 1395–8.

Snajdar, R. M., Dene, H. & Rapp, J. P. (1986). Atrial natriuretic factor in inbred Dahl salt-sensitive and salt-resistant rats. *J. Hypertension* (Suppl.) **4**: S343–7.

Sonnenberg, H. (1987). The physiology of atrial natriuretic factor. *Can. J. Physiol. Pharmacol.* **65**: 2021–3 (review).

Sonneberg, H., Veress, A. T. & Pearce, J. W. (1972). A humoral component of the natriuretic mechanism in sustained blood volume expansion. *J. Clin. Invest.* **51**: 2631–44.

Stasch, J. P., Kazda, S., Hirth, C. & Morich, F. (1987). Role of nisoldipine on blood pressure, cardiac hypertrophy, and atrial natriuretic peptides in spontaneously hypertensive rats. *Hypertension* **10**: 303–7.

Steigerwalt, S., Carretero, O. A. & Beierwaltes, W. H. (1986). A stop-flow study of intrarenal effects of atrial natriuretic factor. *Proc. Soc. Exp. Biol. Med.* **182**: 88–94.

Stewart, R. E., Swithers, S. E. & McCarty, R. (1987). Alterations in binding sites for atrial natriuretic factor in kidneys and adrenal glands of Dahl hypertension-sensitive rats. *J. Hypertension* **5**: 481–7.

Suzuki, M., Almeida, F. A., Nussenzveig, D. R., Sawyer, D. & Maack, T. (1987). Binding and functional effects of atrial natriuretic factor in isolated rat kidney. *Am. J. Physiol.* **253**: F917–28.

Swithers, S. E., Stewart, R. E. & McCarty, R. (1987). Binding sites for atrial natriuretic factor (ANF) in kidneys and adrenal glands of spontaneously hypertensive (SHR) rats. *Life Sci.* 1673–81.

Trippodo, N. C. (1987). An update on the physiology of atrial natriuretic factor. *Hypertension* **10**: I122–7 (review).

Uchida, K., Azukizawa, S., Kamei, M., Yoshida, I., Kigoshi, T., Yamamoto, I., Hosojima, H. *et al.* (1987). Effect of atrial natriuretic factor on aldosterone and its precursor steroid production in adrenal zona glomerulosa cells from spontaneously hypertensive rat. *Clin. Exp. Hypertension: Part A. Theory Pract.* **9**: 2131–42.

Verburg, K. M., Freeman, R. H., Villarreal, D. & Brands, M. W. (1987). Atrial natriuretic factor in dogs with one-kidney, one-clip Goldblatt hypertension. *Am. J. Physiol.* **253**: H1623–7.

Volpe, M., De Luca, N., Atlas, S. A., Camargo, M. J., Indolfi, C., Lembo, G., Trimarco, B. *et al.* (1988). Reduction of atrial natriuretic factor circulating levels by endogenous sympathetic activation in hypertensive patients. *Circulation* **77**: 997–1002.

Volpe, M., Mele, A. F., Indolfi, C., De Luca, N., Lembo, G., Focaccio, A., Condorelli, M. *et al.* (1987). Hemodynamic and hormonal effects of atrial natriuretic factor in patients with essential hypertension. *J. Am. Coll. Cardiol.* **10**: 787–93.

Volpe, M., Mele, A. F., De Luca, N., Golino, P., Bondiolotti, G., Camargo, M. J., Atlas, S. A. *et al.* (1986a). Carotid baroreceptor unloading decreases plasma atrial natriuretic factor in hypertensive patients. *J. Hypertension (Suppl.)* **4**: S519–22.

Volpe, M., Odell, G., Kleinert, H. D., Camargot, M. J., Laragh, J. H., Lewicki, J. A., Maack, T. *et al.* (1984). Antihypertensive and aldosterone-lowering effects of synthetic atrial natriuretic factor in renin-dependent renovascular hypertension. *J. Hypertension* (Suppl.): Andersson *et al.* (1986). S313–15.

Volpe, M., Odell, G., Kleinert, H. D., Muller, F., Camargo, M. J., Laragh, J. H., Maack, T. *et al.* (1985). Effect of atrial natriuretic factor on blood pressure, renin, and aldosterone in Goldblatt hypertension. *Hypertension* **7**: I43–8.

Volpe, M., Sosa, R. E., Muller, F. B., Camargo, M. J., Glorioso, N., Laragh, J. H., Maack, T. *et al.* (1986b). Differing haemodynamic responses to atrial natriuretic factor in two models of hypertension. *Am. J. Physiol.* **250**: H871–8.

Waldman, S., Rapoport, R. M. & Murad, F. (1984). Atrial natriuretic factor selectively activates particulate guanylate cyclase elevates cyclic GMP in rat tissues. *J. Biol. Chem.* **259**: 14332–4.

Wambach, G., Gotz, S., Suckau, G., Bonner, G. & Kaufman, W. (1987). Plasma levels of atrial natriuretic peptide are raised in essential hypertension during low and high sodium intake. *Klin. Wochenschr.* **65**: 232–7.

Weder, A. B., Sekkarie, M. A., Takiyyuddin, M., Schork, N. J. & Julius, S. (1987). Antihypertensive and hypotensive effects of atrial natriuretic factor in men. *Hypertension* **10**: 582–9.

Winquist, R. J., Faison, E. P., Waldman, S. A., Schwartz, K., Murad, F. & Rapoport, R. M. (1984). Atrial natriuretic factor elicits an endothelium-independent relaxation and activates particulate guanylate cyclase in vascular smooth muscle. *Proc. Nat. Acad. Sci. USA* **81**: 7661–4.

Winquist, R. J., Napier, M. A., Vandlen, R. L., Arcuri, K., Keegan, M. E., Faison, E. P. & Baskin, E. P. (1985). Pharmacology and receptor binding of atrial natriuretic factor in vascular smooth muscle. *Clin. Exp. Hypertension: Part A. Theory Pract.* **7**: 869–86.

Wood, P. (1963). Polyuria in paroxysmal tachycardia and paroxysmal atrial flutter and fibrillation. *Br. Heart J.* **25**: 273–82.

Zeidel, M. D. & Brenner, B. M. (1987). Actions of atrial natriuretic peptides on the kidney. *Seminars Nephrol.* **7**: 91–7 (review).

Zeidel, M. D., Silva, P., Brenner, B. M. & Seifter, J. L. (1987). cGMP mediates effects of atrial peptides on medullary collecting duct cells. *Am. J. Physiol.* **252**: 551–9.

Chapter 9
Neutral endopeptidase and atrial natriuretic factor
John M. C. Connell and Alan Jardine

Introduction

Steady-state plasma levels of a hormone are determined by secretion and disposal rates. It is possible, therefore, to alter plasma hormone levels either by increasing secretion rate (or administration of exogenous hormone) or by changing the rate at which the hormone is degraded or excreted. The control of synthesis and release of atrial natriuretic factor (ANF) from cardiac atria have been studied intensively in the last few years (Ballerman & Brenner, 1985; Kenyon & Jardine, 1989) and are considered elsewhere in this monograph. Less is known about disposal of the hormone. This article will consider inactivation of ANF and how alteration of this might be used as a means of harnessing the hormone for therapeutic use.

Two principal mechanisms have been suggested to be of importance in the clearance of ANF. First, the hormone binds to a non-guanylate cyclase linked receptor (the so-called C-receptor), and there is some evidence that this acts as a means of regulating access of the hormone to the numerically less but biologically active B-(guanylate cyclase) receptors (Almeida et al., 1989; Waldman & Murad, 1989). Thus, when C-receptors are blocked by an analogue of ANF which does not bind to the B-receptor, the apparent volume of distribution of the hormone decreases and the effects of ANF at the guanylate cyclase (B) receptor are increased (Maack et al., 1987; Almeida et al., 1989). The fate of the hormone after binding to the C-receptor is not clear and whether this is truly a clearance mechanism for ANF remains uncertain. There are some data which

181

suggest that binding of ANF to C-receptors increases membrane phosphoinositide turnover (Ganguly *et al.*, 1989; Hirata, Chang & Murad, 1989) and it may be that activation of this receptor has some additional physiological function.

Secondly, the hormone is inactivated by enzymatic cleavage. Initial evidence showed that clearance of ANF occurred mainly across the renal circulation. For example, up to 80% of the hormone is cleared from plasma after a single passage through the kidney, while < 20% is cleared by the pulmonary circulation (Weselcouch, Humphrey & Aiken, 1985; Hollister *et al.*, 1989). Initial studies showed that ANF in the kidney is inactivated by enzymatic cleavage (Koehn *et al.*, 1987; Olins *et al.*, 1987). After filtration this inactivation is carried out by the zinc-containing enzyme neutral endopeptidase (EC 3.4.24.11) (Stephenson & Kenny, 1987b; Kenny & Stephenson, 1988) which is present in the brush border of the proximal tubule of the kidney. The relationship between this enzyme and the C-receptor, and their individual contributions to overall clearance of ANP remain obscure. The remainder of this chapter will be devoted to consideration of this enzyme and of its inhibitors, which can alter the clearance of endogenous and exogenous ANF.

Endopeptidase 24.11 (NEP)

NEP is a zinc-containing metalloendopeptidase which was first localized in the brush border of the proximal tubule of the kidney in 1974 (Booth & Kenny, 1974). Since then NEP has been described in a large number of sites and in a variety of species including pig, rat and man (for a review, see Erdos & Skidgel, 1989). Messenger RNA encoding the enzyme has now been cloned allowing the amino-acid sequence to be deduced (Devault *et al.*, 1987; Malfroy *et al.*, 1987, 1988). This shows the enzyme to be a membrane-spanning protein of molecular weight 62 000 Da. There is a very high degree of homology (> 90%) between the published nucleotide sequences (man, pig and rat) with only a few, minor substitutions, indicating marked evolutionary conservation. The predicted protein structure suggests that there is a short intracellular N-terminal domain and a hydrophobic membrane-spanning sequence; the majority of the protein is extracellular. Localized thus, NEP can inactivate extracellular peptide hormones, and so regulate endocrine, paracrine or autocrine actions of its substrates.

NEP shares a highly conserved nucleotide consensus sequence with other metalloendopeptidases which may represent a zinc-binding region close to the active site (Devault *et al.*, 1987). There are six possible glycosylation sites in the predicted protein sequence, although it is not known whether these are differentially glycosylated in the various tissue sites of the enzyme (Malfroy *et al.*, 1988). NEP is usually bound to tissue (including neutrophils), although a soluble form of NEP has been described in patients with adult respiratory distress syndrome (Erdos & Skidgel, 1989). The significance of this latter observation is uncertain. NEP is also present in urine, and is presumed to derive from renal NEP (Skidgel et al., 1987; Ura, Carretero & Erdos, 1987).

Distribution of NEP

NEP is a widely distributed enzyme. In the brain it is found in globus pallidus and substantia nigra and in centres responsible for pain perception, in a distribution similar to that seen for μ- and δ-opiate receptors (Malfroy et al., 1978; Llorens et al., 1982); studies with drugs which inhibit the activity of NEP suggest that this localization is of importance in regulating access of opiate peptides to these receptors (see below). In the kidney, NEP is found in the brush border of the proximal tubule (i.e. the luminal surface) (Booth & Kenny, 1974). The enzyme is also found in the glomerulus, but is present in much lower concentrations elsewhere in the kidney. NEP is also present in other brush border membranes, including the gut and the placenta (Johnson et al., 1985). In the male NEP is present in high concentrations in the seminiferous tubules (and in sperm) (Erdos et al., 1985). NEP is found in pulmonary tissue in alveoli and in association with airways (Johnson et al., 1985). There is little NEP on vascular endothelium but the enzyme is present in high concentrations in circulating neutrophils, where it may be involved in breakdown of chemotactic peptides. Current studies suggest that the protein structures of NEP in different tissue sites is identical. However, there are no data on possible differences in attachment of carbohydrate residues to the enzyme, and it is possible that NEP, like angiotensin-converting enzyme, shows a heterologous pattern of glycosylation in various tissues (Skidgel et al., 1987).

Substrates for NEP

Early studies demonstrated that enkephalins were naturally occurring substrates for NEP, and the localization of NEP to sites in the brain which were rich in opiate receptors suggested that the enzyme was involved in regulation of endogenous opioid analgesic effects (Malfroy et al., 1978; Llorens et al., 1982). Since that time a large number of other peptides have been shown to be substrates for NEP both in vitro and in vivo (Table 9.1) (Erdos & Skidgel, 1989). Most of these peptides have a molecular weight less than 3000 Da, although there is some evidence that NEP may also be involved in degradation of interleukin 1, which has a molecular weight of 17000 Da. The enzyme cleaves peptides at the amino side of hydrophobic bonds. For example, when ANF 99–126 is incubated with the enzyme there is a single cleavage site between cysteine-105 and phenylalanine-106, although it is of interest that when shorter fragments of the peptide (for

Table 9.1 Endogenous substrates for endopeptidase 24.11.

Atrial natriuretic factor
Insulin B chain
Enkephalins
Endorphins
Bradykinin
Substance P
Neurotensin
Oxytocin
LHRH
Angiotensin I and II
Gastrin
Cholecystokinin

example ANF 103–126) are used as substrate further cleavage sites are noted (Olins *et al.*, 1986). The reason for this is uncertain, although it is possible that the C-terminal fragment of ANF 99–126 protects the other cleavage sites. Other vasoactive hormones are also substrates *in vivo* for NEP. Within the kidney angiotensin I and angiotensin II (ANGII) and bradykinin are degraded by the enzyme (Stephenson & Kenny, 1987a). The importance of NEP in overall clearance of angiotensins remains to be determined. Evidence using specific inhibitors of NEP and angiotensin-converting enzyme (which also has kininase activity) suggests that NEP is responsible for more than 60% of kinin inactivation in rat kidney (Ura *et al.*, 1987). Substance P and neurotensin are also substrates for NEP, and this may be of importance in the central nervous system and in pulmonary tissue (Matsas *et al.*, 1983).

Interaction between NEP and ANF

Initial observations showed that ANF was cleared by the kidney, and that incubation of renal tissue with the peptide resulted in the generation of a ring-open form with a single cleavage site between cysteine-105 and phenylalanine-106 (Olins *et al.*, 1987; Stephenson & Kenny, 1987b). Subsequent studies have shown that incubation of ANF with NEP results in an identically cleaved peptide, consistent with the proposal that NEP is the renal enzyme responsible for the initial degradation and inactivation of the hormone. Some enzyme kinetic studies have suggested that the pH optimum for degradation of ANF in the kidney is higher than seen with NEP elsewhere, and it has been proposed that there may be a separate renal enzyme which breaks down ANF (Bertrand & Doble 1988). However, the majority of studies favour the proposal that NEP is the enzyme responsible for degradation of ANF in the kidney.

Within the kidney the concentration of NEP is highest in the luminal border of the proximal renal tubule. NEP is also present in the glomerulus (Shima *et al.*, 1988), and within the kidney most ANF cleavage activity is found within the glomerulus and the proximal tubule. These data suggest that ANF is cleaved after filtration and that the products of cleavage then are excreted in the urine. As most ANF in the circulation is cleared by the kidney, renal NEP is a major mechanism for inactivating the peptide after filtration. The exact mechanisms of the renal actions of ANF remain unresolved, although there is evidence to suggest that ANF acts mainly on the collecting ducts to alter sodium excretion (Leckie, 1987). If this is so, it is possible that inactivation of the peptide 'protects' these distal sites from exposure to filtered ANF, although this hypothesis implies that filtered ANF would have access to its receptors on the contraluminal side of the distal tubule. NEP in other sites may also be involved in the metabolism of ANF. In a study of a specific and potent inhibitor of NEP (UK 69,578) Samuels and colleagues (see below) showed that the half-life of exogenous ANF could be prolonged by administration of the drug to nephrectomized rats, and interpreted these data as showing that NEP in extrarenal sites accounted for a proportion of ANF degradation (Samuels *et al.*, 1989a).

Inhibitors of NEP

Thiorphan was the first drug shown to be a potent and specific inhibitor of NEP (Roques *et al.*, 1980). Early studies showed that administration of the drug to rats had significant antinociceptive action; this seems likely to be a consequence of inhibition of degradation of endogenous enkephalins. Since then, other inhibitors of NEP have been shown to have similar actions (Chipkin *et al.*, 1988). Thiorphan has only weak effects on sodium and water metabolism. Although the drug on its own does not alter sodium excretion, it potentiates the natriuresis caused by exogenous ANF, and this is likely to be a consequence of inhibition of breakdown of the hormone (Koepke *et al.*, 1989; Olins *et al.*, 1989). Another inhibitor of NEP, phosphoramidon, increases renal sodium and water excretion in rats, but does not affect potassium excretion or glomerular filtration rate (GFR) (Ura *et al.*, 1987). Studies of both thiorphan and phosphoramidon have shown that these drugs also inhibit the breakdown of bradykinin, and it was initially proposed that some of the renal effects of inhibition of NEP were due to increased delivery of kinins to the distal renal tubule. It now seems more likely, however, that inhibition of breakdown of ANF accounts for these actions.

A more recent study of an unrelated compound (SQ 29,072) also confirms that the natriuretic and vasorelaxant properties of exogenous ANF are enhanced in volume-expanded rats. In this experiment, cyclic guanyl monophosphate (cGMP) excretion was increased by the drug,

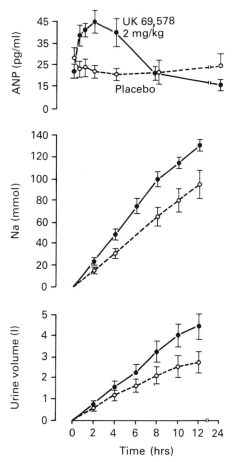

Fig. 9.1 Changes for plasma ANF, urinary sodium excretion and urine volume during administration of UK 69,578 (2 mg/kg intravenously between 0 and 20 min). Eight subjects were studied. Changes in ANF, urine sodium and urine volume were significant ($P < 0.01$) by analysis of variance. Points represent mean standard error of the mean.

consistent with the hypothesis that it acted by increasing availability of ANF to B-receptors (Seymour, Fennell & Swerdel, 1989).

In pulmonary tissue the two bronchoconstrictors, substance P and neurotensin, are both inactivated by NEP (Erdos & Skidgel, 1989). Inhibition of NEP with phosphoramidon or thiorphan causes increased bronchial reactivity, particularly in response to inhaled substance P (Djokic et al., 1989). The bronchoconstrictor response to substance P is increased in animals exposed to the chemical toluene dicyanate. This sensitization is reduced by treatment with phosphoramidon, and it has been suggested that some bronchoconstrictor agents act by altering NEP activity and so indirectly affecting bronchomotor response to endogenous bronchoconstrictors (Kohrogi et al., 1988; Shepperd et al., 1988). NEP inhibition with thiorphan increases the irritant effects of capsaicin on airways, suggesting that the effect of the irritant is mediated via endogenous bronchoconstrictor peptides normally inactivated by NEP (Kohrogi *et al.*, 1988). The net effect of inhibition of NEP on bronchial reactivity remains uncertain. ANF is a relatively potent bronchodilator in both isolated animal airways (Ishii & Murad, 1989) and in human asthmatic subjects (Hulks *et al.*, 1989), and if NEP inhibition increases ANF in pulmonary tissue, it may be that the overall effect of inhibition of NEP on airway tone is neutral.

NEP is present in the gastrointestinal tract, and inhibition of the enzyme with thiorphan increases gut transit time and reduces the laxative effect of irritant cathartics, probably by preventing the breakdown of local opiate peptides (Lecomte *et al.*, 1986). However, other inhibitors of NEP which also have analgesic properties do not affect gut transit time (Chipkin *et al.*, 1988), and there appears to be variability in the tissue actions of these drugs.

Studies with UK 69,578 in animals

A series of specific inhibitors of NEP have been developed by Pfizer Central Research (UK). Of these, UK 69,578 has been extensively tested in animals and, more recently, in human subjects. The drug was first identified in 1986, and initial testing showed it to inhibit the degradation of ANF *in vitro*, and to be natriuretic *in vivo* (Alabaster *et al.*, 1989; Samuels *et al.*, 1989a,b,c). It is a potent and specific inhibitor of EC 3.4.24.11 without significant effects on a range of other endopeptidases including angiotensin-converting enzyme, carboxytrypsin and trypsin. The drug prolongs the half-life of exogenous ANF in rats, and potentiates the natriuretic effect of the peptide. Given in the absence of exogenous ANF, UK 69,578 increases urinary sodium and water excretion, and this effect is abolished by administration of polyclonal antibody to ANF. In nephrectomized rats UK 69,578 also prolongs the half-life of ANF, indicating that inhibition of NEP affects ANF degradation at sites other than the kidney. The finding that the natriuretic and diuretic actions of UK 69,578 are abolished by specific antibodies to ANF suggests that most of the renal effects of this drug are mediated through alteration in ANF metabolism and not by inhibition of other NEP substrate (e.g. kinin) degradation.

Studies with UK 69,578 in man

UK 69,578 was first administered to normal male human subjects. This initial study was designed to test the safety of the drug, to give some indication of its efficacy and to provide information about approximate dose ranges (Jardine *et al.*, 1989; Northridge *et al.*, 1989). Sixteen subjects

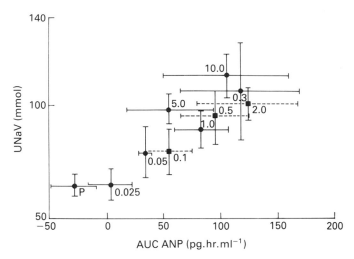

Fig. 9.2   Relationship between plasma ANF during administration of UK 69,578 (dose range 0–10 mg/kg intravenously) and urinary sodium excretion. ANF is expressed as area below the curve during the first 8 h after drug or placebo administration. P represents the placebo study day; points throughout represent mean standard error of the mean. Circular points $n = 41$; square points $n = 8$.

were studied: each received three intravenous doses of UK 69,578 and one of placebo on separate study days at least 1 week apart. Subjects were maintained on a normal sodium (150 mmol) and (70 mmol) potassium intake during each study period. Plasma ANF concentrations rose after administration of UK 69,578. Although the drug was given by intravenous infusion over a 20-min period, plasma levels of the peptide remained high for several hours (Fig. 9.1). Peak plasma levels of ANF after administration of UK 69,578 were not related to dose of the drug but the integrated ANF response (measured as the area below the curve) did show evidence of a dose–response relationship. The rise in plasma ANF was associated with a natriuresis and diuresis, so that at the highest dose of the drug studied (10 mg/kg) urinary sodium excretion increased nearly twofold, and integrated ANF response and urinary sodium excretion following administration of UK 69,578 were positively correlated (Fig. 9.2). Despite the large increase in urinary sodium loss, plasma renin concentration was suppressed during active drug administration when compared with placebo, and similar changes were seen for ANGII and aldosterone (Table 9.2).

Blood pressure and heart rate did not change during or after administration of UK 69,578 or placebo. Glomerular filtration rate was measured in this study by the clearance of inulin (using a constant infusion/steady-state technique) and renal plasma flow by that of para-amino hippuric acid. UK 69,578 did not cause any change in renal plasma flow when compared with placebo, whereas GFR increased (Table 9.2).

Table 9.2   (see text)

Time (h)		0	1	2	4	8	24
Renin	P	36.0±7.2	—	44.8±10.9	—	33.0±9.0	—
(uU/ml)	A	35.6±6.4	—	23.0±4.7*	—	16.8±2.8*	55.1±7.9
A_2 (pg/ml)	P	6.9±2.2	—	9.4±2.8	—	6.2±1.1	11.4±2.0
	A	6.9±1.5	—	6.1±0.7	—	5.6±0.7	11.7±1.3
Aldo (ng/dl)	P	7.6±1.2	—	7.1±1.4	—	5.6±1.0	12.0±1.3
	A	11.0±2.0	—	6.3±1.5	—	6.6±1.4	13.3±1.9
GFR	P	100	130±12	138±14	155±16	—	—
(% basal)	A	100	143±21	177±21*	192±29*	—	—
ERPF	P	100	127±32	137±38	145±53	—	—
(% basal)	A	100	137±24	153±36	147±39	—	—

Changes in renin–angiotensin–aldosterone system and renal function during administration of UK 69,578 ($n = 8$).
P represents placebo study and A administration of 2 ng/kg UK 69,578 by 20-min intravenous infusion at time 0 h.
* $P < 0.05$.

These data are consistent with the proposal that UK 69,578 inhibits the breakdown of endogenous ANF in man, and that the increased availability of the peptide to its receptors in the kidney results in alterations in renal function which are very similar to those observed during low-dose ANF infusion.

In a collaborative pilot study with colleagues at the Department of Cardiology, Western Infirmary, UK 69,578 was given to six subjects with mild cardiac failure, in whom basal ANF levels were slightly elevated or at the upper end of the normal range (Northridge et al., 1989). In all subjects the drug caused a further rise in ANF concentrations, and this was associated with natriuresis and diuresis (Fig. 9.3). There was a small, though significant, fall in right atrial pressure when compared with placebo, and a similar small fall in pulmonary artery wedge pressure (Fig. 9.3). These data suggest that inhibition of NEP in cardiac failure results in increased plasma levels of ANP and that this might cause cardiovascular haemodynamic effects which, if present after chronic dosing, would have therapeutic benefit.

UK 79,300

UK 79,300 is an orally active prodrug which is the indanyl ester of the active enantiomer of UK 69,578. In a preliminary study of oral administration of UK 79,300, 12 subjects with essential hypertension were given 10 mg (four subjects), 50 mg (four subjects), or 200 mg (four subjects) of the drug in a single-dose double-blind placebo controlled

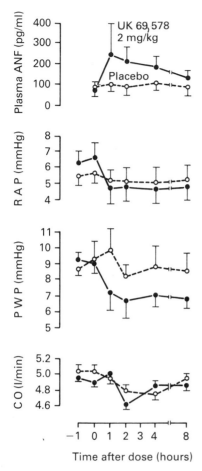

Fig. 9.3 Effect of UK 69,578 (by intravenous infusion for 20 min from time 0) on plasma ANF, right atrial pressure, pulmonary artery wedge pressure and cardiac output in six subjects with mild heart failure. Changes in plasma ANF, right atrial pressure and pulmonary artery wedge pressure during active infusion ($P < 0.05$) by analysis of variants.

manner. In all subjects drug administration caused plasma ANF levels to rise when compared with placebo, and at the highest dose of the drug studied there was a significant increase in urinary sodium excretion (248 ± 81 mmol/12 h vs. 104 ± 9 mmol/12 h). No change in blood pressure or heart rate was seen in this single-dose study (O'Connell *et al.*, 1989).

These three initial studies suggest that the rise in plasma levels of ANF after administration of UK 69,578 (or UK 79,300) results from inhibition of NEP in the kidney (and probably in other sites), and it seems likely that this accounts for the renal effects of the drug. The effect of UK 69,578 on breakdown of other substrates for NEP (such as kinins or angiotensins) in man remains to be studied in detail, and it is possible that some of the effects of the drug are due to alteration in the action of vasoactive peptides other than ANF. However, the close relationship between the change in plasma levels of ANF and urinary sodium loss described above (Fig. 9.2) along with the evidence from animal studies supports the hypothesis that the actions of UK 69,578 are mainly due to inhibition of ANF metabolism.

Other inhibitors of NEP

Thiorphan and other inhibitors of NEP have been studied extensively in animals (see above), although initial studies concentrated on potential analgesic properties (see above). Thiorphan and phosphoramidon both alter renal function, although the effects of thiorphan on its own are relatively minor. These actions were initially felt to be due to alteration in kinin metabolism but it now seems more likely that they reflect inhibition of ANF metabolism. Acetorphan, which is chemically similar to thiorphan, alters ANF levels and renal electrolyte excretion after oral administration to man (Gros *et al.* 1989).

The effects of NEP inhibitors on substrates other than ANF in man are unknown. In view of the wide range of substrates which, *in vitro*, interact with the enzyme it is clearly possible that NEP inhibitors will effect metabolism of not only ANF but also of kinins, substance P and angiotensins. An analogy may be drawn here with angiotensin-converting enzyme inhibitors. Angiotensin-converting enzyme has major effects on kinin (and other substrate) metabolism *in vitro* and the enzyme is very widely distributed in a large number of tissues. The important clinical effects of angiotensin-converting enzyme inhibitors seem, however, to relate principally to inhibition of ANGII generation in vascular and renal tissue. Whether the important clinical actions of NEP inhibitors are mainly due to inhibition of ANF breakdown remains to be studied. Clearly, factors such as drug lipid solubility, and the kinetics of drug–enzyme and substrate–enzyme interaction will determine the *in vivo* effects of particular NEP inhibitors.

Therapeutic implications

Hypertension

ANF infusion in subjects with essential hypertension over a 5-day period causes blood pressure to fall, and this suggests that the peptide may be of therapeutic benefit in hypertension (Janssen *et al.*, 1989). In this study the fall in blood pressure was maximal at 48 h after the start of ANF infusion, although the main natriuretic effects had occurred by 24 h. ANF is not orally available, and drugs which prolong the half-life of ANF by inhibiting its degradation may offer an alternative therapeutic way of modifying the action of the hormone. The effects of ANP inhibitors on blood pressure after chronic dosing are at present unknown and such studies are awaited with interest. Initial evidence (above) shows that UK 69,578, the first available NEP inhibitor for human use, does cause natriuresis without activation of the renin–angiotensin system (effects similar to those seen during ANF infusion), and these actions do suggest that the drug may be of therapeutic use in the treatment of hypertension.

Heart failure

In heart failure, the infusion of ANF results in some beneficial effects, although the resultant natriuresis is probably less than in normal subjects (Serizawa *et al.*, 1988). The preliminary evidence with UK 69,578 in subjects with mild heart failure suggests that a natriuretic effect also occurs after the inhibition of endogenous ANF degradation. If this effect is confirmed and is sustained during chronic dosing, then a therapeutic benefit may well be seen with this class of drugs in chronic heart failure.

Acknowledgements

The support of Pfizer (UK) in the above studies is gratefully acknowledged. Miss J. Doyle provided invaluable technical help, and Sister G. Davidson assisted with the human studies.

References

Alabaster, C. T., Machin, I., Barclay, P. L. & Samuels, G. M. R. (1989). The effect of UK 69,578, an atriopeptidase inhibitor, in a conscious dog model of cardiac insufficiency. *J. Am. Coll. Cardiol.* **13**: 75A.

Almeida, F. A., Suzuki, M., Scarborough, R. M., Lewicki, J. A. & Maack, T. (1989). Clearance function of type-C receptors of atrial natriuretic factor in rats. *Am. J. Physiol.* **256**: R469–75.

Ballerman, B. J. & Brenner, B. M. (1985). Biologically active atrial peptides. *J. Clin. Invest.* **76**: 2041–8.

Bertrand, P. & Doble, A. (1988). Degradation of atrial natriuretic peptides by an enzyme in rat kidney resembling neutral endopeptidase 24.11. *Biochem. Pharmacol.* **37**: 3817–21.

Booth, A. G. & Kenny, A. J. (1974). A rapid method for the preparation of microvilli from rabbit kidney. *Biochem. J.* **142**: 575–81.

Chipkin, R. E., Berger, J. G., Billard, W., Iorio, L. C., Chapman, R. & Barnett, A. (1988). Pharmacology of SCH 34826, an orally active enkephalinase inhibitor. *J. Pharmacol. Exp. Therapeut.* **245**: 829–38.

Devault, A., Lazure, C., Nault, C., Moval, H., Seidah, N. G., Chretein, M., Kahn, P. *et al.* (1987). Amino acid sequence of rabbit kidney neutral endopeptidase 24.11 (enkephalinase) derived from a complementary DNA. *EMBO J.* **6**: 1317–22.

Djokic, T. D., Dusser, D. J., Borson, D. B. & Nadel, J. A. (1989). Neutral endopeptidase modulates neurotensin induced airways contraction. *J. Appl. Physiol.* **66**: 2338–43.

Erdos, E. G., Schulz, W. W., Gafford, J. T. & Defendini, R. (1985). Neutral metallo-endopeptidase in human male genital tract: comparison to angiotensin I converting enzyme. *Lab. Invest.* **52**: 437–47.

Erdos, E. G. & Skidgel, R. A. (1989). Neutral endopeptidase 24.11 (enkephalinase) and related regulators of peptide hormones. *FASEB J.* **3**: 145–51.

Ganguly, A., Chiou, S., West, L. A. & Davis, J. S. (1989). Atrial natriuretic factor inhibits angiotensin-induced aldosterone secretion—not through cGMP or interference with phospho-lipase-C. *Biochem. Biophys. Res. Commun.* **159**: 148–54.

Gros, C., Souque, A., Schwartz, J. C., Duchier, J., Cournot, A., Baumer, P., Lecomte, J. M. (1989). Protection of atrial natriuretic factor against degradation: diuretic and natriuretic responses after *in vivo* inhibition of enkephalinase (EC 3.4.24.11) by Acetorphan. Proc. Nat. Acad. Sci. USA **86**: 7850–4.

Hirata, M., Chang, C. H. & Murad, F. (1989). Stimulatory effects of atrial natriuretic factor on phosphoinositide hydrolysis in cultured bovine aortic smooth muscle cells. *Biochim. Biophys. Acta* **1010**: 346–51.

Hollister, A. S., Rodeheffer, R. J., White, F. J., Potts, J. R., Imada, T. & Inagami, T. (1989). Clearance of atrial natriuretic factor by lung, liver, and kidney in human subjects and the dog. *J. Clin. Invest.* **83**: 623–8.

Hulks, G., Jardine, A., Connell, J. M. C. & Thomson, N. C. (1989). Atrial natriuretic peptide is a bronchodilator in asthmatic subjects. *Br. Med. J.* **299**: 1081–2.

Ishii, K. & Murad, F. (1989). ANP relaxes bovine tracheal smooth muscle and increases cGMP. *Am. J. Physiol.* **256**: C495–500.

Janssen, W. M. T., de Zeeuw, D., Gdalt, K. & de Jong, P. E. (1989). Antihypertensive effect of a five day infusion of atrial natriuretic factor in humans. *Hypertension* **13**: 640–6.

Jardine, A. G., Connell, J. M. C., Dilly, S. G., Cussans, N. J., Northridge, D. B., Leckie, B. J. & Lever, A. F. (1989). Inhibition of ANP degradation by the atriopeptidase inhibitor UK 69,578 in man. *Clin. Sci.* **74** (Suppl. 20): 21P.

Johnson, A. R., Ashton, J., Schulz, W. W. & Erdos, E. G. (1985). Neutral metalloendopeptidase in human lung tissue and cultured cells. *Annu. Rev. Respir. Dis.* **132**: 564–8.

Kenny, A. J. & Stephenson, S. L. (1988). Role of endopeptidase 24.11 in the inactivation of atrial natriuretic peptide. *FEBS Lett.* **232**: 1–8.

Kenyon, C. J. & Jardine, A. J. (1989). Atrial natriuretic peptide: water and electrolyte homeostasis. *Clin. Endocrinol. Metab.* **3**: 431–50.

Koehn, J. A., Norman, J. A., Jones, B. N., Le Sueur, L., Sakane, Y. & Ghai, R. D. (1987). Degradation of atrial natriuretic factor by kidney cortex membranes. *J. Biol. Chem.* **262**: 11 623–7.

Koepke, J. P., Tyler, L. D., Trapani, A. J., Bovy, P. R., Spear, K. L., Olins, G. M. & Blaine, E. H. (1989). Interaction of non-guanylate cyclase-linked atriopeptin receptor ligand and endopeptidase inhibitor in conscious rats. *J. Pharmacol. Exp. Therapeut.* **249**: 172–6.

Kohrogi, H., Graf, P. D., Sekizawa, K., Borson, D. B. & Nadel, J. A. (1988). Neutral endopeptidase inhibitors potentiate substance P- and capsaicin-induced cough in awake guinea pigs. *J. Clin. Invest.* **82**: 2063–8.

Leckie, B. (1987). How the heart rules the kidneys. *Nature* **326**: 644–5.

Lecomte, J. M., Constentin, J., Vlaiculescu, A., Chaillet, P., Marcais-Callado, H., Llorens-Cortez, C., Leboyer, M. *et al.* (1986). Pharmacological properties of acetorphan, a parenterally active enkephalinase inhibitor. *J. Pharmacol. Exp. Therapeut.* **237**: 937–44.

Llorens, C., Malfroy, B., Schwartz, J., Gacel, G., Roques, B. P., Roy, J., Morgat, J. L. *et al.* (1982). Enkephalin dipeptidylcarboxypeptidase (enkephalinase) activity: selective radioassay properties and regional distribution in human brain. *J. Neurochem.* **39**: 1081–9.

Maack, T., Suzuki, M., Almeida, F. A., Nussensveig, D., Scarborough, R. M., McEnroe, G. M. & Lewicki, J. A. (1987). Physiological role of silent receptors of atrial natriuretic factor. *Science* **238**: 675–8.

Malfroy, B., Kuang, W. J., Seeburg, P. H., Mason, A. J. & Schofield, P. R. (1988). Molecular cloning and amino acid sequence of human enkephalinase (neutral endopeptidase). *FEBS Lett.* **229**: 206–10.

Malfroy, B., Schofield, P. R., Kuang, W. J., Seeburg, P. H., Mason, A. J. & Henzel, W. J. (1987). Molecular cloning and amino acid sequence of rat enkephalinase. *Biochem. Biophys. Res. Commun.* **144**: 59–66.

Malfroy, B., Swerts, J. P., Guyson, A., Roques, B. P. & Schwartz, J. (1978). High affinity enkephalin degrading peptidase in brain is increased after morphine. *Nature* **276**: 523–6.

Matsas, R., Fulcher, I. S., Kenny, A. J. & Turner, A. J. (1983). Substance P and Leu-enkephalin are hydrolyzed by an enzyme in pig caudate synaptic membranes that is identical with the endopeptidase of kidney microvilli. *Proc. Nat. Acad. Sci. USA* **80**: 3111–15.

Northridge, D. B., Jardine, A. J., Alabaster, C. T., Barclay, P. L., Connell, J. M. C., Dargie, H. J., Dilly, S. G. *et al.* (1989). Preliminary studies with a novel atriopeptidase inhibitor (UK 69,578) in animals, normal volunteers and heart failure patients. *Lancet* **ii**: 591–3.

O'Connell, J., Jardine, A. J., Davidson, G., Doyle, J., Lever, A. F. & Connell, J. M. C. (1989). UK 79,300, an orally active atriopeptidase inhibitor, raises plasma ANP and is natriuretic in essential hypertension. *J. Hypertension* **7**: 923.

Olins, G. M., Krieter, P. A., Trapani, A. J., Spear, K. L. & Bovy, P. R. (1989). Specific inhibitors of endopeptidase 24.11 inhibit the metabolism of atrial natriuretic peptides *in vitro* and *in vivo*. *Molec. Cell. Endocrinol.* **61**: 201–8.

Olins, G. M., Spear, K. L., Siegel, N. R., Zurcher-Neely, H. A. & Smith, C. E. (1986). Proteolytic degradation of atriopeptin 111 by kidney brush border membranes. *Fed. Proc.* **45**: 427A.

Olins, G. M., Spear, K. L., Siegel, N. R. & Zurcher-Neely, H. A. (1987). Inactivation of atrial natriuretic factor by the renal brush border. *Biochem. Biophys. Acta* **901**: 97–100.

Roques, B. P., Fournie-Zaluskie, M. C., Soroca, E., Lecomte, J. M., Malfroy, B., Llorens, C. & Schwartz, J. C. (1980). The enkephalinase inhibitor thiorphan shows antinocioceptive activity in mice. *Nature* **288**: 286–8.

Samuels, G. M. R., Barclay, P. L., Alabaster, C. T., Peters, C. J. & Ellis, P. (1989a). The preclinical pharmacology of UK 69,578—a novel atriopeptidase inhibitor. *Clin. Sci.* **74** (Suppl. 20): 29P.

Samuels, G. M. R., Barclay, P. L., Ellis, P. & Shepperson, N. B. (1989b). The natriuretic and diuretic efficacy of an orally active atriopeptidase inhibitor (API). *Am. J. Hypertension* **2** (5, part 2): 119A.

Samuels, G. M. R., Barclay, P. L., Shepperson, N. B. & Bennet, J. A. (1989c). The acute and chronic antihypertensive efficacy of atriopeptidase inhibition of rats. *J. Am. Coll. Cardiol.* **13** (2): 76A.

Serizawa, T., Hirata, T., Kohmoto, O., Iizuka, M., Matsuoko, H., Sato, H., Takahashi, T. *et al.* (1988). Acute haemodynamic effects of alpha atrial natriuretic polypeptide in patients with congestive heart failure. *Jap. Heart J.* **29**: 143–9.

Seymour, A. A., Fennell, S. A. & Swerdel, J. N. (1989). Potentiation of renal effects of atrial natriuretic factor by SQ 29,072. *Hypertension* **14**: 87–97.

Shepperd, D., Thomson, J. E., Sycpinski, L., Dusser, D., Nadel, J. A. & Borson, B. (1988). Toluene diisocyanate increases airway responsiveness to substance P and decreases airway neutral endopeptidase. *J. Clin. Invest.* **81**: 1111–15.

Shima, M., Seino, Y., Torikai, S. & Imai, M. (1988). Intrarenal localisation of degradation of atrial natriuretic peptide in isolated glomeruli and cortical nephron segments. *Life Sci.* **43**: 357–63.

Skidgel, R. A., Schulz, W. W., Tam, L.-T. & Erdos, E. G. (1987). Human renal angiotensin I converting enzyme and neutral endopeptidase. *Kidney Int.* **31**: S45–8.

Stephenson, S. L. & Kenny, A. J. (1987a). Metabolism of neuropeptides. *Biochem. J.* **241**: 237–42.

Stephenson, S. L. & Kenny, A. J. (1987b). The hydrolysis of α-human natriuretic peptide by pig kidney microvillar membranes is initiated by endopeptidase 24.11. *Biochem. J.* **243**: 183–7.

Ura, N., Carretero, O. A. & Erdos, E. G. (1987). Role of endopeptidase 24.11 in kinin metabolism *in vitro* and *in vivo*. *Kidney Int.* **32**: 507–13.

Waldman, S. A. & Murad, F. (1989). Atrial natriuretic peptides—receptors and second messengers. *Bio Essays* **10**: 16–19.

Weselcouch, E. O., Humphrey, W. R. & Aiken, J. W. (1985). Effects of pulmonary and renal circulations on activity of atrial natriuretic factor. *Am. J. Physiol.* **249**: R595–602).

Chapter 10
Biologically active atrial natriuretic factor receptors
Michael Chinkers

Introduction

Molecular cloning of a membrane
GC/ANF receptor

Functions of the intracellular domains
of the ANF receptor

A second GC/natriuretic factor
receptor: GC-B

Summary

References

Introduction

Atrial natriuretic factor (ANF) exerts many of its biological effects by stimulating membrane guanylate cyclase (GC) activity, leading to increases in cyclic guanyl monophosphate (cGMP) concentrations in target cells. Biochemical approaches initially identified two types of ANF receptor: a high-molecular-weight ($M_r \sim 130\,000$) (130 kDa) receptor coupled to GC activation, that copurifies with GC activity, and a low-molecular-weight ($M_r \sim 65$ kDa) receptor that does not appear to be coupled to GC activation and does not copurify with GC activity (reviewed in Inagami, 1989). This chapter describes the characterization of high-molecular-weight, GC-coupled ANF receptors through the use of recombinant DNA techniques.

Molecular cloning of a membrane GC/ANF receptor: GC-A (or ANP-A)

Several groups demonstrated that a high-molecular-weight ANF receptor copurified with GC activity (Kuno *et al.*, 1986; Paul *et al.*, 1987; Takayanagi *et al.*, 1987; Meloche *et al.*, 1988). However, since the receptor preparations were not homogeneous, and GC activity in the preparations was not stimulated by ANF, it was not clear whether ANF-activated GC activity was intrinsic to the receptor. To determine whether the ANF receptor contained GC activity, a molecular cloning approach was adopted: complementary DNA (cDNA) clones encoding membrane GCs were isolated and expressed in mammalian cells; it was then determined whether the expressed proteins possessed both GC and ANF-binding activities.

Using as probe a cDNA clone encoding a sea urchin membrane GC, partial-length cDNA clones encoding membrane GCs were isolated from human kidney and placental libraries (Lowe *et al.*, 1989); a partial-length clone was in turn used to isolate a full-length cDNA clone from a rat brain library (Chinkers *et al.*, 1989). Subsequently, the partial-length human cDNA was ligated to appropriate 5' genomic sequences for functional expression (Lowe *et al.*, 1989). Transient expression of the rat or human membrane GC clones in COS-7 cells resulted in dramatic increases in both basal and ANF-stimulated membrane GC activity and in specific ^{125}I-ANF binding to the cells (Chinkers *et al.*, 1989; Lowe *et al.*, 1989). This was the first demonstration that GC activity and ANF-binding activity resided in the same protein. Binding competition studies showed that the recombinant GC/ANF receptor possessed high affinity and specificity for ANF similar to that described for the high-molecular-weight ANF receptor from tissues (Chinkers *et al.*, 1989; Lowe *et al.*, 1989). ^{125}I-ANF was specifically crosslinked to a 130-kDa protein present in cells transfected with the GC cDNA but not in control cells (Chinkers *et al.*, 1989), and competition for this crosslinking with various concentrations of unlabelled ANF or a truncated analogue showed the same high affinity and specificity as for total binding to transfected cells (M. Chinkers and D. L. Garbers, unpublished observations). Thus, both rat and human clones encoded a 130-kDa ANF receptor possessing intrinsic ANF-stimulated GC activity.

The GC/ANF receptor clones each encoded a protein containing an amino-terminal signal sequence, followed by an extracellular domain with homology to the extracellular binding domain of the low-M_r ANF receptor (Fuller *et al.*, 1988; Porter *et al.*, 1989), a single transmembrane domain, an intracellular domain homologous to the catalytic domain of protein kinases, and a COOH-terminal domain homologous to soluble GC (Koesling *et al.*, 1988; Nakane *et al.*, 1988).

Functions of the intracellular domains of the ANF receptor

Conservation of little more than the protein-kinase-like domain between membrane GCs from mammals (Chinkers *et al.*, 1989; Lowe *et al.*, 1989) and one sea urchin species (Singh *et al.*, 1988) implied that this domain contained GC activity. However, conservation of only the COOH-terminal sequences between soluble GC, the GC/ANF receptor, a membrane GC from a second sea urchin species (Thorpe & Garbers, 1989) and a bovine brain adenylate cyclase (Krupinski *et al.*, 1989), suggested that GC activity resided in this COOH-terminal domain. In order to localize the GC catalytic domain, most of either the kinase-like or COOH-terminal sequences were deleted from the rat GC/ANF receptor, and the mutant cDNA clones were expressed in mammalian cells (Chinkers & Garbers, 1989).

While both deletion mutants bound ANF, deletion of the kinase domain yielded an ANF receptor having constitutively high GC activity, whereas deletion of the COOH-terminal domain destroyed GC activity.

Thus, GC catalytic activity resided in the COOH-terminal sequences homologous to soluble GC and to adenylate cyclase. The kinase deletion mutant failed to respond to ANF in intact cells or membrane preparations. In addition, this mutant responded minimally to ATP, which potentiated ANF activation of GC activity in membranes containing the wild-type receptor (Kurose, Inagami & Ui, 1987; Chinkers & Garbers, 1989). The observation that removal of the kinase domain seemed to result in full activation of GC, even in the absence of ANF, suggested that the kinase-like domain ordinarily functions as a negative regulatory element; suppression of GC activity by the kinase-like domain appears to be relieved following binding of ANF.

A second GC/natriuretic factor receptor: GC-B (or ANP-B)

Using GC/ANF receptor cDNA clones as probes, related cDNA clones were isolated from human and rat brain libraries (Chang et al., 1989; Schulz et al., 1989). The overall topology of the proteins encoded by these cDNA clones (designated GC-B) was similar to that of the GC/ANF receptor (designated GC-A), although GC-B diverged significantly from GC-A in the extracellular amino-acid sequence. Like GC-A, the GC-B protein showed guanylate cyclase activity as well as ^{125}I-ANF and ^{125}I-brain natriuretic peptide (BNP) binding activity when expressed in mammalian cells. BNP is a recently described natriuretic peptide similar in structure to ANF and having similar physiological effects (Sudoh et al., 1988). Despite these similarities, stimulation of cGMP formation by ANF and BNP was markedly different in cells transfected with cDNA encoding GC-A or GC-B. GC-B was preferentially stimulated by BNP as compared with ANF; this was not the case for GC-A (Chang et al., 1989; Schulz et al., 1989). However, the requirement for very high, probably non-physiological, concentrations of BNP to obtain even small increases in cGMP concentrations suggested the possibility that another, as-yet-undiscovered, natriuretic peptide may be the natural ligand for GC-B (Schulz et al., 1989).

Summary

Expression of cDNA clones encoding biologically active ANF receptors has permitted a direct demonstration that these receptors contain intrinsic ANF-activated GC activity. Thus, the ANF receptor itself generates the second messenger, cGMP. Deletion mutagenesis experiments have shown that GC activity resides in carboxyl sequences homologous to soluble GC and to adenylate cyclase, while a protein-kinase-like domain appears to function as a regulatory element. Recently, cDNA clones encoding a second membrane GC/natriuretic factor receptor have been identified, suggesting the existence of a family of GC receptors.

References

Chang, M., Lowe, D. G., Lewis, M., Hellmiss, R., Chen, E. & Goeddel, D. V. (1989). Differential activation by atrial and brain natriuretic peptides of two different receptor guanylate cyclases. *Nature* **341**: 68–72.

Chinkers, M. & Garbers, D. L. (1989). The protein kinase domain of the ANP receptor is required for signaling. *Science* **245**: 1392–4.

Chinkers, M., Garbers, D. L., Chang, M.-S., Lowe, D. G., Chin, H., Goeddel, D. V. & Schulz, S. (1989). A membrane form of guanylate cyclase is an atrial natriuretic peptide receptor. *Nature* **338**: 78–83.

Fuller, F., Porter, J. G., Arfsten, A. E., Miller, J., Schilling, J. W., Scarborough, R. M., Lewicki, J. A. *et al.* (1988). Atrial natriuretic peptide clearance receptor: complete sequence and functional expression of cDNA clones. *J. Biol. Chem.* **263**: 9395–401.

Inagami, T. (1989). Atrial natriuretic factor. *J. Biol. Chem.* **264**: 3043–6.

Koesling, D., Herz, J., Gausepohl, H., Niroomand, F., Hinsch, K.-D., Mulsch, A., Bohme, E., *et al.* (1988). The primary structure of the 70-kDa subunit of bovine soluble guanylate cyclase. *FEBS Lett.* **239**: 29–34.

Krupinski, J., Coussen, F., Bakalyar, H. A., Tang, W.-J., Feinstein, P. G., Orth, K., Slaughter, C. *et al.* (1989). Adenylyl cyclase amino acid sequence: possible channel- or transporter-like structure. *Science* **244**: 1558–64.

Kuno, T., Andresen, J. W., Kamisaki, Y., Waldman, S. A., Chang, L. Y., Saheki, S., Leitman, D. C. *et al.* (1986). Co-purification of an atrial natriuretic factor receptor and particulate guanylate cyclase from rat lung. *J. Biol. Chem.* **261**: 5817–23.

Kurose, H., Inagami, T. & Ui, M. (1987). Participation of adenosine 5'-triphosphate in the activation of membrane-bound guanylate cyclase by the atrial natriuretic factor. *FEBS Lett.* **219**: 375–9.

Lowe, D. G., Chang, M.-S., Hellmiss, R., Chen, E., Singh, S., Garbers, D. L. & Goeddel, D. V. (1989). Human atrial natriuretic peptide receptor defines a new paradigm for second messenger signal transduction. *EMBO J.* **8**: 1377–84.

Meloche, S., McNicoll, N., Liu, B., Ong, H. & De Lean, A. (1988). Atrial natriuretic factor R_1 receptor from bovine adrenal zona glomerulosa: purification, characterization, and modulation by amiloride. *Biochemistry* **27**: 8151–8.

Nakane, M., Saheki, S., Kuno, T., Ishii, K. & Murad, F. (1988). Molecular cloning of a cDNA coding for 70 kilodalton subunit of soluble guanylate cyclase from rat lung. *Biochem. Biophys. Res. Commun.* **157**: 1139–47.

Paul, A. K., Marala, R. B., Jaiswal, R. K. & Sharma, R. K. (1987). Coexistence of guanylate cyclase and atrial natriuretic factor receptor in a 180-kD protein. *Science* **235**: 1224–6.

Porter, J. G., Scarborough, R. M., Wang, Y., Schenk, D., McEnroe, G. A., Kang, L.-L. & Lewicki, J. A. (1989). Recombinant expression of a secreted form of the atrial natriuretic peptide clearance receptor. *J. Biol. Chem.* **264**: 14179–84.

Schulz, S., Singh, S., Bellet, R. A., Singh, G., Tubb, D. J., Chin, H. & Garbers, D. L. (1989). The primary structure of a plasma membrane guanylate cyclase demonstrates diversity within this new receptor family. *Cell* **58**: 1155–62.

Singh, S., Lowe, D. G., Thorpe, D. S., Rodriguez, H., Kuang, W.-J., Dangott, L. J., Chinkers, M. *et al.* (1988). Membrane guanylate cyclase is a cell-surface receptor with homology to protein kinases. *Nature* **334**: 708–12.

Sudoh, T., Kangawa, K., Minamino, N. & Matsuo, H. (1988). A new natriuretic peptide in porcine brain. *Nature* **332**: 78–81.

Takayanagi, R., Inagami, T., Snajdar, R. M., Imada, T., Tamura, M. & Misono, K. S. (1987). Two distinct forms of receptors for atrial natriuretic factor in bovine adrenocortical cells: purification, ligand binding, and peptide mapping. *J. Biol. Chem.* **262**: 12104–13.

Thorpe, D. S. & Garbers, D. L. (1989). The membrane form of guanylate cyclase: homology with a subunit of the cytoplasmic form of the enzyme. *J. Biol. Chem.* **264**: 6545–9.

Chapter 11
Atrial natriuretic factor clearance receptors

John McMurray and David B. Northridge

Introduction

The possibility of more than one atrial natriuretic factor (ANF) receptor type began to emerge within a few years of deBold's pioneering observations (deBold *et al.*, 1981). Several groups demonstrated a poor correlation between ANF binding and cyclic guanyl monophosphate (cGMP) stimulation in tissues and a similar disparity between binding affinity and bioactivity of truncated ANF analogues was reported (Leitman *et al.*, 1986, 1988; Scarborough *et al.*, 1986). The first functional differentiation of these speculative binding-subtypes was published in 1987 (Maack *et al.*, 1987).

Structural and ligand differentiation of receptors

Two main ANF receptor types have been generally agreed (though others are in the process of characterization) (Martin & Ballermann, 1989). The first receptor type has a molecular mass of approximately 120–140 kDa under reducing conditions (Misono *et al.*, 1985; Vandlen *et al.*, 1986). This receptor copurifies with guanylate cyclase (GC) and a complementary DNA clone encoding the mammalian ANF receptor/membrane GC has been described (Chinkers *et al.*, 1989; Lowe *et al.*, 1989; Waldman & Murad, 1989). Stimulation of this receptor type leads to cGMP accumulation and biological activity such as vasorelaxation and natriuresis (Waldman & Murad, 1989). The receptor appears to require the carboxyterminal phenylalanine–arginine moiety for binding and competition studies have shown a greater affinity for ANF 99–126 than ANF 103–123 (Martin & Ballermann, 1989; Waldman & Murad, 1989). This GC-linked receptor is a relatively poor binding site for ring-contracted analogues of ANF.

By contrast, a second well-defined receptor exists as a 120–130 kDa disulphide homodimer which can be reduced to 60–70 kDa subunits (Schenk et al., 1985; Fuller et al., 1988; Porter et al., 1989; Uchida et al., 1989b). Purification, DNA cloning and recombinant expression studies suggest that this receptor consists of a large (436-amino-acid) extracellular domain, a single transmembrane anchor domain (23 amino acids) and a short cytoplasmic domain (37 amino acids) (Fuller et al., 1988; Porter et al., 1989). The extracellular domain shows homology with the comparable domain of the GC-linked receptor. Receptor binding activity appears to be resistant to acid, freezing, thawing and freeze–drying but is lost in the absence of univalent ions (Uchida et al., 1989). The receptor is glycosylated (probably 3N-linked oligosaccharides per 70-kDa subunit) though these moieties are not essential for binding (Fuller et al., 1988; Porter et al., 1989; Uchida et al., 1989b). The monomeric and dimeric receptor forms bind ANF equally well suggesting the intersubunit disulphide bond is not necessary for binding (the role of dimerization is unclear) (Porter et al., 1989; Uchida et al., 1989b). Purified preparations of this second receptor do not contain GC and, conversely, purified preparations of particulate GC do not contain the 60–70 kDa receptor subunit (Waldman & Murad, 1989). Receptor stimulation does not lead to cGMP accumulation. Though this receptor binds ANF 99-126 with similar affinity to that of the GC-linked receptor, competition studies have shown that this second receptor type will also bind truncated ANF analogues with high affinity (order: ANF 101–126 > ANF 103–126 > ANF 103–123 ≫ ANF 111–126) (i.e. the phenylalanine–arginine moiety does not seem to be necessary for binding) (Porter et al., 1989; Waldman et al., 1989).

Importantly, this receptor will also bind ring-contracted analogues with high affinity (Maack et al., 1987). These analogues neither stimulate GC nor antagonize ANF-mediated stimulation of GC. This non-GC receptor is the dominant ANF binding site in many tissues (e.g. vascular smooth muscle, lung, endothelial cells and kidney), outnumbering the GC-coupled receptor by 20:1 (Martin & Ballermann, 1989; Waldman & Murad, 1989).

Functional role of the non-GC receptor

Maack and colleagues, in a landmark experiment, suggested a clearance role for non-GC receptors (Maack et al., 1987). Crucial in their study was the synthesis and employment of a 15-amino-acid ANF residue (Fig. 11.1) shortened by 5 amino acids within the disulphide-bridged ring and shortened by 5 amino acids at the carboxy terminal—des (Gln[116], Ser[117],

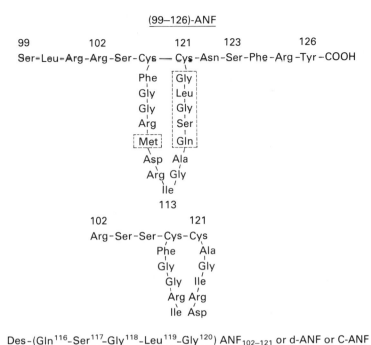

Fig. 11.1 Amino-acid sequence of human–(99–126)–ANF and the ring-deleted analogue.

Gly[118], Leu[119], Gly[120])–ANF$_{102-121}$–NH$_2$ (also called C-ANF and d-ANF). This analogue has a high specificity and affinity for non-GC receptors; it does not stimulate particulate GC nor antagonize the cGMP elevating effect of ANF in cell cultures. Using this ligand, Maack and coworkers were able to show that, whereas its infusion into isolated perfused kidneys had no biological effect, infusion (1 µg/kg/min) into intact anaesthetized rats resulted in a natriuresis ($U_{Na}V$ increased from 1.85 ± 0.63 to 4.22 ± 0.8 µmol/min). Interestingly, there was little, if any, effect on blood pressure. This renal action was associated with a threefold (51.4 ± 9.4 to 141.7 ± 21.1 pg/ml) rise in circulating concentrations of endogenous ANF. A similar increment in ANF, brought about by exogenous infusion (0.02 µg/kg/min), resulted in comparable biological effects. C-ANF (0.3 µg/kg/min) also produces a natriuresis and diuresis in conscious dogs (Gregory *et al.*, 1988). Another specific non-GC receptor ligand, SC 46542 (des (Phe[106], Gly[107], Ala[115], Gln[116])–ANF 103–126), has also been reported to induce a small natriuresis in the anaesthetized rat (Koepke, Tyler & Blaine, 1989a). As a consequence of these findings, Maack *et al.* postulated that the non-GC receptors acted as clearance/storage–binding sites. Occupancy of these receptors by C-ANF would therefore decrease binding of native ANF and increase the circulating concentration of the latter, with the expected biological effects.

The same group (Almeida *et al.* 1989) have tested this hypothesis further using coinfusions of C-ANF and ^{125}I-labelled ANF 99–126 in the rat. If C-ANF competes with native ANF for C-ANF receptors then the volume of distribution of the ANF 99–126 should be decreased and its metabolic clearance rate (MCR) retarded; this is in fact what was found. The apparent volume of distribution at steady state (V_{ss}) decreased from 97 ± 12 ml/100 g body weight (i.e. approximately equal to body weight) to 49 ± 3 (with C-ANF 1 μg/kg/min) and 36 ± 2 (with C-ANF 10 μg/kg/min) (the latter still being in excess of extracellular fluid volume). Similarly the MCR was halved by the lower dose of C-ANF. A reduction in V_{ss} and MCR by one half with C-ANF 1 μg/kg/min might be expected to increase the endogenous ANF concentration approximately twofold, which was equivalent to what was observed in the earlier experiment (suggesting no short-term change in ANF secretion following C-ANF infusion) (Almeida *et al.*, 1989). Interestingly, a delay in the later hydrolytic products of ^{125}I-ANF was also observed with C-ANF leading the authors to suggest that these degradation products reflect ligand–receptor internalization (see below).

Mechanism of clearance of ANF by the non-GC receptor

Several groups have demonstrated ANF internalization in cultured cells (Hirata *et al.*, 1985; Napier, Arcuri & Vandlen, 1986; Murthy, Thibault & Cantin, 1989). Ligand–receptor delivery to lysosomes can be demonstrated autoradiographically (Hirata *et al.*, 1985). Only the ~ 60 kDa receptor type has been shown to be internally sequestrated (Murthy *et al.*, 1989). Studies with lysosomotropic agents such as chloroquine support the occurrence of intralysosomal degradation (Hirata *et al.*, 1985; Napier *et al.*, 1986; Murthy *et al.*, 1989). This process is temperature-dependent (inhibited at 4 °C) and rapid (lysosomal uptake occurs within 5 min). Degradation products are extruded from the cell.

It has been suggested that, because of the high affinity of binding of ANF to non-GC receptors, ligand dissociation will be slow and therefore internalization will predominate over dissociation at physiological concentrations of ANF.

Regulation of the non-GC clearance receptor

It is a well-established principle that a hormone may regulate its own receptor and down-regulation of ANF receptors in cultured cells treated with high concentrations of ANF has been reported. Since the decrease in binding density has not commonly been associated with a decrease in GC activity, selective down-regulation of clearance receptors has been suggested (Martin & Ballermann, 1989). Martin *et al.* (1989) recently addressed this issue in some detail. This group studied ANF receptors in the glomerulus (80 % non-GC coupled) and inner medullary collecting duct (100 % GC coupled) of the rabbit. When a group of rabbits stabilized on a low salt intake were given high-salt drinking water for 14–16 h, a decrease in total glomerular ANF binding site density could be demonstrated. This was also seen with an acute infusion of ANF. However, no change was seen in GC-coupled receptor density in either nephron segment, suggesting that the changes demonstrated above occurred only in the clearance receptor population. Acid washing (to remove bound ligand) of these membrane preparations resulted in an increase in binding, returning the density to that of a control group not given sodium supplementation/ANF infusion. These authors concluded, therefore, that the down-regulation of receptors was only *apparent*, in the sense that it merely reflected occupancy of the 60 kDa clearance receptor by ANF.

It is not clear why this change in clearance receptor occupancy occurs after sodium supplementation or ANF infusion. One possibility is that affinity is somehow altered in the experimental conditions employed by Martin *et al.* (1989). Of relevance here is the finding of Uchida *et al.* (1989) that binding activity of the non-GC-linked receptor is influenced by univalent ion concentration.

There is a very little additional information on clearance receptor regulation. Chabrier *et al.* (1989), in a preliminary communication, have reported that clearance receptors are more sensitive to heterologous regulation (e.g. by angiotensin II (ANG II)) in contrast to biologically active (GC coupled) receptors which are more sensitive to homologous regulation. This group have shown that ANG II decreases total ANF binding in cultured rat vascular smooth muscle cells although it potentiates GC activity, suggesting selective down-regulation of clearance receptors. However their finding that ANF appears to selectively densitize GC activity conflicts with reports from other groups and the effect in other tissues.

Receptor vs. enzymatic clearance of ANF

Clearly one of the most interesting issues to arise from the discovery of the probable clearance role of non-GC receptors is their relationship with neutral endopeptidase (NEP; EC 3.4.24.11) (Kenny & Stephenson, 1988; Shima *et al.*, 1988). Like NEP, non-GC receptors are found in high concentrations in those organs that contribute significantly to the clearance of ANF (Kenny & Stephenson, 1988; Martin & Ballermann, 1989). However within these organs, clearance receptors and NEP may have a different distribution. For example, NEP is located mainly in the proximal tubule luminal membrane; by contrast non-GC receptors are most abundant in the glomerulus.

The interaction between these two clearance mechanisms has been studied in the anaesthetized rat by Koepke *et al.* (1989b). SC-46542 was used as a specific ligand for non-GC binding and thiorphan as an inhibitor of NEP. SC-46542 (16 μg/kg/min) caused a small increase in urine flow rate and sodium excretion (the circulating ANF concentrations did not, however, appear to change: 359 ± 32 vs. 355 ± 28 pg/ml). Thiorphan (30 mg/kg) had no significant effect on renal excretory function (the ANF concentration was unchanged: 382 ± 44 vs. 395 ± 17 pg/ml). SC-46542 *plus* thiorphan, however, caused an impressive diuresis and natriuresis (with a rise in circulating ANF from 325 ± 46 to 676 ± 86 pg/ml). In a second experiment, neither thiorphan nor SC-46542, alone seemed to augment the renal effects of a threshold dose (50 ng/kg/min) of ANF 103–126. However, pretreatment with both blockers considerably enhanced urinary flow rate and natriuresis after ANF 103–126 infusion.

The first of these experiments has led the authors to the interesting speculation that if only one clearance mechanism is blocked the other may compensate. Martin & Ballermann (1989) have also suggested that the NEP mechanism only operates when clearance receptors are overwhelmed. Recent studies, however, have shown that NEP inhibition alone can increase plasma ANF and initiate a natriuresis but the relative importance of these two mechanisms remains undetermined (Northridge *et al.*, 1989).

Physiological and pathophysiological considerations

Non-GC-coupled receptors appear to have a K_D for ANF of between 10^{-12} and 10^{-10} M, suggesting binding at physiological hormone levels (Saheki *et al.*, 1989; Uchida *et al.*, 1989).

In man, platelet ANF binding is modulated by sodium intake (decreased binding sites with high sodium intake) (Schiffrin, Deslongchamps & Thibault, 1986). Platelets do not contain particulate GC, suggesting that this finding reflects physiological regulation of clearance receptors in man in a similar way to that found by Martin *et al.* (1989) in the rabbit.

In chronic heart failure, where ANF levels are elevated, platelet ANF binding density has also been reported to be decreased, again supporting the possibility of clearance receptor modulation (Schiffrin, 1988). Receptor change may also occur in hypertension. In the spontaneously hypertensive rat (SHR), total glomerular ANF binding sites are normal but a marked increase in glomerular ANF binding sites can be detected after acid washing. This increase in binding sites does not involve GC-coupled receptors, which suggests that there may be a greater expression of clearance receptors in the SHR (Martin *et al.*, 1989). This seems a logical response in the SHR because circulating ANF levels are also increased.

Just as the discovery of the role of NEP has had therapeutic implications, so too may the discovery of clearance receptors. One might speculate that, as with nEP inhibitors, clearance receptor blockers might enhance the biological effects of endogenous ANF in a clinically useful way, e.g. lower arterial pressure. Early results in this direction are, however, disappointing. Koepke *et al.* (1989) in a preliminary communication, have reported that SC-46542 (100 μg/kg/h) by continuous intravenous infusion for 10 days failed to alter mean arterial pressure (MAP) in the SHR. SC-46542 plus thiorphan (itself ineffective) did lower MAP in this model but the effect was lost by 9 days with return of MAP to baseline levels. This is a particularly interesting observation as one concern about NEP blockade alone (or clearance receptor blockade alone) is that subsequent chronic elevation of ANF might lead to a compensatory increase in the capacity of the alternative clearance pathway. Koepke and colleagues' report suggests that tolerance can develop even when both mechanisms are blocked.

Outstanding questions

Much more needs to be learned about the fundamental role of clearance receptors—for example, do they feedback to alter ANF secretion? A number of recent, intriguing, observations also need explanation: not all non-GC-linked receptors may be clearance receptors—for example, adrenal receptors appear to be biologically active yet do not stimulate GC (Martin & Ballermann, 1989; Saheki *et al.*, 1989). Conversely some 60-kDa receptors may be coupled to GC. Other subdivisions of the 60-kDa receptor type may exist and subtype switching may occur (Saheki *et al.*, 1989; Uchida *et al.*, 1989a,b). Many interesting developments can be anticipated in this area in the near future.

References

Almeida, F. A., Suzuki, M., Scarborough, R. M., Lewicki, J. A., Maak, T. (1989). Clearance function of type C receptors of atrial natriuretic factor in rats. *Am. J. Physiol.* **256**, R469–R475.

Chabrier, P. E., Roubert, P., Plas, P. & Braquet, P. (1989). Homoregulation and heteroregulation of atrial natriuretic factor receptors in vascular smooth muscle cells. *Am. J. Hypertension* (Suppl.) **2**: 62A.

Chinkers, M., Garbers, D. L., Chang, M. S., Lowe, D. G., Chin, H., Goeddel, D. V. & Schulz, S. (1989). A membrane form of guanylate cyclase is an atrial natriuretic peptide receptor. *Nature* **338**: 78–83.

deBold, A. J., Borenstein, H. B., Veress, A. T. & Sonnenberg, H. (1981). A rapid and potent natriuretic response to intravenous injection of atrial myocardial extract in rats. *Life Sci.* **28**: 89–94.

Fuller, F., Porter, J. G., Arfsten, A. E., Miller, J., Schilling, J. W., Scarborough, R. M., Lewicki, J. A. *et al.* (1988). Atrial natriuretic peptide clearance receptor. *J. Biol. Chem.* **263**: 9395–401.

Gregory, L. C., Scarborough, R. M., Metzler, C. H., McEnroe, G. A., Maack, T. & Lewicki, J.

A. (1988). Effects of acute infusion of a c-ANP receptor specific compound in conscious dog. *J. Cell Biol.* (Suppl.) **12A**: 23.

Hirata, Y., Takata, S., Tomita, M. & Takaichi, S. (1985). Binding, internalisation and degradation of atrial natriuretic peptide in cultured vascular smooth muscle cells of rat. *Biochem. Biophys. Res. Commun.* **132**: 976–84.

Kenny, A. J. & Stephenson, S. L. (1988). Role of endopeptidase-24.11 in the inactivation of atrial natriuretic peptide. *FEBS Lett.* **232**: 1–8.

Koepke, J. P., Tyler, L. D. & Blaine, E. H. (1989a). Chronic infusion of endopeptidase 24.11 inhibitor and non-guanylate cyclase linked atriopeptin receptor ligand on mean arterial pressure in spontaneously hypertensive rats. *Am. J. Hypertension* (Suppl.) **2**: 23A.

Koepke, J. P., Tyler, L. D., Trapani, A. J., Bovy, P. R., Spear, K. L., Olins, G. M. & Blaine, E. H. (1989b). Interaction of non-guanylate cyclase linked atriopeptin receptor ligand and endopeptidase inhibitor in conscious rats. *J. Pharmacol. Exp. Therapeut.* **249**: 172–6.

Leitman, D. C., Andresen, J. W., Catalamo, R. M., Waldman, S. A., Tuan, J. J. & Murad, F. (1988). Atrial natriuretic peptide binding, cross linking and stimulation of cyclic GMP accumulation and particulate guanylate cyclase activity in cultured cells. *J. Biol. Chem.* **263**: 3720–8.

Leitman, D. C., Andresen, J. W., Kuno, T., Kamisaki, Y., Chang, J. K. & Murad, F. (1986). Identification of multiple binding sites for atrial natriuretic factor by affinity cross linking in cultured endothelial cells. *J. Biol. Chem.* **261**: 11650–5.

Lowe, D. G., Chang, M. S., Hellmiss, R., Chen, E., Singh, S., Garbers, D. L. & Goeddel, D. V. (1989). Human atrial natriuretic peptide receptor defines a new paradigm for second messenger signal transduction. *EMBO J.* **8**: 1377–84.

Maack, T., Suzuki, M., Almeida, F. A., Nussen-Zveig, D., Scarborough, R. M., McEnroe, G. A. & Lewicki, J. A. (1987). Physiological role of silent receptors of atrial natriuretic factor. *Science* **238**: 675–8.

Martin, E. R. & Ballermann, B. J. (1989). Atrial natriuretic peptide receptors. In: *Atrial Natriuretic Peptides* (Brenner, B. M. & Stein, J. H., eds). New York: Churchill Livingstone, p. 105–36.

Martin, E. R., Lewicki, J. A., Scarborough, R. M. & Ballermann, B. J. (1989). Expression and regulation of ANP receptor subtypes in rat renal glomeruli and papillae. *Am. J. Physiol.* **257**: F649–57.

Misono, K. S., Grammer, R. T., Rigby, J. W. & Inagami, T. (1985). Photoaffinity labelling of atrial natriuretic factor receptor in bovine and rat adrenocortical membranes. *Biochem. Biophys. Res. Commun.* **130**: 994–1001.

Murthy, K. K., Thibault, G. & Cantin, M. (1989). Binding and intracellular degradation of atrial natriuretic factor by cultured vascular smooth muscle cells. *Molec. Cell. Endocrinol.* **67**: 195–206.

Napier, M. A., Arcuri, K. E. & Vandlen, R. L. (1986). Binding and internalisation of atrial natriuretic factor by high affinity receptors in A10 smooth muscle cells. *Arch. Biochem. Biophys.* **248**: 516–22.

Northridge, D. B., Jardine, A. G., Alabaster, C. T., Barclay, P. L., Connell, J. M. C., Dargie, H. J., Dilly, S. G. et al. (1989). Effects of UK 69578: a novel atriopeptidase inhibitor. *Lancet* **ii**: 591–3.

Porter, J. G., Scarborough, R. M., Wang, Y., Schenk, D., McEnroe, G. A., Kang, L. L. & Lewicki, J. A. (1989). Recombinant expression of a secreted form of the atrial natriuretic peptide clearance receptor. *J. Biol. Chem.* **264**: 14179–84.

Saheki, T., Shimonaka, M., Uchida, K., Mizuno, T. & Hirose, S. (1989). Immunochemical and biochemical distinction of subtypes of atrial natriuretic peptide receptor. *J. Biochem.* **106**: 627–32.

Scarborough, R. M., Schenk, D. B., McEnroe, G. A., Arfsten, A., Kang, L. L., Schwartz, K. & Lewicki, J. A. (1986). Truncated atrial natriuretic peptide analogs. Comparison between receptor binding and stimulation of cyclic GMP accumulation in cultured vascular smooth muscle cells. *J. Biol. Chem.* **261**: 12960–4.

Schenk, D. B., Phelps, M. N., Porter, J. G., Scarborough, R. M., McEnroe, G. A. & Lewicki, J. A. (1985). Identification of the receptor for atrial natriuretic factor on cultured vascular cells. *J. Biol. Chem.* **260**: 14887–90.

Schiffrin, E. L. (1988). Decreased density of binding sites for atrial natriuretic peptide on platelets with severe congestive heart failure. *Clin. Sci.* **74**: 213–18.

Schiffrin, E. L., Deslongchamps, M. & Thibault, G. (1986). Platelet binding sites for atrial natriuretic factor in humans. Characterization and effects of sodium intake. *Hypertension* **8** (Suppl. II): II6–10.

Shima, M., Seino, Y., Torikai, S. & Imai, M. (1988). Intrarenal localisation of degradation of atrial natriuretic peptide in isolated glomeruli and cortical nephron segments. *Life Sci.* **43**: 357–63.

Uchida, K., Mizuno, T., Shimonaka, M., Sugiura, N., Hagiwara, H. & Hirose, S. (1989a). Subtype switching of ANP receptors during *in vitro* culture of vascular cells. *Am. J. Physiol.* **256**: H311–14.

Vahida, K., Mizuno, T., Shimonaka, M., Sugiura, N., Nara, K., Ling, N., Hagiwara, H. *et al.* (1989b). Purification and properties of active atrial natriuretic peptide receptor (type C) from bovine lung. *Biochem. J.* **263**: 671–8.

Vandlen, R. L., Arcuri, K. E., Hupe, L., Keegan, M. E. & Napier, M. A. (1986). Molecular characteristics of receptors for atrial natriuretic factor. *FASEB J.* **45**: 2366–70.

Waldman, S. A. & Murad, F. (1989). Atrial natriuretic peptides: receptors and second messengers. *Bio Essays* **10**: 16–20.

Waldman, S., Rapoport, R. M., Fiscus, R. R., Leitman, D. C., Chang, L. Y. & Murad, F. (1989). Regulation of particulate guanylate cyclase by atriopeptins: relation between peptide structure, receptor binding and enzyme kinetics. *Biochim. Biophys. Acta* **999**: 157–62.

Chapter 12
Urodilatin (hANF 95–126)—characteristics of a new atrial natriuretic factor peptide

Stephan M. Feller, Hans-Jürgen Mägert, Peter Schulz-Knappe and Wolf-Georg Forssmann

Summary

Urodilatin (URO) is a 32-amino-acid peptide isolated from human urine. Its amino-acid sequence is identical to the 32 C-terminal amino acids of the cardiac peptide hormone named atrial natriuretic factor (ANF). Synonyms for ANF are for instance atrial natriuretic peptide (ANP), atriopeptin (AP) or cardiodilatin (CDD). According to the official nomenclature for ANF (introduced by WHO, ISH and AHA) urodilatin should be named human atrial natriuretic factor 95–126 (hANF 95–126). Interestingly, some results suggest that urodilatin is synthesized in the kidney, despite the fact that no gene expression of the hANF gene was detected using the method of selective amplification by polymerase chain reaction. Although urodilatin could be derived from a different gene, its origin remains to be defined.

The aim of this review is to summarize the results with regards to the origin, molecular form, metabolism and bioactivity of urodilatin in comparison to other natriuretic peptides. According to the data available the bioactivity of urodilatin is in general similar to that of hANF 99–126. As a major contrast, urodilatin is very stable against proteolytic cleavage by endopeptidase 24.11, the major hANF 99–126 degradating activity in the kidney. A high concentration of this enzyme is present in renal tubular membranes. Recent degradation experiments show that porcine brain natriuretic peptide 26, a natriuretic peptide with partial sequence homology to ANF peptides, is cleaved into several fragments by renal

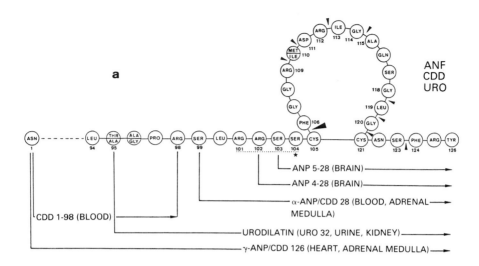

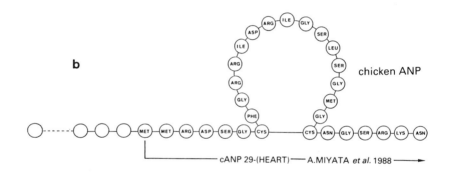

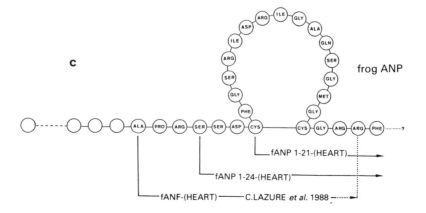

cortex membranes containing endopeptidase 24.11 activity. Considering the high activity of this enzyme in renal proximal tubules, physiological concentrations of circulating hANF 99–126 (and possibly also circulating BNP peptides) are likely to be inactivated during their passage through early parts of the nephron, suggesting that under physiological conditions hANF 99–126 does not reach the functional ANF receptors in the luminal membrane of renal collecting ducts. This idea is supported by the increasing number of studies demonstrating that hANF 99–126 is not a potent natriuretic substance *in vivo* in a physiological dose range. Immunohistochemical data show the presence of urodilatin-immunoreactive (IR) cells in renal distal tubules or collecting ducts depending on the species analysed. If these IR cells secrete urodilatin into the nephron lumen, urodilatin and not hANF 99–126 may be the relevant activator of renal collecting duct ANF receptors *in vivo*.

Introduction

Since the demonstration of a natriuretic activity in rat atrial extracts (Sonnenberg *et al.*, 1980; deBold *et al.*, 1981), an increasing number of natriuretic peptides have been identified in several tissues including heart ventricles, brain, adrenal glands, lung and different vessels (for review see e.g. Forssmann *et al.*, 1989a). During initial attempts to isolate the atrial natriuretic factor (ANF), a variety of bioactive fragments was isolated and sequenced. The full sequences of the human, rat and porcine ANF prohormones, isolated from atrial tissue, were published in 1984 (reviewed by e.g. Forssmann, 1986). Later, the native molecular forms of extra-atrial ANF in body fluids and ANF synthesizing organs were identified (summarized in Fig. 12.1a; for review see Forssmann *et al.*, 1989b).

All these mammalian ANF peptides show a remarkable sequence

Fig. 12.1 (a) Molecular forms of ANF peptides in different organs (for review see Forssmann *et al.*, 1989b). In the heart, the storage form is almost exclusively the 126-amino-acid ANF prohormone (ANF 1–126). Costorage of ANF 1–126 and ANF 99–126 was demonstrated in the chromaffin granules of the adrenal medulla. Two ANF peptides of 24 and 25 amino acids (ANF 102–126, ANF 103–126) have been isolated from porcine brain. Urodilatin (hANF 95–126) is the major form in human urine. In porcine kidney two peptides eluting similar to synthetic ANF 99–126 and ANF 95–126 were detected (Feller *et al.*, 1989d). Of the 30 C-terminal amino acids of the ANF prohormone 1–126 only position 110 differs among all mammalian species analysed to date. Arrowheads indicate the enzymatic cleavage sites that have been reported in studies with ANF 99–126 or shorter ANF peptides. (b) 'Chicken ANP' (Miyata *et al.*, 1988). A 29-amino-acid peptide has been isolated from chicken heart. The chicken ANP sequence is more closely related to BNP peptides than to the mammalian ANF peptides. No information on the nucleic-acid sequence of chicken ANP is available. (c) 'Frog ANP' (Lazure *et al.*, 1988; Sakata, Kangawa & Matsuo, 1988). Three fragments consisting of 21, 24 and 26 amino acids have been isolated so far. Like chicken ANP, frog ANP shows a higher homology to the C-terminus of the presently known mammalian BNP peptides than to the mammalian ANF peptides. The cDNA sequence is not known so far.

homology at the C-terminal region of the prohormone. Additionally, a variety of sequentially related natriuretic peptides (brain natriuretic peptides (BNPs), iso-rat atrial natriuretic peptide, chicken ANF and frog ANF; see Fig. 12.1b and c, Fig. 12.2a–c and Fig. 12.3a for sequences and references) were isolated from mammalian and non-mammalian heart and brain. These peptides are derived from mRNAs with relatively weak homology to the mammalian ANF-mRNAs. It appears that only the size of the ring structure generated by an intramolecular disulphide bond and small epitopes of the molecule are conserved in all cases. A schematic drawing of the 'general structure' of the presently known ANF-type peptides is shown in Fig. 12.3b.

Renal sites with receptors for natriuretic peptides

The initial studies of A. J. deBold and H. Sonnenberg (deBold et al., 1981; Sonnenberg et al., 1982) indicated that the kidney is an important target organ for ANF peptide(s). As early as 1984, shortly after the first ANF sequence data were available, high-affinity ANF binding sites for synthetic ANF were demonstrated in membrane preparations from renal cortex of rat and rabbit and in the porcine renal cell line LLC-PK$_1$ (Napier et al., 1984). This publication also demonstrated that the binding affinity of different ANF analogues correlates with their natriuretic potency in vivo. Further investigations showed the location of binding sites in the basolateral membrane of the renal cortex (Hori et al., 1985). C. C. Yip and colleagues purified a protein, migrating as a 140-kDa band from the renal cortex of rat, with the capacity to bind ANF specifically (Yip, Laing & Flynn, 1985).

Since then, by means of autoradiography and other methods, binding sites have been localized and partly characterized as functional receptors in renal arterial vasculature, glomeruli, proximal tubules and inner medullary collecting ducts (IMCDs) (Murphy et al., 1985; Healy & Fanestil, 1986; Bianchi et al., 1987; Shimonaka et al., 1987; Yamamoto, Ogura & Ota, 1987; Brucksch et al., 1988; Gunning et al., 1988), suggesting multiple sites of action for ANF within the kidney. The existence of different types of receptors has also been documented. Almost 99 % of the renal receptors seem to be clearance receptors (Maack et al., 1987).

Renal actions of natriuretic peptides

Today it is generally accepted that natriuretic peptides of the ANF-type increase sodium chloride, and urea excretion, and multiple sites of action have been detected (for review see Genest & Cantin 1988; Goetz, 1988; and article, this volume). Our idea is that other natriuretic peptides apart from circulating ANF 99–126 interact with natriuretic peptide receptors in the kidney.

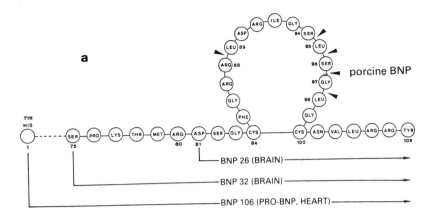

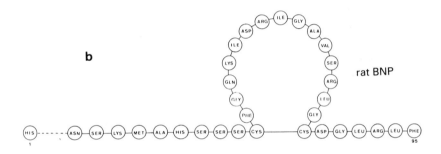

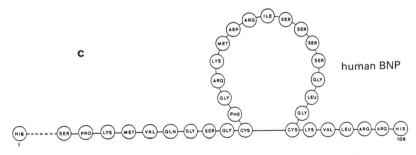

Fig. 12.2 Brain natriuretic peptides (BNPs). (a) Porcine BNP. The 26-amino-acid form from brain was the first BNP peptide known (Sudoh *et al.*, 1988a). Later, a 32-amino-acid peptide and a prohormone of 106 amino acids were isolated from the porcine heart (Minamino, Kangawa & Matsuo, 1988; Sudoh *et al.*, 1988b). As deduced from the cDNA sequences (Maekawa *et al.*, 1988; Porter *et al.*, 1989), this prohormone is generated by the removal of a 25-amino-acid signal peptide from the initially synthesized preprohormone of 131 amino acids. (b,c) At present, the BNP peptide sequences from rat (b) and man (c) can only be deduced from the cloned cDNA sequences (Kojima *et al.*, 1989; Sudoh *et al.*, 1989). However, rat BNP is very similar to iso-rat-ANP, a peptide isolated very recently by Flynn *et al.* (1989) (see Fig. 12.3).

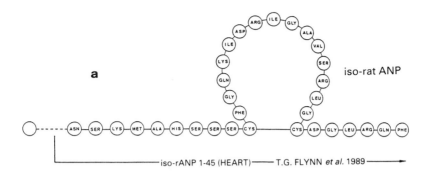

iso-rat ANP

iso-rANP 1-45 (HEART) ——— T.G. FLYNN *et al.* 1989 ———▶

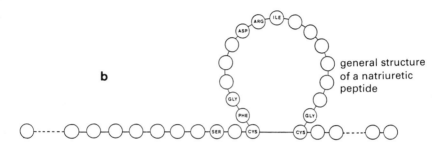

general structure
of a natriuretic
peptide

Fig. 12.3 (a) 'Iso-rat-ANP', a new natriuretic peptide, was recently isolated from rat atria (Flynn *et al.*, 1989). It has to be determined whether the 45-amino-acid peptide that has been published is a native molecular form or a fragment of a longer molecule that is stored in the atria. Iso-rat-ANP is almost identical to the rat BNP deduced from the nucleotide sequence of a cloned rat cDNA (Kojima *et al.*, 1989). Only two different amino acids appear between rat BNP and iso-rat-ANP (in positions 6 and 44 of iso-rat-ANP). Thus it seems very likely that the peptides named 'iso-rat-ANP' and 'rat BNP' are identical. Further sequence studies of peptides and DNA sequences are necessary to decide whether an incorrect sequencing or a natural variability (which could possibly be detected as a restriction fragment length polymorphism) explain these differences. (b) General structure of an 'ANF-type' natriuretic peptide. As far as we know, all ANF-type natriuretic peptides are derived from a preprohormone of approximately 120–150 amino acids from which a signal peptide and a large N-terminal peptide are removed during the processing into a native natriuretic and vasorelaxant molecule. Although a relatively large variation occurs in the amino-acid sequences, the derived C-terminal peptides share some striking similarities which could be explained by a conservation of the native receptors. However, only nine of the C-terminal amino acids in the presently known ANF-type natriuretic peptides are conserved throughout all mammalian and non-mammalian species. The number of amino acids in the ring structure formed by a disulphide bond is always constant and a C-terminal elongation of the peptide for at least five amino acids after this loop structure appears. Thus it seems likely that the ANF-type peptides are derived from a common ancestor peptide. The detection of ANF-IR in an invertebrate organism and the presence of vasorelaxant activity in partially purified peptide extracts from this IR tissue (Nehls *et al.*, 1985) indicates that an ANF-type natriuretic peptide may have existed before the first vertebrate appeared.

The structural and sequential similarity of ANF and BNP indicate that circulating brain natriuretic peptides are additional candidates for an interaction with natriuretic peptide receptors in the kidney. A recent study demonstrated the competitive binding of rANF 103–126 and porcine BNP 26 in heart and kidney (Oehlenschlager *et al.*, 1989).

ANF peptides have been reported to decrease renin release *in vivo*, but not in isolated afferent arterioles (Itoh *et al.*, 1987). ANF was shown to dilatate these arterioles, while postglomerular arterioles are constricted (Marin-Grez, Fleming & Steinhausen, 1986). This may explain at least in part the increase of the glomerular filtration rate that has been observed in many studies. Additionally, other glomerular sites of action have been reported (see, e.g. Meyer-Lehnert *et al.*, 1988). In proximal tubules ANF inhibits angiotensin-stimulated reabsorption of sodium and water (Harris, Thomas & Morgan, 1987) and the resorption of phosphate (Hammond, Haramati & Knox, 1985; Nakai *et al.*, 1988; Yusufi *et al.*, 1989). Despite an enormous number of publications on renal actions of ANF, there is still a lot of controversy about the function and major renal action site of endogenous, circulating ANF *in vivo*. Many functional studies have been carried out with pharmacological ANF doses or with isolated kidneys, renal vessels and nephron segments, some of them with truncated analogues of the circulating ANF 99–126. Thus many studies do not present data which are relevant to ANF 99–126 *in vivo*.

In contrast, in some studies ANF infused in low doses has increased plasma ANF in a physiological and pathophysiological range (e.g. Anderson *et al.*, 1987; Banks, 1988; Firth, Raine & Ledingham, 1988). Although these results are controversial to some extent, in all these studies relatively small effects on natriuresis, diuresis, renal haemodynamics and nephron transport mechanisms were detected. Several recent reports cast doubt on the hypothesis that circulating ANF 99–126 has a major effect on the regulation of natriuresis and diuresis (Brown, 1988; Goetz, 1988).

The natriuretic effects of atrial extracts on the collecting duct had been demonstrated by microcatheterization in 1982 (Briggs *et al.*, 1982; Sonnenberg *et al.*, 1982). Subsequently, an ANF-mediated inhibition of the IMCD sodium transport (Sonnenberg *et al.*, 1986), and an increase of cGMP levels by ANF up to 20-fold was demonstrated in IMCD (Nonoguchi, Knepper & Manganiello, 1987; Nonoguchi, Sands & Knepper, 1988). In isolated IMCD cells a single class of specific high-affinity receptors of 130 kDa is present on the cellular surface (Gunning *et al.*, 1988). In these cells Na^+-transport-dependent O_2 consumption is inhibited (Zeidel *et al.*, 1988) and intracellular cGMP is increased (Zeidel *et al.*, 1987) by ANF. With the patch clamp technique it was demonstrated that either 10^{-5} M dibutyryl-cGMP or 10^{-11} M ANF inhibit single-ion channels in the apical membrane of IMCD cells (Light *et al.*, 1989). Chronic heart failure reduces the ANF binding of the renal medulla

(Tsunoda *et al.*, 1988). Hildebrandt & Banks (1987) have reported that a functional renal papilla does not seem to be required for the action of ANF peptides, while others (e.g. Borenstein *et al.*, 1983; Fried, Osgood & Stein, 1988) have reported effects of atrial extracts or ANF peptides on papillary collecting ducts. However, the high concentration of ANF 99–126 degradating activity in renal proximal tubules suggest that only vascular effects of ANF could occur in the renal papilla and collecting duct rather than any direct tubular effects at these sites.

ANF peptides and urodilatin in kidney and urine

Renal ANF-immunoreactive material (ANF-IR) was first analysed in rats by Sakamoto *et al.* (1985). A relatively large amount of ANF-IR (approximately 5 ng/g tissue, predominantly in the cortex) was detected, but the renal ANF-IR eluted like rANF 99–126 and no high-molecular-weight ANF-IR was detectable. Thus an extra renal origin of the ANF-IR was suggested. Similarly, the localization of ANF-IR cells in intercalating cells of rat renal collecting ducts (McKenzie *et al.*, 1985) has contributed to the idea that renal collecting ducts contain ANF-responsive cells or a non-specific uptake of ANF might occur. Flügge, Inagami & Fuchs (1987) detected ANF-IR in the straight part of renal distal tubules in inner cortex and outer medulla of the tree shrew (Tupaia belangeri). Smaller amounts were found in the perinuclear region of collecting duct cells.

The first quantitative analysis and partial biochemical characterization of ANF-IR in the urine of healthy volunteers were published by Marumo *et al.* and Greenwald, McLaughlin & Needleman in 1986. In these studies no difference between the major plasma form of ANF-IR or synthetic hANF 99–126 and urinary ANF-IR, which eluted as a single peak on a gelfiltration column, was observed. Thus Greenwald *et al.* (1986) suggested an excretion of circulating hANF 99–126 into the urine. However, no correlation between the ANF-IR levels in plasma and urine was detected by RIA (Marumo *et al.*, 1987; Mißbichler *et al.*, 1988). In contrast to the study with healthy volunteers (Marumo *et al.*, 1986), the presence of high-molecular-weight ANF-IR in urine of patients with renal diseases (Marumo *et al.*, 1987) was reported. A new 32-amino-acid ANF peptide was isolated as bioactive ANF-IR from human urine (Schulz-Knappe *et al.*, 1988). It was named urodilatin (URO) and is the main, and maybe only, molecular form of ANF-IR in human urine.

Several groups have identified circulating forms of ANF peptides from blood (Arendt *et al.*, 1985; Miyata *et al.*, 1985, 1987; Schwartz *et al.*, 1985; Thibault *et al.*, 1985; Ogawa *et al.*, 1987; Theiss *et al.*, 1987; Yandle *et al.*, 1987) or haemofiltrate (Forssmann *et al.*, 1986), but up to now this 32-amino-acid peptide has not been detected in blood. Although it is possible to separate urodilatin (hANF 95–126) from hANF 99–126 by cation exchange HPLC and RP-HPLC (Dörner et al., 1989b), its elution pattern from most columns used in the characterization of the circulating ANF forms are very similar. Thus it seems unlikely that a circulating hANF 95–126 peptide would not have been detected during the isolation if it were present in more than trace amounts. These results, together with the immunohistochemical data from different species (McKenzie et al., 1985; Flügge et al., 1987; Feller et al., 1988a) and the lack of correlation between ANF-IR concentration in plasma and urine (Marumo et al., 1987) raised the possibility that an intrarenal source of ANF-like peptide(s) existed.

Studies to identify the origin of urodilatin

Our approach to identify the origin of urodilatin followed different strategies. Immunohistochemical studies on renal sections of different mammals were performed with segment-specific antibodies against N-terminal and C-terminal epitopes of the ANF prohormone. A polyclonal antiserum against a heptapeptide representing the N-terminus of urodilatin was raised and used for immunohistochemistry. Very recently, a radioimmunoassay which seems to be capable of discriminating between hANF 99–126 and hANF 95–126 has been established using this antiserum (unpublished data). ANF-IR from porcine kidney was extracted and highly purified. The bioactivity of the ANF-IR was controlled during the purification by a vascular smooth muscle relaxation assay. A 40 mer oligonucleotide labelled with high specific activity was used for blot hybridizations to poly(A)$^+$RNA from human renal cortex and medulla/papilla. Just before this manuscript was completed, poly(A)$^+$RNA blots were hybridized with a random-prime-labelled human cDNA probe and a combination of cDNA synthesis and sequence-specific cDNA amplification by the polymerase chain reaction technique (PCR) was applied to poly(A)$^+$RNA from porcine kidney. The obtained PCR fragments were isolated, cloned and sequenced.

With the antibody against the C-terminus of the ANF prohormone we obtained an immunohistochemical staining of distal tubular cells or collecting ducts depending on the species analysed (Feller et al., 1988b, 1989d). Antibodies directed against the N-terminal region of ANF 1–126 gave a much weaker staining, indicating that—if renal synthesis occurs—the prohormone is not a major storage form. Using the urodilatin (ANF 95–126) antiserum, a staining similar to that obtained with the C-terminal antibody was detected (Feller et al., 1989d). As mentioned above, this antiserum was reported to discriminate between hANF 99–126 and hANF 95–126. During the purification of ANF-IR, which occurs at a concentration of approximately 1 pmol/g tissue in porcine kidney, trace amounts of IR material eluting with a higher molecular weight than ANF 99–126 and urodilatin were detected (Feller et al., 1989d). After several purification steps the low-molecular-weight ANF-IR was separated on an analytical ion exchange HPLC column able to separate synthetic ANF 99–126 from ANF 95–126.

Radioimmunoassay of the obtained fractions demonstrated two peaks of ANF-IR. The major peak, representing at least 75% of the total ANF-IR, eluted like synthetic ANF 95–126, the minor peak like ANF 99–126 (Feller et al., 1989d). Isolation of poly(A)$^+$RNA from human kidney and hybridization with a 40-mer oligonucleotide complementary to the part of the ANF-mRNA which codes for the C-terminus of the prohormone gave signals on dot blots (Feller et al., 1988b). However, the intensity was very low and no signals were seen on northern blots.

This result was contributed to by the lower detection sensitivity of the northern blot method. Thus, after first-strand cDNA synthesis with poly(A)$^+$RNA from auricle and kidney, we used the PCR method to amplify ANF-related cDNA sequences. Two 22-mer oligonucleotides coding for regions in the DNA sequences representing the N-terminal and C-terminal amino acids of the preprohormone and some nucleotides of the untranslated 3′- and 5′-mRNA region were used as primers. The PCR was performed with different primer annealing temperatures and the PCR products were then separated on an agarose gel. The annealing temperature was increased until no PCR products appeared anymore. The obtained bands were excised, the DNA was extracted, cloned into pUC 19 and sequenced. Surprisingly, even in the PCR with the highest annealing temperature only DNA sequences not related to the known ANF sequences were identified in porcine kidney (H. J. Mägert et al., unpublished data). This result indicates that the ANF gene is not expressed in the kidney. However, the presence of PCR products when using ANF–mRNA complementary primers might explain the obtained blot hybridization signals. This leaves the origin of the urodilatin-IR in the kidney, and urine, still to be established.

Renal degradation of hANF 99–126 and urodilatin

The function of the different natriuretic peptides in the activation of renal receptors cannot be determined without an analysis of their renal catabolism. At present, degradation experiments have been carried out with hANF 99–126 and shorter ANF molecules (reviewed by, e.g. Gagelmann et al., 1989), urodilatin (Gagelmann, Hock & Forssmann, 1988) and with porcine brain natriuretic peptide (pBNP 26; Vogt-Schaden et al., 1989).

Tang et al. (1984) documented that the kidney has the highest ANF degradating activity when compared to liver, lung, heart and plasma. An extensive degradation of hANF 99–126 by renal brush border membranes was reported by Hori et al. (1985). Further studies indicated that proteolytic degradation rather than excretion accounts for a large proportion of ANF clearance in the kidney (Luft et al., 1986). A detailed

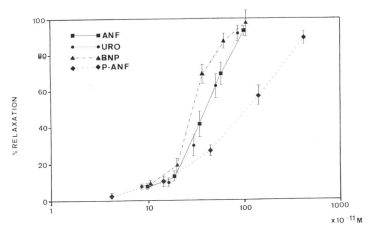

Fig. 12.4 Vasodilatory activity of urodilatin and other natriuretic peptides. To determine the vasorelaxant potency of urodilatin in comparison to ANF 99–126 and other peptides, vascular strips of rabbit thoracic aorta were equilibrated in a physiologic solution with a pretension of 2 g. Different doses of test substances were applicated ($x =$ 5–10) after the precontraction induced by norepinephrine (10^{-7} M) had reached a plateau. The vasodilatative potency (% relaxation, results given as mean $\pm$ s.d.) is defined as the antagonization of the norepinephrine-induced contraction (defined as 100%). According to our results hANF 99–126 (abbreviated as ANF in the explanation of symbols) and urodilatin are equipotent, while porcine BNP 26 (BNP) tends to be slightly more potent. Phosphorylation of Ser 104 in ANF 99–126 (P-ANF) strongly diminishes the vasodilatative potency. This has also been demonstrated for urodilatin (see text).

study on the degradation of hANF 103–126 (atriopeptin III) detected cleavage in several positions (Olins *et al.*, 1986).

In contrast, HPLC analysis in similar experiments with hANF 99–126 and rANF 99–126 showed a single, newly generated peak representing the vast majority of peptide. This material turned out to be a 'full-size' molecule with a cleaved Cys[105]–Phe[106] bond but an intact disulphide bridge (Koehn *et al.*, 1987; Olins *et al.*, 1987; Stephenson & Kenny, 1987a; Bertrand & Doble, 1988). This cleavage between Cys and Phe opens the loop structure which is essential for the bioactivity of ANF peptides. Inhibition studies suggested a metalloendoprotease with an alkaline pH optimum as the cleaving enzyme (Koehn *et al.*, 1987). Similar results were obtained with purified endopeptidase 24.11 (EC 3.4.24.11; Stephenson & Kenny, 1987a). In addition, minor cleavage products and products of secondary degradation steps which take place after the initial attack on the Cys–Phe bond have also been characterized (Stephenson & Kenny, 1987a; Kenny & Stephenson, 1988; Vanneste *et al.*, 1988).

Endopeptidase 24.11 (or enkephalinase; see Hersh, 1986) is present in renal proximal tubules in a high concentration and is thought to play a key role in the inactivation of several bioactive peptides (Stephenson & Kenny, 1987b). This is also the case for the inactivation of circulating ANF 99–126 (Sonnenberg *et al.*, 1988; Gagelmann *et al.*, 1989). A detailed investigation of the ANF degradation sites in the nephron has been presented by Berg *et al.* (1988). These experiments show that the proximal tubules are in fact the major site of renal ANF catabolism. The recent publication of Olins *et al.* (1989) has shown that specific inhibition of endopeptidase 24.11 decreases the elimination of exogenous ANF 103–126 from the circulation. The arrow heads in Fig. 12.1a point out the cleavage sites of ANF 99–126 or shorter ANF peptides that have been reported so far (see also Gagelmann *et al.*, 1989). Porcine BNP (pBNP 26) is the only BNP peptide analysed in degradation experiments to date. Renal cortical membranes with endopeptidase 24.11 activity cleave pBNP 26 at several sites (Vogt-Schaden *et al.*, 1989; cleavage sites are indicated by the arrowheads in Fig. 12.2a).

In summary, hANF 99–126 is most likely cleared from the luminal fluid in the early parts of the nephron (Kenny & Stephenson, 1988) and thus does not seem to be of significant importance for the activation of luminal receptors in the renal medulla. This may also be true for circulating BNP peptides. Furthermore, it seems unlikely that the ANF-IR identified in urine can be attributed to an excretion of circulating hANF 99–126. The isolation of urodilatin from human urine (Schulz-Knappe *et al.*, 1988) suggested that this ANF peptide might pass through the kidney and be stable against endopeptidase 24.11. In fact urodilatin is not activated when incubated with renal membrane preparations which cleave hANF 99–126 similar to endopeptidase 24.11 (Gagelmann *et al.*, 1988). Thus, urodilatin may be the physiological activator of luminal natriuretic peptide receptors in the renal IMCDs.

Biological properties of urodilatin in comparison with other natriuretic peptides

Parallel to the approaches to identify the origin of urodilatin, we have undertaken different studies to compare the biological activities of urodilatin with other natriuretic peptides. Besides the degradation experiments (Gagelmann *et al.*, 1988) mentioned above, we have analysed the effects of urodilatin *in vivo* on haemodynamic and renal parameters, plasma, hormone levels, urodilatin receptor binding and the activation of guanylate cyclase in isolated membranes and tissues.

First details of the bioactivity of urodilatin *in vivo* have been investigated in dogs with and without congestive heart failure (Riegger *et al.*, 1988, 1989, 1990). The haemodynamic effects of hANF 99–126 and urodilatin are very similar, but in contrast to hANF 99–126, urodilatin did not suppress renin and aldosterone secretion. A 2.4-fold increase of urine flow and sodium excretion occurred in dogs with congestive heart failure after urodilatin. These effects were not seen with hANF 99–126. The greater natriuretic and diuretic activity of urodilatin may be explained by

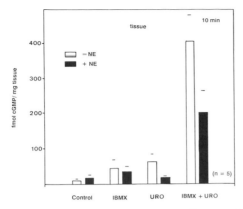

Fig. 12.5 Effects of urodilatin on cyclic guanosine monophosphate in aortic tissue. Urodilatin induces a rapid increase of cGMP in vascular tissue of rabbit thoracic aorta. The maximum increase is observed after approximately 2 min and a partial decrease of cGMP response (in the range of 20 %) occurs if the endothelium is detroyed (data not shown). 3-isobutyl-1-methyl-xanthine (IBMX, 10^{-4} M) a phosphodiesterase inhibitor, decreases the breakdown of cGMP but has only minor effects on cAMP. It is therefore a useful tool to study the cGMP response of small tissue samples. The cGMP increase induced by urodilatin (10^{-7} M) is reduced by the addition of norepinephrine (NE, 10^{-7} M). Results are shown as mean $\pm$ s.d.

the low sensitivity of urodilatin against endopeptidase 24.11, which could enable this substance to reach luminal medullary collecting duct receptors in bioactive concentrations.

The vasodilatory effects of urodilatin and hANF 99–126 are almost identical (Feller *et al.*, 1989a,b,c; see also Fig. 12.4). Like other natriuretic peptides, physiological (10^{-10} M) and pharmacological doses of urodilatin increase cGMP rapidly and in a dose-dependent manner (Feller *et al.*, 1989a). We have used rabbit aortic tissue rather than primary cultures of vascular smooth muscle cells because a receptor subtype switch during culture has been reported in these cells (Uchida *et al.*, 1989). The cGMP increase is diminished by norepinephrine (see Fig. 12.5) or phosphorylation of serine 104 (Dörner *et al.*, 1989a) in urodilatin. Furthermore, ANF receptors which are not human platelet coupled to guanylate cyclase show a single binding site for urodilatin and no difference between the binding affinities of ANF 99–126 and urodilatin (Heim *et al.*, 1989). In contrast to this, bovine adrenal cortex membranes containing predominantly guanylate cyclase coupled receptors bind urodilatin with higher affinity (K_d: 30 pM) than hANF 99–126 (K_d: 52 pM), but the resulting stimulatory effect on cGMP generation is similar (Heim *et al.*, 1989).

Suggestions on the function of urodilatin (hANF 95–126)

At the present state of knowledge only speculations on the origin and function of urodilatin *in vivo* are possible. This is, however, to a large extent also the case for circulating hANF 99–126. The intrarenal localization of urodilatin IR cells, together with the presence of urodilatin in urine indicate a luminal secretion into the nephron. Its stability against endopeptidase 24.11 and its similarity in most cases to the biological activity of hANF 99–126 makes it a good candidate as the natural substance to activate luminal medullary collecting duct receptors for natriuretic peptides. The apparent activity in dogs suffering CHF could enable urodilatin to play a future role in the treatment of patients with fluid and sodium retention due to congestive heart failure.

References

Anderson, J. V., Donckier, J., Payne, N. N., Beacham, J., Slater, J. D. H. & Bloom, S. R. (1987). Atrial natriuretic peptide: Evidence of action as a natriuretic hormone at physiological plasma concentrations in man. *Clin. Sci.* **72**: 305–12.

Arendt, R. M., Stangl, E., Zähringer, J., Liebisch, D. C. & Herz, A. (1985). Demonstration and characterization of alpha-human atrial natriuretic factor in human plasma. *FEBS Lett.* **189**: 57–61.

Banks, R. O. (1988). Effects of a physiological dose of ANP on renal function in dog. *Am. J. Physiol.* **255**: F907–10.

Berg, J. A., Hayashi, M., Fujii, Y. & Katz, A. I. (1988). Renal metabolism of atrial natriuretic peptide in the rat. *Am. J. Physiol.* **255**: F466–73.

Bertrand, P. & Doble, A. (1988). Degradation of atrial natriuretic peptides by an enzyme in rat kidney resembling neutral endopeptidase 24.11. *Biochem. Pharmacol.* **37**: 3817–21.

Bianchi, C., Gutkowska, J., Garcia, R., Thibault, G., Genest, J. & Cantin, M. (1987). Localization of ¹²⁵I-atrial natriuretic factor (ANF)-binding sites in rat renal medulla. A light and electron microscope autoradiographic study. *J. Histochem. Cytochem.* **35**: 149–53.

Borenstein, H. B., Cupples, W. A., Sonnenberg, H. & Veress, A. T. (1983). The effect of a natriuretic atrial extract on renal hemodynamics and urinary excretion in anaesthetized rats. *J. Physiol.* **334**: 133–40.

Briggs, J. P., Steipe, B., Schubert, G. & Schnermann, J. (1982). Micropuncture studies of the renal effects of atrial natriuretic substance. *Pflügers Arch.* **395**: 271–6.

Brown, J. (1988). Is α-ANP primarily a natriuretic hormone? *Trends Pharmacol. Sci.* **9**: 312–14.

Bruksch, A., Gröne, H. J., Talartschik, J. & Fuchs, E. (1988). Binding sites of atrial natriuretic peptide in human renal tissue—Quantification by *in vitro* receptor autoradiography. *Klin. Wochenschr.* **66**: 303–7.

deBold, A. J., Borenstein, H. B., Veress, T. & Sonnenberg, H. (1981). A rapid and potent natriuretic response to intravenous injection of atrial myocardial extracts in rats. *Life Sci.* **28**: 89–94.

Dörner, Th., Gagelmann, M., Feller, S., Herbst, F. & Forssmann, W. G. (1989a). Phosphorylation and dephosphorylation of the natriuretic peptide urodilatin (CDD/ANP-95-126) and the effect on the biological activity. *Biochem. Biophys. Res. Commun.* **163**: 830–5.

Dörner, Th., Gagelmann, M., Hock, D., Herbst, F. & Forssmann, W. G. (1989b). Separation of synthetic cardiodilatin/atrial natriuretic factor and related peptides by RP-HPLC. *J. Chromatogr.* **490**: 411–17.

Feller, S. M., Bub, A., Gagelmann, M. & Forssmann, W. G. (1989a). Natriuretic peptides from heart brain and kidney: Localization, processing, vasoactivity and proteolytic degradation. In: *Heart Failure—Mechanisms and Management* (Kimchi, A. & Lewis, B. S., eds). (in press).

Feller, S. M., Christmann, M., Bub, A., Dörner, Th. & Forssmann, W. G. (1989b). Vasorelaxation of rabbit arteries by different natriuretic peptide hormones and their derivatives. *Eur. J. Cell Biol.* **48** (Suppl. 26): 18.

Feller, S. M., Christmann, M., Dörner, Th., Bub, A., Gagelmann, M. & Forssmann, W. G. (1989c). Characteristics and mechanisms of vasodilatation induced by natriuretic peptides. *J. Vasc. Biol. Med.* **1**: 169.

Feller, S. M., Gagelmann, M. & Forssmann, W. G. (1989d). Urodilatin: a newly described member of the ANP family. *Trends Pharmacol. Sci.* **10**: 93–4.

Feller, S. M., Meyer, M., Hock, D. & Forssmann, W. G. (1988a). Extraaurilüläre lokalisationen von cardiodilatin. *Acta Anatom.* **132**: 80.

Feller, S. M., Schulz-Knappe, P. & Forssmann, W. G. (1988b). The kidney, a paracrine, urodilatin-producing organ. *Circulation* **78** (Suppl. II): II429.

Firth, J. D., Raine, A. E. G. & Ledingham, J. G. G. (1988). Low concentrations of ANP cause pressure-dependent natriuresis in the isolated kidney. *Am. J. Physiol.* **255**: F391–6.

Flügge, G., Inagami, T. & Fuchs, E. (1987). Atrial natriuretic peptide detected by immunocytochemistry in peripheral organs of Tupaia belangeri. *Histochemistry* **86**: 479–83.

Flynn, T. G., Brar, A., Tremblay, L., Sarda, I., Lyons, C. & Jennings, D. B. (1989). Isolation and characterization of iso-rANP, a new natriuretic peptide from rat atria. *Biochem. Biophys. Res. Commun.* **161**: 830–7.

Forssmann, W. G. (1986). Cardiac hormones. I. Review on the morphology, biochemistry and molecular biology of the endocrine heart. *Eur. J. Clin. Invest.* **16**: 439–51.

Forssmann, K., Hock, D., Herbst, F., Schulz-Knappe, P., Talartschik, J., Scheler, F. & Forssmann, W. G. (1986). Isolation of the circulating human cardiodilatin (alpha ANP). *Klin. Wochenschr.* **64**: 1276–80.

Forssmann, W. G., Feller, S. M., Meyer, M. & Schulz-Knappe, P. (1989a). Morphology of the myoendocrine cardiac cell and extra-auricular systems producing cardiac hormones. In: *Endocrinology of the heart* (Kaufmann, W. & Wambach, G., eds). Heidelberg, Tokyo, New York: Springer-Verlag, pp. 3–26 (in press).

Forssmann, W. G., Nokihara, K., Gagelmann, M., Hock, D., Feller, S., Schulz-Knappe, P. & Herbst, F. (1989b). The heart is the center of a new endocrine, paracrine and neuroendocrine system. *Arch. Histol. Cytol.* **52** (Suppl.) 293–315.

Fried, T. A., Osgood, R. W. & Stein, J. H. (1988). Tubular site(s) of action of atrial natriuretic peptide in the rat. *Am. J. Physiol.* **255**: F313–16.

Gagelmann, M., Feller, S., Hock, D., Schulz-Knappe, P. & Forssmann, W. G. (1989). Biochemistry of the differential release, processing and degradation of cardiac and related peptide hormones. In: *Endocrinology of the Heart* (Kaufmann, W. & Wambach, G., eds). Heidelberg, Tokyo, New York: Springer-Verlag, pp. 27–40.

Gagelmann, M., Hock, D. & Forssmann, W. G. (1988). Urodilatin (CDD/ANP 95–126) is not biologically inactivated by a peptidase from dog kidney cortex membranes in contrast to atrial natriuretic peptide/cardiodilatin (α-hANP/CDD-99–126). *FEBS Lett.* **233**: 249–54.

Genest, J. & Cantin, M. (1988). The atrial natriuretic factor: its physiology and biochemistry. *Rev. Physiol. Biochem. Pharmacol.* **110**: 1–145.

Goetz, K. L. (1988). Physiology and pathophysiology of atrial peptides. *Am. J. Physiol.* **254**: E1–15.

Greenwald, J., McLaughlin, L. & Needleman, P. (1986). Atriopeptide excretion in human urine. *Fed. Proc.* **45**: 912.

Gunning, M. E., Ballermann, B. J., Silva, P., Brenner, B. M. & Zeidel, M. L. (1988). Characterization of ANP receptors in rabbit inner medullary collecting duct cells. *Am. J. Physiol.* **255**: F324–30.

Hammond, T. G., Haramati, A. & Knox, F. G. (1985). Synthetic atrial natriuretic factor decreases renal tubular phosphate reabsorption in rats. *Am. J. Physiol.* **249**: F315–18.

Harris, P. J., Thomas, D. & Morgan, T. O. (1987). Atrial natriuretic peptide inhibits angiotensin-stimulated proximal tubular sodium and water reabsorption. *Nature* **326**: 697–8.

Healy, D. P. & Fanestil, D. D. (1986). Localization of atrial natriuretic peptide binding sites within the rat kidney. *Am. J. Physiol.* **250**: F573–8.

Heim, J.-M., Kiefersauer, S., Fülle, H.-J. & Gerzer, R. (1989). Urodilatin and β-ANF: Binding properties and activation of particulate guanylate cyclase. *Biochem. Biophys. Res. Commun.* **163**: 37–41.

Hersh, L. B. (1986). Nomenclature for enkephalin degrading peptidases. *Life Sci.* **38**: 1151–3.

Hildebrandt, D. A. & Banks, R. O. (1987). Effect of atrial natriuretic factor on renal function in rats with papillary necrosis. *Am. J. Physiol.* **252**: F977–80.

Hori, R., Inui, K.-I., Saito, H., Matsukawa, Y., Okumura, K., Nakao, K., Morii, N. *et al.* (1985). Specific receptors for atrial natriuretic polypeptide on basolateral membranes isolated from rat renal cortex. *Biochem. Biophys. Res. Commun.* **129**: 773–9.

Itoh, S., Abe, K., Nushiro, N., Omata, K., Yasujima, M. & Yoshinaga, K. (1987). Effect of atrial natriuretic factor on renin release in isolated afferent arterioles. *Kidney Int.* **32**: 493–7.

Kenny, A. J. & Stephenson, S. L. (1988). Role of endopeptidase-24.11 in the inactivation of atrial natriuretic peptide. *FEBS Lett.* **232**: 1–8.

Koehn, J. A., Norman, J. A., Jones, B. N., LeSueur, L., Sakane, Y. & Ghai, R. D. (1987). Degradation of atrial natriuretic factor by kidney cortex membranes. *J. Biol. Chem.* **262**: 11 623–7.

Kojima, M., Minamino, N., Kangawa, K. & Matsuo, H. (1989). Cloning and sequence analysis of a cDNA encoding a precursor for rat brain natriuretic peptide. *Biochem. Biophys. Res. Commun.* **159**: 1420–6.

Lazure, C., Ong, H., McNicoll, N., Netchitailo, P., Chretien, M., De Lean, A. & Vaudry, H. (1988). The amino acid sequence of frog heart atrial natriuretic-like peptide and mammalian ANF are closely related. *FEBS Lett.* **238**: 300–6.

Light, D. B., Schwiebert, E. M., Karlson, K. H. & Stanton, B. A. (1989). Atrial natriuretic peptide inhibits a cation channel in renal inner medullary collecting duct cells. *Science* **243**: 383–5.

Luft, F. C. *et al.* (1986). Atriopeptin III kinetics and pharmacodynamics in normal and anephric rats. *J. Pharmacol. Exp. Therapeut.* **236**: 416–18.

McKenzie, J. C., Tanaka, I., Misono, K. S. & Inagami, T. (1985). Immunocytochemical localization of atrial natriuretic factor in the kidney, adrenal medulla, pituitary and atrium of rat. *J. Histochem. Cytochem.* **33**: 828–32.

Maack, T., Suzuki, M., Almeida, F. A., Nussenzweig, D., Scarborough, R. M., McEnroe, G. A. & Lewicki, J. A. (1987). Physiological role of silent receptors of atrial natriuretic factor. *Science* **238**: 675–8.

Maekawa, K., Sudoh, T., Furusawa, M., Minamino, N., Kangawa, K., Ohkubo, H., Nakanishi, S. *et al.* (1988). Cloning and sequence analysis of cDNA encoding a precursor for porcine brain natriuretic peptide. *Biochem. Biophys. Res. Commun.* **157**: 410–16.

Marin-Grez, M., Fleming, J. T. & Steinhausen, M. (1986). Atrial natriuretic peptide causes pre-glomerular vasodilatation and post-glomerular vasoconstriction in rat kidney. *Nature* **324**: 473–6.

Marumo, F., Sakamoto, H., Ando, K., Ishigami, T. & Kawakami, M. (1986). A highly sensitive radioimmunoassay of atrial natriuretic peptide (ANP) in human plasma and urine. *Biochem. Biophys. Res. Commun.* **137**: 231–6.

Marumo, F., Umetani, N., Sakamoto, H., Ando, K. & Ishigami, T. (1987). Characterization of atrial natriuretic peptide (ANP) in plasma and urine in renal diseases. *Kidney Int.* **31**: 278.

Meyer-Lehnert, H., Tsai, P., Caramelo, C. & Schrier, R. W. (1988). ANF inhibits vasopressin-induced Ca^{2+} mobilization and contraction in glomerular mesangial cells. *Am. J. Physiol.* **255**: F771–80.

Minamino, N., Kangawa, K. & Matsuo, H. (1988). Isolation and identification of a high molecular weight brain natriuretic peptide in porcine cardiac atrium. *Biochem. Biophys. Res. Commun.* **157**: 402–9.

Mißbichler, A., Pittner, F., Hartter, E. & Wolozczuk, W. (1988). Direkter quantitativer nachweis von humanem atrialem natriuretischem peptid (hANP) im harn mittels HPLC. *Biol. Chem. Hoppe–Seyler* **369**: 878.

Miyata, A., Kangawa, K., Toshimori, T., Hatoh, T. & Matsuo, H. (1985). Molecular forms of atrial natriuretic polypeptides in mammalian tissues and plasma. *Biochem. Biophys. Res. Commun.* **129**: 248–55.

Miyata, A., Minamino, N., Kangawa, K. & Matsuo, H. (1988). Identification of a 29-amino acid natriuretic peptide in chicken heart. *Biochem. Biophys. Res. Commun.* **155**: 1330–7.

Miyata, A., Toshimori, T., Hashiguchi, T., Kangawa, K. & Matsuo, H. (1987). Molecular forms of atrial natriuretic polypeptides circulating in human plasma. *Biochem. Biophys. Res. Commun.* **142**: 461–7.

Murphy, K. M. M., McLaughlin, L. L., Michener, M. L. & Needleman, P. (1985). Autoradiographic localization of atriopeptin III receptors in rat kidney. *Eur. J. Pharmacol.* **111**: 291–2.

Nakai, M., Fukase, M., Kinoshita, Y. & Fujita, T. (1988). Atrial natriuretic factor inhibits phosphate uptake in opossum kidney cells as a model of renal proximal tubules. *Biochem. Biophys. Res. Commun.* **155**: 1416–20.

Napier, M. A., Vandlen, R. L., Albers-Schonberg, G., Nutt, R. T., Brady, S., Lyle, T., Winquist, R. *et al.* (1984). Specific membrane receptors for atrial natriuretic factor in renal and vascular tissues. *Proc. Nat. Acad. Sci. USA* **81**: 5946–50.

Nehls, M., Reinecke, M., Lang, R. E. & Forssmann, W. G. (1985). Biochemical and immunological evidence for a cardiodilatin-like substance in the snail neurocardiac axis. *Proc. Nat. Acad. Sci. USA* **82**: 7762–6.

Nonoguchi, H., Knepper, M. A. & Manganiello, V. C. (1987). Effects of atrial natriuretic factor on cyclic guanosine monophosphate and cyclic adenosine monophosphate accumulation in microdissected nephron segments from rat. *J. Clin. Invest.* **79**: 500–7.

Nonoguchi, H., Sands, J. M. & Knepper, M. A. (1988). Atrial natriuretic factor inhibits vasopressin-stimulated osmotic water permeability in rat inner medullary collecting duct. *J. Clin. Invest.* **82**: 1383–90.

Oehlenschlager, W. F., Baron, D. A., Schomer, H. & Currie, M. M. (1989). Atrial and brain natriuretic peptides share binding sites in the kidney and heart. *Eur. J. Pharmacol.* **161**: 159–64.

Ogawa, K., Smith, A. I., Hodsman, G. P., Jackson, B., Woodcock, E. A. & Johnston, C. I. (1987). Plasma atrial natriuretic peptide: Concentrations and circulating forms in normal man and patients with chronic renal failure. *Clin. Exp. Pharmacol. Physiol.* **14**: 95–102.

Olins, G. M., Krieter, P. A., Trapani, A. J., Spear, K. L. & Bovy, P. R. (1989). Specific inhibitors of endopeptidase 24.11 inhibit the metabolism of atrial natriuretic peptides *in vitro* and *in vivo*. *Molec. Cell. Endocrinol.* **61**: 201–8.

Olins, G. M., Spear, K. L., Siegel, N. R. & Zurcher-Neely, H. A. (1987). Inactivation of atrial natriuretic factor by the renal brush border. *Biochim. Biophys. Acta* **901**: 97–100.

Olins, G. M., Spear, K. L., Siegel, N. R., Zurcher-Neely, H. A. & Smith, C. E. (1986). Proteolytic degradation of atriopeptin III by rabbit kidney brush border membranes. *Fed. Proc.* **45**: 427.

Porter, J. G., Arfsten, A., Palisi, T., Scarborough, R. M., Lewicki, J. A. & Seilhammer, J. J. (1989). Cloning of a cDNA encoding porcine brain natriuretic peptide. *J. Biol. Chem.* **264**: 6689–92.

Riegger, G. A. J., Elsner, D., Schulz-Knappe, P., Forssmann, W. G. & Kromer, E. P. (1988). The new peptide urodilatin (ANP-95–126) in dogs with and without heart failure. *Circulation* **78** (Suppl. II): II429.

Riegger, A. J. G., Elsner, D., Schulz-Knappe, P., Forssmann, W. G. & Kromer, E. P. (1989). Urodilatin (ANP-95–126) vor und nach induktion einer kongestiven herzinsuffizienz am hund. *Zeitschr. Kardiol.* **78** (Suppl. 1): 23.

Riegger, G. A. J., Elsner, D., Schulz-Knappe, P., Forssmann, W. G., Kromer, E. P. & Kochsiek, K. (1990). Hemodynamic, hormonal and renal effects of a new natriuretic peptide (ANP-95–126) in control dogs and dogs with congestive heart failure. *Circulation* (submitted).

Sakamoto, M., Nakao, K., Kihara, M., Morii, N., Sugawara, A., Suda, M., Shimokura, M. *et al.* (1985). Existence of atrial natriuretic polypeptide in kidney. *Biochem. Biophys. Res. Commun.* **128**, 1281–7.

Sakata, J.-I., Kangawa, K. & Matsuo, H. (1988). Identification of new atrial natriuretic peptides in frog heart. *Biochem. Biophys. Res. Commun.* **155**: 1338–45.

Schulz-Knappe, P., Forssmann, K., Herbst, F., Hock, D., Pipkorn, R. & Forssmann, W. G. (1988). Isolation and structural analysis of "urodilatin", a new peptide of the cardiodilatin-(ANP)-family, extracted from human urine. *Klin. Wochenschr.* **66**: 752–9.

Schwartz, D., Geller, D. M., Manning, P. T., Siegel, N. R., Fok, F. K., Smith, C. E. & Needleman, P. (1985). Ser–Leu–Arg–Arg–atriopeptin III: The major circulating forms of atrial natriuretic peptide. *Science* **229**: 397–400.

Shimonaka, M., Saheki, T., Hagiwara, H., Hagiwara, Y., Sono, H. & Hirose, S. (1987). Visualization of ANP receptor on glomeruli of bovine kidney by use of a specific antiserum. *Am. J. Physiol.* **253**: F1058–62.

Sonnenberg, H., Cupples, W. A., deBold, A. J. & Veress, A. T. (1982). Intrarenal localization of the natriuretic effect of cardiac atrial extracts. *Can. J. Physiol. Pharmacol.* **60**: 1149–52.

Sonnenberg, H., Honrath, U., Chon, C. K. & Wilson, D. R. (1986). Atrial natriuretic factor inhibits sodium transport in medullary collecting duct. *Am. J. Physiol.* **250**: F963–6.

Sonnenberg, J. L., Sakane, Y., Jeng, A. Y., Koehn, J. A., Ansell, J. A., Wennogle, L. P. & Ghai, R. D. (1988). Identification of protease 3.4.24.11 as the major atrial natriuretic factor degrading enzyme in the rat kidney. *Peptides* **9**: 173–80.

Sonnenberg, H., Veress, A. T., Borenstein, H. B. & deBold, A. J. (1980). Rapid and potent natriuretic response to intravenous injection of atrial myocardial extract in rats. *Physiologist* **23**: 13.

Stephenson, S. L. & Kenny, A. J. (1987a). The hydrolysis of α-human atrial natriuretic peptide by pig kidney membranes is initiated by endopeptidase 24.11. *Biochem. J.* **243**: 183–7.

Stephenson, S. L. & Kenny, A. J. (1987b). Metabolism of neuropeptides. *Biochem. J.* **241**: 237–41.

Sudoh, T., Kangawa, K., Minamino, N. & Matsuo, H. (1988a). A new natriuretic peptide from porcine brain. *Nature* **332**: 78–81.

Sudoh, T., Maekawa, K., Kojima, M., Minamino, N., Kangawa, K. & Matsuo, H. (1989). Cloning and sequencing of cDNA encoding a precursor for human brain natriuretic peptide. *Biochem. Biophys. Res. Commun.* **159**: 1427–34.

Sudoh, T., Minamino, N., Kangawa, K., & Matsuo, H. (1988b). Brain natriuretic peptide-32: N-terminal six amino acid extended form of brain natriuretic peptide identified in porcine brain. *Biochem. Biophys. Res. Commun.* **155**: 726–32.

Tang, G. J., Webber, R. J., Chang, D., Chang, J. K., Kiang, J. & Wei, E. T. (1984). Depressor and natriuretic activities of several atrial peptides. *Regul. Peptides* **9**: 53–9.

Theiss, G., John, A., Morich, F., Neuser, D., Schröder, W., Stasch, J.-P. & Wohlfeil, S. (1987). α-h-ANP is the only form of circulating ANP in humans. *FEBS Lett.* **218**: 159–62.

Thibault, G., Lazure, C., Schriffin, E. L., Gutkowska, J., Chartier, L., Garcia, R., Seidah, N. G. *et al.* (1985). Identification of a biologically active circulating form of rat atrial natriuretic factor. *Biochem. Biophys. Res. Commun.* **130**: 981–6.

Tsunoda, K., Mendelsohn, F. A. O., Sexton, P. M., Chai, S. Y., Hodsman, G. P. & Johnston, C. I. (1988). Decreased atrial natriuretic peptide binding in rat renal medulla in rats with chronic heart failure. *Circulation Res.* **62**: 155–61.

Uchida, K., Mizuno, T., Shimonaka, M., Sugiura, N., Hagiwara, H. & Hirose, S. (1989). Subtype switch of ANP receptors during *in vitro* culture of vascular cells. *Am. J. Physiol.* **256**: H311–14.

Vanneste, Y., Michel, A., Dimaline, R., Najdovski, T. & Deschodt-Lanckman, M. (1988). Hydrolysis of α-human natriuretic peptide *in vitro* by human kidney membranes and purified endopeptidase-24.11. *Biochem. J.* **254**: 531–7.

Vogt-Schaden, M., Gagelmann, M., Hock, D., Herbst, F. & Forssmann, W. G. (1989). Degradation of porcine brain natriuretic peptide (pBNP-26) by endoprotease-24.11 from kidney cortical membranes. *Biochem. Biophys. Res. Commun.* **161**: 1177–83.

Yamamoto, I., Ogura, T. & Ota, Z. (1987). *In vitro* macro- and micro-autoradiographic localization of atrial natriuretic peptide in the rat kidney. *Res. Commun. Chem. Pathol. Pharmacol.* **56**: 185–98.

Yandle, T., Crozier, I., Nicholls, G., Espiner, E., Carne, A. & Brennan, S. (1987). Amino acid sequence of atrial natriuretic peptides in human coronary sinus plasma. *Biochem. Biophys. Res. Commun.* **146**: 832–9.

Yip, C. C., Laing, L. P. & Flynn, T. G. (1985). Photoaffinity labelling of atrial natriuretic factor receptors of rat kidney cortex plasma membranes. *J. Biol. Chem.* **260**: 8229–32.

Yusufi, A. N. K., Berndt, T. J., Moltaji, H., Donovan, V., Dousa, T. P. & Knox, F. G. (1989). Rat atrial natriuretic factor (ANP-III) inhibits phosphate transport in brush border membrane from superficial and juxtamedullary cortex. *Proc. Soc. Exp. Biol. Med.* **190**: 87–90.

Zeidel, M. L., Kikeri, D., Silva, P., Burrowes, M. & Brenner, B. M. (1988). Atrial natriuretic peptides inhibit conductive sodium uptake by rabbit inner medullary collecting duct cells. *J. Clin. Invest.* **82**: 1067–74.

Zeidel, M. L., Silva, P., Brenner, B. M. & Seifter, J. L. (1987). cGMP mediates effects of atrial peptides on medullary collecting duct cells. *Am. J. Physiol.* **252**: F551–9.

Chapter 13
Brain natriuretic peptide
A. D. Struthers

Introduction

The discovery of ANF has inevitably led to a search for other peptides with natriuetic activity. This search has led to two major new peptides, i.e. brain natriuretic peptide (BNP) (discussed below) and iso-rat-atrial natriuretic peptide (iso-rat-ANP) which is a 45-amino-acid peptide (Flynn *et al.*, 1989). Both BNP and iso-rat-ANP are structurally distinct from atrial natriuretic factor (ANF) although both show a remarkable sequence homology to ANF and to each other.

With regard to BNP, Sudoh *et al.* (1988a) originally isolated this peptide from porcine brain. BNP has 26 amino-acid residues and resembles ANF in having a 17-amino-acid ring structure closed by a disulphide bridge. In the ring structure, 13 of the 17 amino-acid residues are identical between BNP and ANF (Fig. 13.1). Furthermore, at the C-terminus, both BNP and ANF 1–126 share the same Arg–Tyr sequence.

Subsequent to identifying BNP itself, Sudoh *et al.* (1988b) have now isolated a different form of BNP from porcine brain. This consists of the original 26-residue BNP with an additional six amino acids attached at the N-terminus and has been designated BNP-32 in order to distinguish it from BNP itself. Of the six additional amino acids, two are homologous with ANF 1–126 (Fig. 13.2). Human BNP from atrial tissue has 32 amino acids with a disulphide bridge (Kambayashi *et al.* 1990).

Location of BNP

A pattern is gradually being built up of the location of BNP within the body. Naturally enough the CNS was the main focus of attention and Ueda *et al.* (1988) have compared the concentrations of immunoreactive BNP (ir-BNP) and immunoreactive ANF (ir-ANF). The results, shown in Table 13.1, show marked differences between BNP and ANF in the CNS. Overall, there was 13 times more BNP than ANF in porcine brain, with

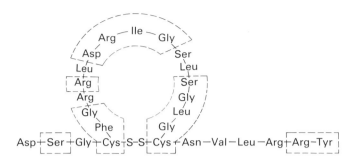

Fig. 13.1 Amino-acid structure of BNP. Dotted lines indicate identical residues with ANF 1–126.

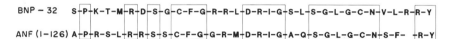

Fig. 13.2 Amino-acid sequences of BNP-32 and ANF 1–126 using one-letter amino-acid notation.

Table 13.1 Distribution of immunoreactive BNP and ANF in porcine CNS.

	ir-BNP (pmol/g wet wt)	ir-ANF (pmol/g wet wt)
Spinal cord	1.81	0.06
Whole brain	0.63	0.05
Medulla—pons	1.59	0.14
Striatum	1.44	< 0.04
Hypothalamus	1.13	0.26
Midbrain—thalamus	0.51	0.17
Cortex	0.50	< 0.04
Myocardial atrial extract	65.1	5910

its highest concentration in the medulla, a crucial area for central cardiovascular control. Moreover, the regional distribution of ir-BNP was found to be different from ir-ANF, which suggests that the BNP–neuronal system is distinct from the ANF–neuronal system. This differential localization of BNP and ANF has been confirmed immunohistochemically in the rat (Saper *et al.*, 1989). Immunoassay techniques have now been extended to other species (Itoh *et al.*, 1989). Although ir-BNP was found in both the porcine and canine brain and also at its highest concentration in the medulla in both species, these authors did not detect any ir-BNP in the human, monkey or rat brain (Itoh *et al.*, 1989).

With regard to the cardiovascular system, Togashi *et al.* (1989) recently reported that BNP circulates in normal man in its 1–126 form and at a plasma concentration of 1.5 pmol/l. Extending these observations, ir-BNP has been detected in porcine atrial extract and porcine plasma but not in ventricular tissue (Saito *et al.*, 1989). A large precursor BNP molecule was detected in atria, which suggests that atria synthesize BNP and secrete BNP into the circulation. Therefore the concentration of BNP in atrial tissue is about 100 times that of BNP in whole brain, although this same high atrial concentration of BNP represents only 2% of the corresponding atrial concentration of ANF (Table 13.1) (Minamino *et al.*, 1988a). In absolute terms, the tissue concentrations are in the order of atrial ANF $\gg$ atrial BNP $\gg$ brain BNP > brain ANF. As for the clearance of BNP, Vogt-Schaden *et al.* (1989) have recently shown that kidney endopeptidase-24.11 is capable of cleaving BNP. While this enzyme cleaves ANF mainly at one site, BNP appears to be cleaved at several different sites.

BNP precursor molecules

Although large amounts of ir-BNP occur in the atrium, only 15% exists as the low-molecular-weight forms BNP and BNP-32. Most of the atrial ir-BNP exists as high-molecular-weight storage forms (Minamino *et al.*, 1988a). There appear to be two major storage forms of BNP in porcine cardiac atrium (Fig. 13.3):

1 a 131-amino-acid precursor called preproBNP (Maekawa *et al.*, 1988);
2 a 106-amino-acid precursor called γ-BNP (Minamino *et al.*, 1988b).

Both preproBNP and γ-BNP have BNP itself at their C-terminus. Clearly it seems likely that preproBNP becomes γ-BNP by removal of a 25-residue signal peptide at its N-terminus (Porter *et al.*, 1989). γ-BNP is, like ANF 1–126, the major tissue form in porcine cardiocytes. Thereafter, γ-BNP is cleaved, particularly in brain tissue, in order to produce BNP itself and BNP-32, which are the major tissue forms of BNP in brain tissue. In many respects, this sequence of biosynthesis and processing for BNP is very similar to that of ANF where the precursor is preproANF (now correctly known as preANF 1–126), the atrial tissue form is γ-ANF or proANF (now correctly called ANF 1–126) and the predominant brain peptides are ANF 102–126 and ANF 103–126. Despite this similarity in the processing, ANF 1–126 and γ-BNP themselves have only 31% sequence homology, which mostly occurs in the region of BNP-32. Therefore BNP and ANF have structurally very different precursor molecules although curiously their processing involves cleavage at similar places within these precursor molecules.

The above processing steps for BNP have been established for porcine BNP. There is, however, strong evidence to suggest that, unlike ANF, there are major species variations in the structure of mammalian BNPs. In order to determine the amino-acid sequence of human BNP, Sudoh *et al.*

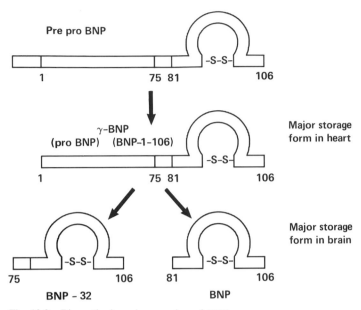

Fig. 13.3   Biosynthesis and processing of BNP.

(1989) constructed a human cardiac atrium cDNA library and then screened for clones hybridizing with porcine BNP cDNA. A human preproBNP has been so identified, with 134-amino-acid residues and a C-terminus which is highly homologous to BNP-32. Similarly, for the rat, a 121-amino-acid residue precursor has recently been identified (Kojima *et al.*, 1989). Human BNP has 32 amino acids with a disulphide bridge (Kambayashi *et al.* 1990).

Biological activity

In the original paper describing BNP, Sudoh *et al.* (1988a) showed that BNP had biological effects similar to ANF, i.e. it has natriuretic–diuretic, hypotensive and chick rectum relaxant activities. Since then, many investigators have examined further the spectrum of biological activity of BNP and it is proving to be very similar to ANF. The hypotensive and vasodilatory activity of BNP in rats has been confirmed in normotensive rats, spontaneously hypertensive rats and in DOCA-salt rats (Kita *et al.*, 1989a,b; Tang *et al.*, 1989). At a receptor level, Hirata *et al.* (1988) showed convincingly that BNP and ANF interact with the same receptor site in rat vascular smooth muscle cells and that in so doing they both activate guanylate cyclase. Similar results have also been obtained for rat glomeruli, rat heart, cultured endothelial cells and cultured aortic smooth muscle cells (Oehlenschlager *et al.*, 1989; Song, Kohse & Murad, 1988). In the kidney, BNP was shown to produce cyclic guanyl monophosphate (cGMP) accumulation in an epithelial cell line (Iwata *et al.*, 1989). Interestingly, the simultaneous addition of BNP and ANF at their maximally effective concentrations did not have an additive effect, which again suggests that BNP and ANF may share the same receptor.

Similar data exist for the adrenal cortex to suggest that BNP binds to a receptor which recognizes both BNP and ANF equally (Hashiguchi *et al.*, 1988). Furthermore, porcine BNP inhibits aldosterone production whether stimulated by angiotensin II (ANGII) or ACTH and also inhibits ACTH-induced cortisol secretion (Higuchi *et al.*, 1989). BNP also appears to have effects on the autonomic nervous system. Not only are there biologically active receptors for BNP in cervical ganglia but BNP has complex resetting effects on the baroreflexes which influence heart rate and renal nerve activity (Morita *et al.*, 1989; Torda, Nazarali & Saavedra, 1989).

At a molecular level, two distinct guanylate cyclase linked receptors have been identified. One (GC-A) responds equally to both ANF and BNP while the other (GC-B) is preferentially stimulated by BNP (see Chapter 10).

Since both BNP and ANF are present in the central nervous system, it is not surprising that both substances appear also to exert major CNS effects. Intracerebroventricular (i.c.v.) injection of ANF suppresses water intake, salt appetite, pressor responses and the secretion of vasopressin in conscious rats. A picture is being built up for BNP which is very similar. Although i.c.v. injection of BNP did not affect blood pressure by itself, it did attenuate the pressor response to i.c.v. ANGII in a dose-dependent manner (Shirakami *et al.*, 1988). As with the pressor responses, i.c.v. BNP itself did not alter spontaneous water intake in rats but it did attenuate the water drinking induced by i.c.v. ANGII (Itoh *et al.*, 1988). When it comes to vasopressin (AVP), i.c.v. BNP inhibits both basal AVP secretion and AVP secretion induced by ANGII (Yamada *et al.*, 1988).

The normal plasma level of BNP at around 0.9 pmol/litre is only 16% of normal plasma ANF level in man. Plasma BNP is elevated in the same diseases as ANF, especially chronic heart failure where BNP is increased 200-fold as opposed to 20-fold for ANF (Mukoyama *et al.* 1990).

Conclusions

Progress with BNP research is proving extremely rapid, mainly due to the elegant and detailed work of Matsuo and colleagues. A picture is being built up for BNP which has elements which are similar to and elements which are dissimilar to ANF (Table 13.2). Despite some differences, it is interesting that the biological activity of BNP and ANF is almost identical. It is too early to make judgements about the physiological or pathophysiological relevance of BNP but this early work suggests that

Table 13.2   Comparison of BNP and ANF.

Similarities	Dissimilarities
Structure of BNP/ANF	
Processing of precursors	Structure of BNP/ANF precursors
Biological activity:	Species variations
CNS	Regional distribution within CNS
natriuretic	Sites of cleavage by endopeptidase-24.11
vasodilator	
adrenal	
cGMP effect	
Peptide levels elevated in heart failure	
Receptor population stimulated	

BNP deserves as much, if not more, attention from research in the future as ANF has in the past. Furthermore, the discovery of both BNP and iso-rat-ANP suggests that there is indeed a family of natriuretic peptides. It is therefore likely that further peptides will be described in the near future.

References

Chang, M., Lowe, D. G., Lewis, M., Hellmiss, R., Chen, E., Goeddel, D. V. (1989) Differential activation by atrial and brain natriuretic peptides of two different receptor guanylate cyclases. *Nature* **341**: 68–72.

Flynn, T. G., Brar, A., Tremblay, L., Sarda, I., Lyons, C. & Jennings, D. B. (1989). Isolation and characterisation of iso-rANP, a new natriuretic peptide from rat atria. *Biochem. Biophys. Res. Commun.* **161**: 830.

Hashiguchi, T., Higuchi, K., Ohashi, M., Minamino, N., Kangawa, K., Matsuo, H. & Nawata, H. (1988). Porcine brain natriuretic peptide, another modulator of bovine adrenocortical steroidogenesis. *FEBS Lett.* **235** (2): 455.

Higuchi, K., Hashiguchi, T., Ohashi, M., Takayanagi, R., Haji, M., Matsuo, H. & Nawata H. (1989). Porcine brain natriuretic peptide receptor in bovine adrenal cortex. *Life Sci.* **44**: 881.

Hirata, Y., Schichiri, M., Emori, T., Marumo, F., Kangawa, K. & Matsuo, H. (1988). Brain natriuretic peptide interacts with atrial natriuretic peptide receptor in cultured rat vascular smooth muscle cells. *FEBS Lett.* **238** (2): 415.

Itoh, H., Nakao, K., Saito, Y., Yamada, T., Shirakami, G., Mukoyama, M., Arai, H. *et al.* (1989). Radioimmunoassay for brain natriuretic peptide (BNP). Detection of BNP in canine brain. *Biochem. Biophys. Res. Commun.* **155**: 733.

Itoh, H., Nakao, K., Yamada, T., Shirakami, G., Kangawa, K., Minamino, N., Matsuo, H. *et al.* (1988). Antidipsogenic action of a novel peptide, 'brain natriuretic peptide', in rats. *Eur. J. Pharmacol.* **150**: 193.

Iwata, T., Inui, K., Nakao, K., Imura, H., Matsuo, H., & Hori, R. (1989). Effect of brain natriuretic peptide on cyclic GMP accumulation in a kidney epithelial cell line (LLC-PKI). *Eur. J. Pharmacol.* **159**: 321.

Kambayashi, Y., Nakao, K., Mukoyama, M., Saito, Y., Ogawa, Y., Shiono, S., Inouye, K., Yoshida, N. & Imura, H., (1990). Isolation and sequence determination of human brain natriuretic peptide in human atrium. *FEBS Letters* **259**, 341.

Kita, T., Kida, O., Kato, J., Nakamura, S., Eto, T., Minamino, N., Kangawa, K. *et al.* (1989a). Natriuretic and hypotensive effects of brain natriuretic peptide in anaesthetised DOCA-salt hypertensive rats. *Clin. Exp. Pharmacol. Physiol.* **16**: 185.

Kita, T., Kida, O., Kato, J., Nakamura, S., Eto, T., Minamino, N., Kangawa, K. *et al.* (1989b). Natriuretic and hypotensive effects of brain natriuretic peptide (BNP) in spontaneously hypertensive rats. *Life Sci.* **44**: 1541.

Kojima, M., Minamino, N., Kangawa, K. & Matsuo, H. (1989). Cloning and sequence analysis of cDNA encoding a precursor for rat brain natriuretic peptide. *Biochem. Biophys. Res. Commun.* **159**: 1420.

Maekawa, K., Sudoh, T., Furusawa, M., Minamino, N., Kangawa, K., Ohkubo, H., Nakanishi, S. *et al.* (1988). Cloning and sequence analysis of cDNA encoding a precursor for porcine brain natriuretic peptide. *Biochem. Biophys. Res. Commun.* **157**: 410.

Minamino, N., Aburaya, M., Ueda, S., Kangawa, K. & Matsuo, H. (1988a). The presence of brain natriuretic peptide of 12000 daltons in porcine heart. *Biochem. Biophys. Res. Commun.* **155**: 740.

Minamino, N., Kangawa, K. & Matsuo, H. (1988b). Isolation and identification of a high molecular weight brain natriuretic peptide in porcine cardiac atrium. *Biochem. Biophys. Res. Commun.* **157**: 402.

Morita, H., Nishida, Y., Motochigawa, H., Kangawa, K., Minamino, N., Matsuo, H. & Hosomi, H. (1989). Effects of brain natriuretic peptide on renal nerve activity in conscious rabbits. *Am. J. Physiol.* **256**: R792.

Mukoyama, M., Nakao, K., Saito, Y., Ogawa, Y., Hosoda, K., Suga, S., Shirakami, G., Jougasaki, M. & Imura, H. (1990). Human brain natriuretic peptide, a novel cardiac hormone. *Lancet* **335**, 801.

Oehlenschlager, W. F., Baron, D. A., Schomer, H. & Currie, M. G. (1989). Atrial and brain natriuretic peptides share binding sites in the kidney and heart. *Eur. J. Pharmacol.* **161**: 159.

Porter, J. G., Arfsten, A., Palisi, T., Scarborough, R. M., Lewicki, J. & Seilhamer, J. J. (1989). Cloning of a cDNA encoding porcine brain natriuretic peptide. *J. Biol. Chem.* **264**: 6689.

Saito, Y., Nakao, K., Itoh, H., Yamada, T., Mukoyoma, M., Arai, H., Hosoda, K. *et al.* (1989). Brain natriuretic peptide is a novel cardiac hormone. *Biochem. Biophys. Res. Commun.* **158**: 360.

Saper, C. B., Hurley, K. M., Moga, M. M., Holmes, H. R., Adams, S. A., Leahy, K. M. & Needleman, P. (1989). Brain natriuretic peptides: differential localization of a new family of neuropeptides. *Neurosci. Lett.* **96** (1): 29.

Shirakami, G., Nakao, K., Yamada, T., Itoh, H., Mori, K., Kangawa, K., Minamino, N. *et al.* (1988). Inhibitory effect of brain natriuretic peptide on central angiotensin II stimulated pressor response in conscious rats. *Neurosci. Lett.* 77.

Song, D. L., Kohse, K. P. & Murad, F. (1988). Brain natriuretic factor. Augmentation of cellular cyclic GMP, activation of particulate guanylate cyclase and receptor binding. *FEBS Lett.* **232**: 125.

Sudoh, T., Kangawa, K., Minamino, N. & Matsuo, H. (1988a). A new natriuretic peptide in porcine brain. *Nature* **332**: 78.

Sudoh, T., Maekawa, K., Kojima, M., Minamino, N., Kangawa, K. & Matsuo, H. (1989). Cloning and sequence analysis of cDNA encoding a precursor for human brain natriuretic peptide. *Biochem. Biophys. Res. Commun.* **159**: 1427.

Sudoh, T., Minamino, N., Kangawa, K. & Matsuo, H. (1988b). Brain natriuretic peptide -32: N-terminal six amino acid extended form of brain natriuretic peptide identified in porcine brain. *Biochem. Biophys. Res. Commun.* **155**: 726.

Tang, C. S., Cui, H., Yuan, Q. X. & Tang, J. (1989). Haemodynamic responses to BNP in rats. *Eur. J. Pharmacol.* **159**: 327.

Togashi, K., Hirata, Y., Ando, K., Takei, Y., Kawakami, M. & Marumo, F. (1989). Brain natriuretic peptide-like immunoreactivity is present in human plasma, *FEBS Lett.* **250**: 235.

Torda, T., Nazarali, A. J. & Saavedra, J. M. (1989). Brain natriuretic peptide receptors in the rat peripheral sympathetic ganglia. *Biochem. Biophys. Res. Commun.* **159**: 1032.

Ueda, S., Minamino, N., Sudoh, T., Kangawa, K. & Matsuo, H. (1988). Regional distributions of immunoreactive brain natriuretic peptide in porcine brain and spinal cord. *Biochem. Biophys. Res. Commun.* **155**: 733.

Vogt-Schaden, M., Gagelmann, M., Hock, D., Herbst, F. & Forssmann, W. G. (1989). Degradation of porcine brain natriuretic peptide (pBNP-26) by endoprotease-24.11 from kidney cortical membranes. *Biochem. Biophys. Res. Commun.* **161**: 1177.

Yamada, T., Nakao, K., Itoh, H., Shirakami, G., Kangawa, K., Minamino, N., Matsuo, H. *et al.* (1988). Intracerebroventricular injection of brain natriuretic peptide inhibits vasopressin secretion in conscious rats. *Neurosci. Lett.* **95**: 223.

Chapter 14
Release of atrial natriuretic factor
A. E. G. Raine

Introduction

The existence of atrial natriuretic factor (ANF) was first demonstrated by
the classic studies of deBold and colleagues in 1981. Although these
showed clearly that an extract of rat atrial tissue was capable of producing
a natriuresis, diuresis, fall in blood pressure and increase in haematocrit
when injected into a test animal, they did not prove that ANF was released
into the circulation from atrial tissue, nor did they identify the factors
controlling its release. These issues awaited the development of suitable
assays for measurement of tissue and plasma ANF concentrations, and it
was only in 1985 that firm evidence emerged in both animals (Lang *et al.*,
1985) and man (Sugawara *et al.*, 1985) concerning the status of ANF as
a circulating hormone.

Since then, some issues relating to cardiac release of ANF have been
resolved, but many more remain unanswered. The aim of this chapter will
be to discuss what is known of the mechanism of ANF release from the
left and right atrium, and its relationship to atrial pressure and stretch in
animals and in man. Other influences on release of ANF, including
frequency of atrial contraction will be considered, together with the still
controversial role of neural, humoral and paracrine factors.

Cellular synthesis, storage and release of ANF

The presence of specific granules in atrial tissue was first recognized over
three decades ago (Kisch, 1955) and these granules were noted to have

235

secretory characteristics morphologically (Jamieson & Palade, 1964). Several studies subsequently confirmed alterations in appearance of atrial granules with changes in fluid and electrolyte balance; for example deBold (1979) showed that water and sodium deprivation in rats led to an increase in atrial granularity. Gel fractionation studies of atrial extracts demonstrated high- and low-molecular-weight forms of ANF (Trippodo, MacPhee & Cole, 1983), which were subsequently shown by sequence analysis and molecular biology techniques to be a prohormone peptide, ANF 1–126, and a circulating 28-amino-acid peptide, ANF 99–126 (Kangawa & Matsuo, 1984) derived from the C-terminus of the prohormone (Atlas et al., 1984; Flynn, deBold & deBold, 1984; Oikawa et al., 1984).

The localization of proANF within atrial granules has been confirmed by specific staining of the granules with antisera raised against several regions of the proANF sequence (Zisfein et al., 1986; Thibault et al., 1987). Similarly, isolation of the granules by fractionation and characterization of their contents by several different antibodies have confirmed that the major storage form of ANF in atrial granules is the 126-amino-acid prohormone (Thibault et al., 1987).

The precise mechanism of the cleavage of ANF 99–126 from its prohormone and release have not been established. Generation of the 28-amino-acid peptide requires breaking of an Arg–Ser peptide bond in proANF, and a seryl protease which may serve this function has recently been identified in atrial tissue (Imada, Takayanagi & Inagami, 1988). The subcellular localization of the cleavage, and mechanism of subsequent secretion of ANF remain controversial. Although atrial cells in culture may secrete the prohormone into the culture medium (Bloch et al., 1985), studies in perfused hearts demonstrated release only of the low-molecular-weight atrial peptide, assessed by bioassay (Currie et al., 1984) and of the 28-amino-acid form of ANF measured by radioimmunoassay (Thibault et al., 1986). Similarly, analysis of coronary sinus blood in man showed no evidence of proANF secretion (Suguwara et al., 1985). Thus, it is likely that cleavage of proANF occurs after secretion from the storage granule, but within the atrial myocyte, by a seryl protease present within the microsomal fraction, which has the capability of specific cleavage of the arginyl peptide bond between Arg^{98} and Ser^{99} in the prohormone, but not bonds involving a double basic residue sequence such as Arg^{101}–Arg^{102}–Ser^{103} (Imada et al., 1988).

Recent studies have established that the N-terminal 1–98 fragment of proANF is cosecreted with ANF 99–126 into the circulation, and it may achieve plasma concentrations 10–20-fold those of C–terminal ANF in normal subjects and in patients with end-stage renal failure (Buckley et al., 1989). Whether there is one-to-one stoichiometry of release of the 1–98 and 99–126 fragments of the prohormone is not confirmed. It is also unclear whether the N-terminal fragment exerts significant physiological effects, although N-terminal fragments are known to be capable of antagonizing noradrenaline-induced vasoconstriction of aortic tissue *in vitro* (Vesely *et al.*, 1987).

Little is known of the subcellular mechanisms transducing peptide secretion in response to myocyte stretch. It is likely that calcium-activated protein kinase C is involved, however. ANF release from isolated perfused hearts was stimulated by both the calcium ionophore A 23187 and the phorbol ester TPA (Ruskoaho, Toth & Lang, 1985), and by the calcium channel agonist BAY K 8644 (Saito *et al.*, 1986). Consistent with these observations, it is now established that ANF secretion is highly dependent on increases in intracellular free calcium concentration (Matsubara *et al.*, 1988). The ANF release process is strongly temperature-dependent; a reduction in temperature from 37° to 21.5°C reduced ANF release *in vitro* by 85% (Bilder, Schofield & Blaine, 1986).

Although the lack of natriuretic activity of ventricular myocardial extract was employed as a control in deBold's initial studies (1981), it is now clear that the ability to synthesize ANF is present also in ventricular myocytes. Ventricular tissue expresses mRNA for ANF (Nemer *et al.*, 1986), although quantitatively at a much lower level than in the atria. ANF of ventricular origin is not stored in granules, but is continuously released (Bloch *et al.*, 1986). The physiological importance of these small quantities of ANF derived from ventricular tissue remains uncertain. In experimental volume overload, ventricular ANF mRNA increases (Lattion *et al.*, 1986) raising the intriguing possibility that in pathological states ventricular ANF may assume importance. Similar increases in ventricular mRNA expression have been observed in myopathic hamsters (Franch *et al.*, 1988), in experimental heart failure in rats (Mendez *et al.*, 1987) and in right ventricular hypertrophy produced by chronic hypoxia in rats (Stockmann *et al.*, 1988).

Atrial pressure, atrial stretch and release of ANF

The knowledge that atrial extracts possessed natriuretic properties and that the density of specific atrial granules was sensitive to changes in volume status led rapidly to speculation that cardiac release of ANF might be responsive to changes in intravascular circulating volume. Early evidence supporting this concept came from Dietz (1984), who demonstrated that release of a cardiac natriuretic substance, as assessed by response of bioassay anaesthetized rats, was stimulated by increase of venous return in an isolated rat heart–lung preparation. The first unequivocal demonstration that ANF was a hormone released in response to increase in circulating volume was provided by Lang *et al.* (1985). These workers employed a radioimmunoassay for ANF to show that volume expansion in anaesthetized rats by infusion of 2- or 8-ml saline caused 2.3-fold and 6.0-fold increases respectively in plasma ANF concentrations, in association with right atrial pressure increases of 1 and 5 mmHg. They also showed a doubling of ANF release from the Langendorff-perfused isolated heart when right atrial pressure was raised by 1 mmHg.

The importance of atrial stretch as a primary stimulus in triggering the release of ANF was rapidly confirmed when strips of atrial tissue were superfused at low and high tension *in vitro*, and increases in ANF perfusate concentration measured by radioimmunoassay (deBold, deBold & Sarda 1985; Schiebinger & Linden, 1986a). Raising or lowering resting tension caused increases or decreases, respectively, in ANF release, and this tension-release relationship was present in both quiescent and beating atria.

The frequency of atrial contraction also influences release of ANF, although there may be a threshold for this effect. deBold *et al.* (1985) observed no effect of changes in pacing frequency between 0 and 2 Hz on release of ANF from atrial strips, whereas increases in pacing rate from 2 to 4 Hz with constant tension doubled ANF release *in vitro* (Schiebinger & Linden, 1986b). Further frequency-related increments in ANF release were observed up to 8 Hz.

Most experimental studies *in vivo* of control of release of ANF have measured right or left atrial pressures, interpreting relationships observed to be equivalent to demonstration of an atrial myocyte stretch–ANF release relationship. This extrapolation is probably not entirely valid. Hintze *et al.* (1989) have pointed out that mean atrial pressure may not provide an accurate measure of atrial filling and the importance of atrial stretch, not atrial pressure, in determining the release of ANF has been emphasized in studies in which atrial transmural pressure was maintained constant (Edwards *et al.*, 1988). Several studies have now measured both atrial pressures and dimensions simultaneously, thus enabling calculation of atrial wall stress, a product of transmural atrial pressure and dimensions. During induction of volume expansion and tachycardia in dogs, Christensen *et al.* (1988) found that systolic wall stress was an important determinant of ANF release. In contrast, studies employing volume expansion in conscious dogs have indicated that diastolic wall stress was most closely related to peptide release (Hintze *et al.*, 1989). Thus, atrial myocyte stretch is undoubtedly a sufficient stimulus for triggering ANF secretion. However, since *in vivo* the atria are hollow chambers, both transmural pressure and atrial diameter may variably influence atrial wall stress and ultimate peptide secretion.

Left and right atrial secretion

Initial studies of the pressure–secretion relationship concentrated on changes in right atrial filling pressure and peptide release (Dietz, 1984;

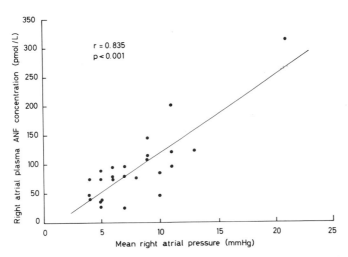

Fig. 14.1 Relation between mean right atrial pressure and right atrial plasma concentrations of ANF in 25 patients at rest.

Lang *et al.*, 1985). In reality, a more complex situation exists. Both atria contain proANF, and thus ANF secreted from either the left or right atrial tissue will ultimately enter the right atrium through the coronary sinus. Clearly, plasma ANF concentration measured in the coronary sinus or at any point downstream in the circulation will represent a mixture of ANF derived from both left and right atrial myocytes.

In rats, measurements of atrial tissue ANF showed an approximately twofold higher peptide concentration in right than in left atrial tissue (Gutkowska *et al.*, 1984; Tanaka, Misono & Inagami, 1984). Despite this difference, very similar quantities of ANF were released from isolated left or right atria of rats in response to either continuous or repetitive stretch (Bilder, Schofield & Blaine, 1986). In rabbits, tissue ANF concentration is approximately 50% higher in the left than right atrium, and in this species the pressure–release relationship, assessed in isolated atria, is steeper for the left than right atrium (Synhorst & Gutkowska, 1988).

Experimentally, selective increase in either right (Lang *et al.*, 1985) or left (Ledsome *et al.*, 1985) atrial pressure is capable of stimulating specific atrial release of ANF. Nevertheless, commonly in pathophysiological situations such as hypervolaemia, combined increases in both left and right atrial pressure occur, and the consequent increment in circulating ANF concentration represents the sum of secretions from left and right atrial tissue.

Atrial pressure and ANF release in man

Early studies in man demonstrated that the plasma concentration of ANF was elevated in conditions associated with increase in atrial pressure, such as supraventricular tachycardia (Yamaji *et al.*, 1985) and congestive heart failure (Tikkanen *et al.*, 1985). A relationship between atrial pressure and ANF release in man was soon confirmed in studies of patients with varying degrees of heart failure who were undergoing cardiac catheterization (Raine *et al.*, 1986). Right atrial plasma concentration of ANF was closely related to mean right atrial pressure (Fig. 14.1) and an equally close relationship existed between pulmonary wedge pressure and the systemic arterial concentration (Fig. 14.2). Quantitatively very similar findings were obtained by other workers (Burnett *et al.*, 1986; Richards *et al.*, 1986). These studies indicated a close parallelism in the pressure–release relationship in man and in animals. In isolated rat hearts, a 1 mmHg increase in right atrial pressure invoked a 38 % increase in ANF release (Lang *et al.*, 1985). In man, a 1 mmHg increase in right atrial pressure was associated with a 36 % increase in right atrial plasma ANF concentration (Raine *et al.*, 1986).

Acute changes in atrial pressure in man are also associated with corresponding changes in plasma ANF concentration. Accordingly, a relationship is present between increases in right atrial pressure and plasma ANF concentration during dynamic exercise (Muller *et al.*, 1986; Nishikimi *et al.*, 1986), during augmentation of venous return by elevation of the legs (Rodeheffer *et al.*, 1986), and during volume expansion by rapid infusion of intravenous saline (Anderson *et al.*, 1986a). Head-out water immersion, which increases central blood volume, is also associated with an increase in plasma ANF concentration (Epstein *et al.*, 1987; Muller *et al.*, 1986). Conversely, ANF release in man is reduced acutely in association with a fall in right atrial pressure by manoeuvres which reduce venous return such as placement of occlusion cuffs around the thighs (Muller *et al.*, 1986), and by reduction of blood volume by venesection (Cannella *et al.*, 1988).

It is less easy in man than in animals to prove that both left and right atrial myocytes may independently contribute to circulating peptide concentration. Nevertheless, patients with pure right heart failure, as in pulmonary hypertension, have elevated plasma ANF concentrations in proportion to the level of pulmonary arterial pressure and pulmonary vascular resistance (Adnot *et al.*, 1987). In addition, greatly elevated plasma ANF concentrations have been described in patients with pure left heart failure, with grossly elevated pulmonary wedge pressure but normal right atrial pressure (Raine *et al.*, 1986).

Demonstration in man that ANF release is related primarily to atrial stretch is also less easy than in laboratory studies. Echocardiographic investigations have shown a positive but weak correlation between left atrial dimension and circulating ANF concentration in subjects with normal renal function (Crozier *et al.*, 1986). In end-stage renal failure. basal plasma ANF concentrations are greatly elevated (Anderson *et al.*, 1986c; Raine *et al.*, 1989) and these patients are subject to considerable

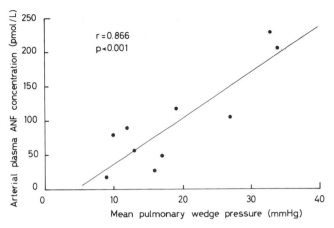

Fig. 14.2 Relation between mean pulmonary wedge pressure and ANF concentrations in arterial plasma of 10 patients.

increases in circulating volume between dialysis treatments. In this group, the relationship is clearer between atrial dimension, assessed echocardiographically, and plasma ANF concentration (Cannella *et al.*, 1987).

More compelling evidence that atrial stretch is the primary stimulus for ANF release in man comes from observations in patients with cardiac tamponade. The high atrial pressure but reduced atrial diameter resulting from tamponade due to pericardial blood or effusion is associated with low plasma ANF concentrations. Relief of tamponade by aspiration or surgery results in a fall in atrial pressure, an increase in atrial dimensions, and an increase in plasma ANF concentration (Koller, Grekin & Nicklas, 1987; Northridge *et al.*, 1989).

ANF release in heart failure and tachycardia in man

High plasma concentrations of ANF in patients with heart failure are best explained by a high rate of release of the peptide, in view of its short plasma half-life (Yandle *et al.*, 1986). Conceivably, depletion of atrial stores of peptide might ensue, and this possibility is supported by observations that in patients with heart failure, exercise-induced increments in plasma ANF were blunted compared with normal subjects, despite greater increases in atrial pressure with exercise in the heart failure group (Raine *et al.*, 1986). Parallel observations are available from animal studies. The cardiomyopathic B104.6 hamster has diminished atrial concentrations of ANF (Chimosky *et al.*, 1984). Edwards *et al.* (1986) have confirmed in this model that atrial granularity decreases as plasma ANF concentration increases. The decrease in atrial tissue immunoreactive ANF is associated with increased atrial ANF mRNA and plasma

ANF (Mendez *et al.*, 1987; Franch *et al.*, 1988). In dogs with pacing-induced heart failure, ultrastructural changes are observed which indicate massive stimulation of the ANF secretory process (Riegger *et al.*, 1988).

As in isolated atrial tissue (Schiebinger & Linden, 1986b), increase in frequency of atrial contraction in man leads to elevation of plasma ANF concentrations, whether as a result of spontaneous (Yamaji *et al.*, 1985; Nicklas *et al.*, 1986) or induced supraventricular tachycardia (Anderson *et al.*, 1986b) or as a response to rapid atrial pacing (Crozier *et al.*, 1985). It is likely that the augmented release of ANF which occurs during tachycardia partly accounts for the polyuria and natriuresis which may be seen during atrial tachycardia and fibrillation in man (Wood, 1963).

Factors modulating cardiac release of ANF

Demonstrations that a pressure–release relationship for ANF exists in the isolated perfused heart (Lang *et al.*, 1985) show that atrial stretch is a sufficient stimulus for ANF release, as such preparations are devoid of neural or hormonal influences. Similarly, plasma ANF concentrations are normal or even elevated in subjects who have undergone cardiac transplantation (Singer *et al.*, 1986) and appropriate increases in plasma ANF concentration occur when venous return is augmented in cardiac transplant recipients (Wilkins *et al.*, 1988).

Autonomic modulation

The possibility remains that a number of neural and hormonal factors may be able to modulate the release of ANF. Several studies have considered whether sympathetic or parasympathetic activation might affect peptide release. Early work employing bioassay suggested that both adrenaline and acetylcholine could increase release of ANF *in vitro* (Sonnenburg & Veress, 1984). In contrast, Naruse *et al.* (1986) incubated atrial tissue *in vitro*, and observed no effect of adrenaline, noradrenaline or isoprenaline in concentrations from 10^{-12} to 10^{-6} M on ANF release, as assessed by radioimmunoassay. However, both Arg-vasopressin and acetylcholine increased ANF release dose-dependently. Other workers have found no effect of either adrenergic or cholinergic agonists (Garcia *et al.*, 1986). Schiebinger & Linden (1986a,b) observed that enhanced peptide release *in vitro* in response to increased tension or frequency of contraction was not blocked by the antagonists, propranolol, phen-tolamine, and atropine in high concentrations and concluded that tension and rate-mediated effects on ANF release were not mediated by endogenous adrenergic or cholinergic neurotransmitters. In contrast, the same group (Schiebinger, Baker & Linden, 1987) have more recently shown that peptide secretion from isolated rat left atria was increased 2.5-fold by 10^{-5} M noradrenaline, and by 10^{-7} M isoprenaline. The cholinergic agonist, methacholine, exerted no basal effect on ANF secretion but attenuated noradrenaline-stimulated secretion. The conclusion was that ANF release is increased by cardiac β-adrenergic activation and reduced by parasympathetic activation.

However, interpretation of these findings must be tempered by the fact that unphysiologically high concentrations of the agonists were used. Other authors have observed no effect of sympathetic stimulation *in vivo* on ANF release in the anaesthetized dog (Ledsome *et al.*, 1986) and have reported increments in ANF release in response to acetylcholine (Sonnenburg & Veress, 1984; Ruskuaho, Toth & Lang, 1985; Naruse *et al.*, 1986). Studies *in vivo* in the anaesthetized rat have shown that vasopressin, dDAVP, phenylephrine and angiotensin II (ANG II) may all increase plasma ANF (Katsube, Schwartz & Needleman, 1985), but that in the doses employed all these agents exerted marked haemodynamic actions, with consequently a considerable increase in atrial pressure. It was not possible to determine whether they exerted any independent effect on release of ANF. Similarly, in the conscious rat, ANG II infusion provokes ANF release as a direct consequence of its haemodynamic action (Lachance & Garcia, 1988).

Other factors

In addition to adrenergic and cholinergic agonists, ANG II and vasopressin, several other factors have been suggested to modulate ANF release. Zamir *et al.* (1987) showed that hypophysectomy altered the release of the peptide in response to stimuli, concluding that the anterior pituitary gland exerted an important modulating influence. Hypoxia increases ANF release in animals (Baertschi, Adams & Sullivan, 1988) and in man (Kawashima *et al.*, 1989), although it is likely this effect is secondary to hypoxic pulmonary vasoconstriction and consequent increase in right atrial pressure.

The recently discovered vasoconstrictor peptide, endothelin, produced a marked enhancement of ANF secretion in cultured rat atrial myocytes (Fukuda *et al.*, 1988). The occurrence of this effect *in vitro*, independent of the haemodynamic actions of endothelin, implies that it may directly affect ANF secretion. This potentially important conclusion is supported also by more recent studies (Garcia, Lachance & Thibault, 1990), and it may be explained by the ability of endothelin to increase intracellular free calcium concentration (Marsden *et al.*, 1989), as this is a potent stimulus for ANF release (Matsubara *et al.*, 1988).

The possible role of osmolarity in modulating secretion of ANF is disputed. Several studies have shown that an increase in plasma osmolality *in vivo* increases plasma ANF levels (Kimura *et al.*, 1986; Salazar *et al.*, 1986) but such experiments are accompanied by intravascular volume expansion, which may completely explain the observed increase in plasma ANF (Salazar *et al.*, 1986). *In vitro* studies have yielded conflicting results, some reporting increased ANF release with a rise in osmolality (Arjamaa & Vuolteenaho, 1985), whereas others do not (Dietz, 1987).

Dissociations between atrial pressure and ANF release in man

Recent clinical obsrvations have suggested that, at times, dissociations may occur between atrial pressure and stretch and ANF release, supporting the possibility that peptide release may be modified by factors external to the heart. In a study of patients paced at normal heart rate in sequential and then ventricular mode, in subjects who maintained systolic pressure during ventricular pacing, plasma ANF concentration more than doubled. In contrast, in patients in whom ventricular pacing produced hypotension, ANF plasma concentration fell by 75%, despite increased atrial pressure. Plasma noradrenaline also increased in these latter patients (Raine *et al.*, 1987; Erne *et al.*, 1987). The conclusion was that when acute cardiac decompensation occurred, ANF release might be suppressed, despite increased atrial pressure, by negative feedback mechanisms possibly involving the baroreflex reflex and autonomic nervous system (Erne *et al.*, 1987).

The possibility of dissociation between atrial pressure and ANF release is supported also by a study by Volpe and colleagues (1986) who showed that carotid baroreceptor unloading and reflex sympathetic activation induced by neck pressure in hypertensive patients caused a fall of 66% in plasma ANF concentrations, despite no change in atrial pressure. In addition, recent animal studies have shown that sino-aortic denervation in rats, which increases sympathetic activity (Alexander *et al.*, 1980) leads to a decrease in both basal plasma ANF levels and those stimulated by volume loading (Morris & Alexander, 1988). The existence of a tonic inhibitory influence on ANF release *in vivo* by basal sympathetic activity might explain why plasma ANF concentrations are markedly increased in cardiac transplant recipients (Singer *et al.*, 1986).

In summary, it remains unclear whether autonomic reflexes may influence release of ANF; studies *in vitro* and *in vivo* in animals and clinical observations have given conflicting results. Nevertheless, it is clear that studies performed to date investigating factors which might influence cardiac release have been hampered by two problems. First, it is well-nigh impossible to administer an agent such as a catecholamine *in vivo* without at the same time altering atrial pressure through haemodynamic effects. Secondly, *in vitro* studies employing atrial tissue are confounded both by the loss of the atrial pressure–stretch relationship, and the difficulty of simulating basal physiological atrial filling pressures.

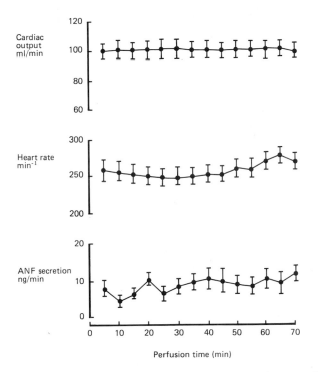

Fig. 14.3 Cardiac output, heart rate and ANF secretion rate of isolated working rat hearts perfused at constant left atrial filling pressure (15 cMH$_2$O) and aortic pressure (100 cMH$_2$O). ANF secretion rate remained constant despite large increases in the ANF concentration in the recirculating perfusate.

Cardiac ANF receptors and ANF release

It is now established that in addition to the existence of ANP-A and ANP-B receptors mediating the biological actions of the hormone, there is a separate class of ANP-C clearance receptors, which are biologically silent and act to remove ANF from the circulation (Maack *et al.*, 1987). Recent radioligand binding studies combined with cDNA amplification have shown that ANP-A and ANP-B receptors are expressed in rat myocardial tissue (Nunez & Brown, 1990). The role of these receptors is unclear. Although very large doses of synthetic peptide have been reported to reduce peak rate of left ventricular pressure rise in anaesthetized rats (Dunn *et al.*, 1986), in most studies no significant effects on contractility have been observed (Bergey & Kotler, 1985; Hiwatari *et al.*, 1986).

Conceivably, myocardial ANP-A receptors might mediate a negative feedback inhibition of ANF release, or possibly cardiac ANP-C receptors might remove ANF from the circulation. Against this possibility, recent studies (unpublished observations) have shown that ANF release from the isolated working rat heart, perfused at unchanging left atrial pressure and afterload, remains constant during 60 min of perfusion, during which period ANF concentration in the recirculating perfusate increased to 1500 pmol/l or more (Fig. 14.3). Studies employing C-receptor blockade (Maack *et al.*, 1987) will be required to elucidate the possible role of myocardial ANF receptors.

Conclusions

A wealth of evidence in both animals and man has established clearly the close relationship between atrial pressure and distension and the consequent release of ANF from storage granules in atrial cardiocytes. Despite this, many questions remain unanswered. The possible role of the 1–98 N-terminal fragment of proANF, which is cosecreted with the active 99–126 peptide, remains unknown. The precise interrelationships between atrial distension, myocyte stretch and atrial wall stress and ANF secretion require further elucidation. The cellular mechanism of release of ANF is as yet poorly understood, beyond a knowledge that release, as with many other hormones, is activated by increased cytosolic calcium concentration. The potential importance of beat-to-beat changes in myocyte stretch and tension and intracellular calcium concentration in relation to ANF release has not yet been approached. Lastly, considerable evidence points to the likelihood that autonomic, neural and possibly endocrine influences may, under certain circumstances, markedly modulate ANF secretion. The mechanisms of these potentially important interactions remains unknown, but when understood will provide a more complete knowledge of overall integration of cardiocirculatory control.

References

Adnot, S., Chabrier, P.E., Andrivet, P., Voissat, I., Piquet, J., Brun-Buisson, C., Gutkowska, Y. & Braquet, P. (1987). Atrial natriuretic peptide concentrations and pulmonary haemodynamics in patients with pulmonary artery hypertension. *Am. Rev. Respir. Dis.* **136**: 951–6.

Alexander, N., Velasquez, M.R., de Cuir, M. & Maronde, R.F. (1980). Indices of sympathetic activity in the sinoaortic denerved rat. *Am. J. Physiol.* **238**: H521.

Anderson, J.V., Donckier, J., McKenna, W.J. & Bloom, S.R. (1986a). The plasma release of atrial natriuretic peptide in man. *Clin. Sci.* **71**: 151–5.

Anderson, J.V., Gibbs, S.R., Woodruff, P.W.R., Greco, C., Rowland, E. & Bloom, S.R. (1986b). The plasma atrial natriuretic peptide response to treatment of acute cardiac failure, spontaneous supraventricular tachycardia and induced re-entrant tachycardia in man. *J. Hypertension* **4** (Suppl. 2): S137–41.

Anderson, J.V., Raine, A.E.G., Proudler, A., Ghatei, M.A. & Bloom, S.R. (1986c). Effect of haemodialysis on plasma concentrations of atrial natriuretic peptide in adult patients with chronic renal failure. *J. Endocrinol.* **110**: 193–6.

Arjamaa, D. & Vuolteenaho, O. (1985). Sodium ion stimulates the release of atrial natriuretic peptide (ANP) from rat atria. *Biochem. Biophys. Res. Commun.* **132**: 375–81.

Atlas, S.A., Kleinert, H.D., Camargo, M.J. *et al.* (1984). Purification, sequencing and synthesis of natriuretic and vasoactive rat atrial peptide. *Nature* **309**: 717–19.

Baertshi, A.J., Adams, J.M. & Sullivan, M.P. (1988). Acute hypoxemia stimulates atrial natriuretic factor secretion *in vivo*. *Am. J. Physiol.* **256** (*Heart Cir. Physiol.* **24**): H295–300.

Bergey, J.L. & Kotler, D. (1985). Effects of atriopeptins I, II and III on atrial contractility, sinus nodal rate (guinea pig) and agonist-induced tension in rabbit aortic strips. *Eur. J. Pharmacol.* **110**: 277–81.

Bilder, G.E., Schofield, T.L. & Blaine, E.H. (1986). Release of atrial natriuretic factor. Effects of repetitive stretch and temperature. *Am. J. Physiol.* **251** (*Renal fluid Electrolyte Physiol.* **20**): F817–21.

Bloch, K.D., Scott, J.A., Zisfein, J.B., Fallon, J.T., Margolies, M.N., Seidman, C.E., Matsueda, G.R., Homcy, C.J., Graham, R.M. & Seidman, J.G. (1985). Biosynthesis and secretion of proatrial natriuretic factor by cultured rat cardiocytes. *Science* **230**: 1168–71.

Bloch, K.D., Seidman, J.G., Maftalin, J.D. & Seidman, C.E. (1986). Neonatal atria and ventricles secrete atrial natriuretic factor via tissue-specific secretory pathways. *Cell* **47**: 695–702.

Buckley, M.G., Sagnella, G.A., Markandu, N.D., Singer, R.J. & MacGregor, G.A. (1989). Immunoreactive N-terminal pro-atrial natriuretic peptide in human plasma: plasma levels and comparisons with α-human atrial natriuretic peptide in normal subjects, patients with essential hypertension cardiac transplant, and chronic renal failure. *Clin. Sci.* **77**: 573–9.

Burnett, J.C., Kao, P.C., Ju D.E. *et al.* (1986). Atrial natriuretic peptide elevation in congestive heart failure in the human. *Science* **231**: 1145–7.

Cannella, G., Ghielmi, S., Assanelli, D., Gaggiotti, M., Rodella, A., Sandrini, M. & Maijorca, R. (1987). Evidence for the existence of positive feed-backs between intravascular volume load (IVL), atrial distention (AD) and atrial natriuretic peptide (ANP) in dialysed uraemic (DU) man. *Xth International Congress of Nephrology*, p. 208 (abstract).

Cannella, G., Ghielmi, S., Sandrini, M. *et al.* (1988). Effect of reduction of blood volume on plasma immunoreactive atrial natriuretic factor concentrations in normal man. *Nephrol. Dial. Transplant* **3**: 601–3.

Chimoskey, J.E., Spielman, W.S., Brandt, M.A. & Heideman, S.R. (1984). Cardiac atria of BIO 14.6 hamsters are deficient in natriuretic factor. *Science* **223**: 820–2.

Christensen, G., Ilebekk, A., Aakeson, I. & Kiil, F. (1988). The release mechanism for atrial natriuretic factor during blood volume expansion and tachycardia in dogs. *Acta Physiol. Scand.* **19** (Suppl. 68): 1–230.

Crozier, I.G., Nicholls, M.G., Ikram, H., Espiner, E.A., Yandle, T.G. & Jans, S. (1985). Atrial natriuretic peptide in humans. production and clearance by various tissues. *Hypertension* **8** (Suppl. II): 11–15.

Crozier, I.G., Nicholls, M.G., Ikram, H. & Espiner, E.A. (1986). Relation between left atrial diameter and plasma atrial natriuretic peptide, renin and vasopressin. *Am. J. Cardiol.* **58**: 1134–6.

Currie, M.G., Sukin, D., Geller, D.M., Cole, B.R. & Needleman, P. (1984). Atriopeptin release from the isolated perfused rabbit heart. *Biochem. Biophys. Res. Commun.* **124**: 711–17.

deBold, A.J. (1979). Heart atria granularity effects of changes in water-electrolyte balance. *Proc. Soc. Exp. Biol. Med.* **161**: 508–11.

deBold, A.J., Borenstein, H.B., Veress, A.T. & Sonnenberg, H. (1981). A rapid and potent natriuretic response to intravenous injection of atrial myocardial extracts in rats. *Life Sci.* **28**: 89–94.

deBold, A.J., deBold, M.L. & Sarda, I.R. (1986). Functional morphological studies on *in vitro* cardionatrin release. *J. Hypertension* **4**: (Suppl 2): S3–7.

Dietz, J.R. (1984). Release of atrial natriuretic factor from rat heart–lung preparation by atrial distension. *Am. J. Physiol.* (*Regul. Integr. Comp. Physiol.* **16**): R1093–6.

Dietz, J.R. (1987). Control of atrial natriuretic factor release from a rat heart–lung preparation. *Am. J. Physiol.*: R498–502.

Dunn, B.R., Ichikawa, I. Pfeffer, J.M., Troy, J.L. & Brenner, B.M. (1986). Renal and systemic haemodynamic effects of synthetic atrial natriuretic peptide in the anaesthetized rat. *Circ. Res.* **59**: 237–46.

Edwards, B.S., Ackerman, D.M., Schwab, T.R., Heublein, D.M., Edwards, W.D., Wold, L.E. & Burnett, J.C. Jr. (1986). The relationship between atrial granularity and circulating atrial natriuretic peptide in hamsters with heart failure. *Mayo Clin. Proc.* **61**: 557–63.

Edwards, B.S., Zimmerman, R.S., Schwab, T.R., Heublein, D.M. & Burnett, J.C. Jr. (1988). Atrial stretch, not pressure, is the principal determinant controlling the acute release of atrial natriuretic factor. *Circulation Res.* **62**: 191–5.

Epstein, M., Loutzenhiser, E., Friedland, R.M., Aceto, M., Camargo, M.J. & Atlas, S.A. (1987). Relationship of increased plasma atrial natriuretic factor and renal sodium handling during immersion-induced central hypervolemia in normal humans. *J. Clin. Invest.* **79**: 738–45.

Erne, P., Raine, A.E.G., Burgisser, E., Gradel, E., Burkart, F. & Buhler, F.R. (1987), Paradoxical inhibition of atrial natriuretic peptide release during pacing-induced hypotension. *Clin. Sci.* **73**: 459–62.

Flynn, T.G., deBold, M.L. & deBold, A.J. (1983). The amino acid sequence of an atrial peptide with potent diuretic and natriuretic properties. *Biochem. Biophys. Res. Commun.* **117**: 859–65.

Franch, H.A., Dixon, R.A.F., Blaine, E.H. & Siegl, P.K.S. (1988). Ventricular atrial natriuretic factor in the cardiomyopathic hamster model of congestive heart failure. *Circulation Res.* **62**, 31–6.

Fukuda, Y., Hirata, Y., Yoshimi, H., *et al.* (1988). Endothelin is a potent secretagogue for atrial natriuretic peptide in cultured rat atrial myocytes. *Biochem. Biophys. Res. Commun.* **115**: 167–72.

Garcia, R., Lachance, D. & Thibault, G. (1990). Positive inotropic action, natriuresis and atrial natriuretic factor release induced by endothelin in the conscious rat. *J. Hypertension* (in press).

Garcia, R., Lachance, D., Thibault, G., Cartin, M. & Gutkowska, J. (1986). Mechanisms of release of atrial natriuretic factor. II Effect of chronic administration of alpha- and beta-adrenergic and cholinergic agonists on plasma and atrial ANF in the rat. *Biochem. Biophys. Res. Commun.* **136**: 510–20.

Gutkowska, J., Thibault, G., Januszewicz, P., Cantin, M. & Genest, J. (1984). Direct radioimmunoassay of atrial natriuretic factor. *Biochem. Biophys. Res. Commun.* **122**: 593–601.

Hintze, T., McIntyre, J.J., Patel, M.B., Shapiro, J.T., Deleonardis, M., Zeballos, G. & Loud, A.V. (1989). Atrial wall function and plasma atriopeptin during volume expansion in conscious dogs. *Am. J. Physiol.* **256**: H713–19.

Hiwatari, M., Satoh, K., Angus, J.A. & Johnston, C.I. (1986). No effect of atrial natriuretic factor on cardiac rate, force and transmitter release. *Clin. Exp. Pharmacol. Physiol.* **13**: 163–8.

Imada, T., Takayanagi, R. & Inagami, T. (1988). Atrioactivase, a specific peptidase in bovine atria for the processing of pro-atrial natriuretic factor. *J. Biol. Chem.* **263** (19): 9515–19.

Jamieson, J.D. & Palade, G.E. (1964). Specific granules in atrial muscle cells. *J. Cell Biol.* **23**: 151–72.

Kangawa, K. & Matsuo, H. (1984). Purification and complete amino acid sequence of a-human atrial natriuretic polypeptide (a-hANP). *Biochem. Biophys. Res. Commun.* **118**: 131–9.

Katsube, N., Schwartz, D. & Needleman, P. (1985). Release of atriopeptin in the rat by vasoconstrictors or water immersion correlates with changes in right atrial pressure. *Biochem. Biophys. Res. Commun.* **133**: 937–44.

Kawashima, A., Kubo, K., Hirai, K., Yoshikawa, S., Matsizawa, Y. & Kobayashi, T. (1989). Plasma level of natriuretic peptide under acute hypoxia in normal subjects. *Respir. Physiol.* **76**: 79–92.

Kimura, T., Abe, K., Ota, K., Omata, K., Shosi, M., Kudo, K., Matsui, K., Inour, M., Vasujima, M. & Voshinga, L. (1986). Effects of acute water load, hypertonic saline infusion and furosemide administration on atrial natriuretic peptide and vasopressin release in humans. *Clin. Endocrinol. Metab.* **62**: 1003–10.

Kisch, B. (1955). Studies in comparative electron microscopy of the heart II: Guinea pig and rat. *Exp. Med. Surg.* **13**: 404–28.

Koller, P.T., Grekin, R.J. & Nicklas, J.M. (1987). Paradoxical response of plasma atrial natriuretic hormone to pericardiocentesis in cardiac tamponade. *Am. J. Cardiol.* **59**: 491–2.

Lachance, D. & Garcia, R. (1988). Atrial natriuretic factor release by angiotensin II in the conscious rat. *Hypertension* **11**: 502–8.

Lang, R.E., Tholken, H., Ganten, D., Luft, F.C., Ruskoaho, H. & Unger, T. (1985). Atrial natriuretic factor — a circulating hormone stimulated by volume loading. *Nature* **314**: 264–6.

Lattion, A.L., Michel, J.B., Arnauld, E., Corvol, P. & Soubrier, F. (1986). Myocardial recruitment during ANF mRNA increase with volume overload in the rat. *Am. J. Physiol.* **251**: H890–6.

Ledsome, J.R., Wilson, N., Courneya, C.A. & Rankin, A.J. (1985). Release of atrial natriuretic peptide by atrial distension. *Can. J. Physiol. Pharmacol.* **63**: 739–42.

Ledsome, J.R., Wilson, N., Rankin, A.J. & Courneya, C.A. (1986). Time course of release of atrial natriuretic peptide in the anaesthetized dog. *Can. J. Physiol. Pharmacol.* **64**, 1017–22.

Maack, T., Suzuki, M., Almeida, F.A., Nussenzveig, D., Scarborough, R.M., McEnroe, G.A. & Lewicki, J.A. (1987). Physiological role of silent receptors of atrial natriuretic factor. *Science* **238**: 675–8.

Marsden, P.A., Danthuluri, N.R., Brenner, B.M., Ballermann, B.J. & Brock, T.A. (1989). Endothelin action on vascular smooth muscle involves inositol triphosphate and calcium mobilization. *Biochem. Biophys. Res. Commun.* **158**: 86–93.

Matsubara, H., Hirata, Y., Yoshimi, H., *et al.* (1988). Role of calcium and protein kinase C in ANF secretion by cultured rat cardiocytes. *Am. J. Physiol.* **255**: H405–9.

Mendez, R.E., Pfeffer, J.M., Ortola, F.V., Bloch, K.D., Anderson, S., Seidman, J.G. & Brenner, B.M. (1987). Atrial natriuretic peptide transcription, storage and release in rats with myocardial infarction. *Am. J. Physiol.* **253**: H1449–55.

Morris, M. & Alexander, N. (1988). Baroreceptor influences on plasma atrial natriuretic peptide (ANP): sinoaortic denervation reduces basal levels and the response to an osmotic challenge. *Endocrinology* **122**: 373.

Muller, F.B., Erne, P., Raine, A.E.G., Bolli, P., Linder, L., Resink, T.J., Cottier, C. & Buhler, F.R. (1986). Atrial antipressor natriuretic peptide: release mechanisms and vascular action in man. *J. Hypertension* **4** (Suppl. 2): S109–14.

Naruse, K., Naruse, M., Obana, K., Brown, A.B., Shibasaki, T., Demura, H., Shizume, K. & Inagami, T. (1986). Right and left atrium share a similar mode of secreting atrial natriuretic factor *in vitro* in rats. *J. Hypertension* **4** (Suppl. 6): S497–9.

Nemer, M., Lavigne, J.-P., Drouin, J., Thibault, G., Gannon, M. & Antalky, T. (1986). Expression of atrial natriuretic factor gene in heart ventricular tissue. *Peptides* **7**: 1147–52.

Nicklas, J.M., diCarlo, L.A., Koller, P.T., Morady, F., Diltz, E.A., Shenker, Y. & Grekin, R.J. (1986). Plasma levels of immunoreactive atrial natriuretic factor increase during supraventricular tachycardia. *Am. Heart J.* **112**, 923–7.

Nishikimi, T., Kohno, M., Marsuura, K., Akioka, M., Teragaki, M., Yasuda, H., Oku, K., Takeuchi, K. & Takeda, T. (1986). Effect of exercise on circulating atrial natriuretic polypeptide in valvular heart disease. *Am. J. Cardiol.* **58**: 1119–20.

Northridge, D.B., McMurray, J., Ray, S., Jardine, A. & Dargie, H.J. (1989). Release of atrial natriuretic factor after pericardiocentesis for malignant pericardial effusion. *Br. Med. J.* **299**: 603–4.

Nunez, D.J. & Brown, M.J. (1990). Atrial natriuretic factor guanylate cyclase and 'C' type receptor mRNAs in the rat heart. *Clin. Sci.* **78** (Suppl. 22): IP.

Oikawa, S., Imai, M., Ueno, A. *et al.* (1984). Cloning and sequence analysis of cDNA encoding a precursor for human atrial natriuretic polypeptide. *Nature* **309**: 724–6.

Raine, A.E.G., Bock, A., Muller, F.B., Brunner, F. & Buhler, F.R. (1989). Comparative effects of haemodialysis and haemofiltration on plasma atrial natriuretic peptide. *Nephrol. Dial. Transplant* **4**: 222–7.

Raine, A.E.G., Erne, P., Burgisser, E. & Buhler, F.R. (1987). Dissociation between atrial natriuretic peptide release and atrial pressure during cardiac pacing in man. In: *Biologically Active Atrial Peptides*, Eds Brenner, B.M. *et al.* Raven Press, New York, pp. 473–6.

Raine, A.E.G., Erne, P., Burgisser, E., Muller, F.B., Bolli, P., Burkart, F. & Buhler, F.R. (1986). Atrial natriuretic peptide and atrial pressure in patients with congestive heart failure. *New Engl. J. Med.* **315**: 533–7.

Richards, A.M., Cleland, J.G.F., Tonolo, G., McIntyre, G.D., Leckie, B.J., Dargie, H.J., Ball, S.G. & Robertson, J.I.S. (1986). Plasma atrial natriuretic peptide in cardiac impairment. *Br. Med. J.* **293**, 409–12.

Riegger, G.A.J., Elsner, D., Kromer, E.P., Daffner, C., Forssmann, W.G., Muders, F., Pascher, E.W. & Kochsiek, K. (1988). Atrial natriuretic peptide in congestive heart failure in the dog: plasma levels, cyclic guanosine monophosphate, ultrastructure of atrial myoendocrine cells, and hemodynamic, hormonal and renal effects. *Circulation* **77**: 398–406.

Rodeheffer, R.J., Tanaka, I., Imada, T., Hollister, A.S., Robertson, D. & Inagami, T. (1986). Atrial pressure and secretion of atrial natriuretic factor into the human central circulation. *J. Am. Coll. Cardiol.* **8**: 18–26.

Ruskoaho, H., Toth, M. & Lang, R.E. (1985). Atrial natriuretic peptide secretion: synergistic effect of phorbol ester and A23187. *Biochem. Biophys. Res. Commun.* **133**: 581–8.

Saito, Y., Nakao, K., Morii, N., Sugawara, A., Shiono, S., Yamada, T., Itoh, H., Sakamoto, M., Kurahashi, K., Fujiwara, M. & Imura, H. (1986). BAY K 8644, a voltage-sensitive calcium channel agonist facilitates secretion of atrial natriuretic polypeptide from isolated perfused rat hearts. *Biochem. Biophys. Res. Commun.* **138**: 1170–6.

Salazar, F.J., Granger, J.P., Joyce, M.L.M., Burnett, J.C. Jr., Bove, A.A. & Romero, J.C. (1986). Effects of hypertonic saline infusion and water drinking on atrial peptide. *Am. J. Physiol.* **251**: R1091–4.

Schiebinger, R.J., Baker, M.Z. & Linden, J. (1987). Effect of adrenergic and muscarinic cholinergic agonists on atrial natriuretic peptide secretion by isolated rat atria. *J. Clin. Invest.* **80**: 1687–91.

Schiebinger, R.J. & Linden, J. (1986a). The influence of resting tension on immunoreactive atrial natriuretic peptide secretion by rat atria superfused *in vitro*. *Circulation Res.* **59**: 105–9.

Schiebinger, R.J. & Linden, J. (1986b). Effect of atrial contraction frequency on atrial natriuretic peptide secretion. *Am. J. Physiol.* **25**: H1095–9.

Singer, D.R., Buckley, M.G., MacGregor, G.A., Khaghani, A., Banner, N.R. & Yacoub, M.H. (1986). Raised concentrations of plasma atrial natriuretic peptide in cardiac transplant recipients. *Br. Med. J.* **293**: 1391–2.

Sonnenberg, H. & Veress, A.T. (1984). Cellular mechanism of release of atrial natriuretic factor. *Biochem. Biophys. Res. Commun.* **124**: 443–9.

Stockmann, P.T., Will, D.H., Sides, S.D., Brunnert, S.R., Wilner, G.D., Leahy, K.M., Wiegand, R.C. & Needleman, P. (1988). Reversible induction of right ventricular atriopeptin synthesis in hypertrophy due to hypoxia. *Circulation Res.* **63**: 207–13.

Suguwara, A., Nakao, K., Morii, N., Sakamoto, M., Suda, M., Shimokura, M., Kiso, Y., Kihara, M., Yamori, Y., Nishimura, K., Soneda, J., Ban, T. & Imura, H. (1985). Human atrial natriuretic polypeptide is released from the heart and circulates in the body. *Biochem. Biophys. Res. Commun.* **129**: 439–46.

Synhorst, D.P. & Gutkowska, J. (1988). Atrial distension of isolated rabbit hearts and release of atrial natriuretic factor. *Am. J. Physiol.* **255**: R232–6.

Takayanagi, R., Imada, T. & Ingami, T. (1987). Synthesis and presence of atrial natriuretic factor in rat ventricle. *Biochem. Biophys. Res. Commun.* **142**: 483–8.

Tanaka, I., Misono, K.S. & Inagami, T. (1984). Atrial natriuretic factor in rat hypothalamus, atria and plasma: determination by specific radioimmunoassay. *Biochem. Biophys. Res. Commun.* **124**: 663–8.

Thibault, G., Garcia, R., Gutkowska, J., Bilodeau, J., Lazure, C., Seidah, N., Chreitien, M., Genest, J. & Cantin, M. (1987). The propeptide Asn[1]–Tyr[126] is the storage form of rat atrial natriuretic factor. *Biochem. J.* **241**: 265–72.

Thibault, G., Garcia, R., Gutkowska, J., Lazure, C., Seidah, N.G., Chreitien, M., Genest, J. & Cantin, M. (1986). Identification of the released form of atrial natriuretic factor by the perfused rat heart. *Proc. Soc. Exp. Biol. Med.* **182**: 137–41.

Tikkanen, I., Fyhrquist, F., Metsarinne, K. & Leidenius, R. (1985). Plasma atrial natriuretic peptide in cardiac disease and during infusion in healthy volunteers. *Lancet* **ii**: 66–9.

Trippodo, N.C., MacPhee, A.A. & Cole, F.E. (1983). Partially purified human and rat atrial natriuretic factor. *Hypertension* **5** (Suppl. I): I81–8.

Vesely, D.L., Norris, J.S., Walters, J.M., Hespersen, R.R. & Baeyens, D.A. (1987). Atrial natriuretic prohormone peptides 1–30, 31–67 and 79–98 vasodilate the aorta. *Biochem. Biophys. Res. Commun.* **148**: 1540–8.

Volpe, M., Mele, A.F., de Luca, N., Golino, P., Bondiolotti, G., Camargo, M.J., Atlas, S.A. & Trimarco, B. (1986). Carotid baroreceptor unloading decreases plasma atrial natriuretic factor in hypertensive patients. *J. Hypertension* **4**: S519–22.

Wilkins, M.R., Gammage, M.D., Lewis, H.M., Bun Tan, L. & Weissberg, P.L. (1988). The effect of lower-body positive-pressure on blood pressure, plasma ANP concentration and sodium and water excretion in healthy volunteers and cardiac transplant recipients. *Cardiovasc. Res.* **22**, 231–5.

Wood P. (1963). Polyuria in paroxysmal tachycardia and paroxysmal atrial flutter and fibrillation. *Br. Heart J.* **25**: 273–82.

Yamaji, T., Ishitashi, M., Nakaoka, H., Imatako, K., Amano, M. & Fujii, J. (1985). Possible role for atrial natriuretic peptide in polyuria associated with paroxysmal atrial arrhythmias. *Lancet* **i**: 1211.

Yandle, T.G., Espiner, E.A., Nicholls, M.G. & Duff, H. (1986). Radioimmunoassay and a characterization of atrial natriuretic peptide in human plasma. *J. Clin. Endocrinol. Metab.* **63**: 72–9.

Zamir, N., Haass, M., Dave, J.R. & Zukowska-Grojec, Z. (1987). Anterior pituitary gland modulates the release of atrial natriuretic peptides from cardiac atria. *Proc. Nat. Acad. Sci. USA* **84**: 541–5.

Zisfein, J.B., Matsueda, G.R., Fallon, J.T., Bloch, K.D., Seidman, C.E., Seidman, J.G., Homcy, C.J. & Graham, R.M. (1986). Atrial natriuretic factor: assessment of its structure in atria and regulation of its biosynthesis with volume depletion. *J. Molec. Cell Cardiol.* **18**: 917–29.

Concluding remarks

A. D. Struthers

This book serves mainly to review our current knowledge about ANF. In this last section, I would like to look to the future.

Atrial natriuretic factor (ANF) has so far fulfilled its expectation as a natriuretic substance which is responsive to changes in blood volume. It has also served to revive interest in the physiology and pathophysiology of renal sodium handling and blood volume regulation. Even more importantly it has served as a focus for the modern techniques of molecular biology and molecular genetics to be applied in seeking the answers to many long-standing yet fundamental questions.

The renin–angiotensin–aldosterone system (RAAS) was for a long time thought to be a system of circulating hormones. More recently it has become established that the RAAS exerts an important paracrine role. ANF is still thought of as a circulating hormone but there are clues that it may, like the RAAS, come to be regarded in addition as a paracrine local modulator. The first clue in this regard is the presence of ANF mRNA in many extra-atrial locations, some of which are near cardiovascular regulatory structures. Secondly, the presence of urodilatin as a potent renally active substance which may be synthesized within the kidney suggests that it fulfils a paracrine rather than an endocrine function.

Almost inevitably, more natriuretic peptides will be discovered. ANF may be the prototype natriuretic peptide but already similar yet distinct peptides like brain natriuretic peptide (BNP) and iso-rat-ANP have been well described and studied. It may even be that ANF is a fairly minor component in a large family of natriuretic peptides. It is interesting that a second and distinct biologically active receptor (ANP-B or GC-B) has now been sequenced. The endogenous ligand for this receptor has not yet been identified but may be BNP or some as yet unknown member of this 'natriuretic family'. It is also interesting to realize that the traditional path of identifying a substance first and then its receptor has been reversed with this GC-B receptor.

We know more about the mechanisms involved in the release of ANF than we do about its metabolic breakdown. Indeed, the latter process seems to involve not only special clearance receptors but also endopeptidase enzymes. The relationship between these two is far from clear but there is now greater urgency to understand this since the advent of endopeptidase inhibitors suggests that manipulating the breakdown of ANF may be a useful therapeutic avenue.

Chronic heart failure is a disease of increasing focus. It is over 200 years since digoxin was first used in this condition and we have now come to realize that the best available treatment is a 'diuretic/ACE inhibitor' combination. Around the same time as this was realized, an endogenous 'diuretic/RAAS inhibitor' substance in the form of ANF was discovered. ANF may be of value in chronic heart failure in two ways. First, plasma levels of ANF might be used as a measure of disease progress, of prognosis or as an objective measure to assist in optimizing therapy in chronic heart failure. Secondly, ANF may be of therapeutic value. The major problem of how to orally administer a 28-amino-acid peptide has largely been overcome by the recent advent of endopeptidase inhibitors. How these drugs work should now be a major focus of attention. Their effects may be due to elevating ANF but it is quite possible that they are due to elevating other natriuretic peptides, such as BNP or even other peptides which have not yet been identified.

The future for both basic and clinical research for ANF is indeed rosy. There is much more to learn from investigators with all types of expertise from molecular genetics to epidemiology. There is also now the distinct possibility that ANF will produce drugs of therapeutic value. This last point should convince all hitherto doubters that ANF investigators are indeed answering questions of importance to mankind.

Postscript

Very recently another new member of this natriuretic peptide family has been described (C-type natriuretic peptide of CNP) (*Biochemical and Biophysical Research Communications* 1990, **168**, 863.)

Index